Handbook of
NURSE
ANESTHESIA

Handbook of
NURSE
ANESTHESIA

John J. Nagelhout, PhD, CRNA
Director, School of Anesthesia
Kaiser Permanente
Pasadena, California

Karen L. Zaglaniczny, PhD, CRNA
Associate Director and Co-Chair
Henry Ford Hospital/University of Detroit Mercy Program of
Nurse Anesthesia
Henry Ford Hospital
Detroit, Michigan
and
Assistant Professor
University of Detroit Mercy College of Health Professions
Detroit, Michigan

Valdor L. Haglund, Jr., MS, CRNA
Detroit Receiving Hospital
Wayne State University
Detroit, Michigan

W.B. SAUNDERS COMPANY
A Division of Harcourt Brace & Company
Philadelphia   London   Toronto   Montreal   Sydney   Tokyo

W.B. SAUNDERS COMPANY
A Division of Harcourt Brace & Company

The Curtis Center
Independence Square West
Philadelphia, Pennsylvania 19106

Library of Congress Cataloging-in-Publication Data

Nagelhout, John J.
Handbook of nurse anesthesia / John J. Nagelhout, Karen L. Zaglaniczny,
Valdor L. Haglund, Jr.

p. cm.

ISBN 0–7216–6694–9

1. Anesthesiology—Handbooks, manuals, etc. 2. Nurse
   anesthetists. I. Zaglaniczny, Karen L. II. Haglund, Valdor L. III. Title.
   [DNLM: 1. Nurse Anesthetists—handbooks. 2. Anesthesia—nurses'
   instruction—handbooks. 3. Anesthetics—nurses'
   instruction—handbooks. WY 49 N147h 1997]

RD82.2.N34 1997   617.9'6—dc20

DNLM/DLC   96-20547

HANDBOOK OF NURSE ANESTHESIA   ISBN 0–7216–6694–9

Printed in the United States of America.

Last digit is the print number: 9   8   7   6   5   4   3   2

PREFACE

The complexity of clinical anesthesia practice continues to increase as new procedures and drugs are introduced and as our methods of conceptualizing and managing diseases evolve. Anesthetists must stay abreast of current practices in a variety of disciplines, since our patients may arrive with an array of medical problems and surgical needs. When selecting the format of this handbook, we chose not to simply produce a condensed version of our text, *Nurse Anesthesia*. We felt that there is a need for a single comprehensive source containing information on common diseases, procedures, and drugs, and that such a source, in a handbook format, would complement the larger text. Today, many clinicians practice at more than one facility, and thus may be called upon to provide anesthesia care in a broader spectrum of operative and diagnostic situations. An up-to-date reference guide is an essential tool for hands-on management in the modern operating suite.

We compiled the *Handbook of Nurse Anesthesia* as a single source that provides

- a thorough overview of the *common diseases* encountered in surgical patients

- a *procedure manual* and guidelines for anesthesia management for a wide variety of diagnostic and surgical procedures

- a convenient and comprehensive *drug reference* for clinical use.

The standardized format was designed and customized for use throughout each of the three individual sections of the *Handbook*. Several appendices at the end of the *Handbook* offer the clinician easy access to the difficult airway algorithm, ACLS Algorithms, hemodynamic formulas, pulmonary function testing, preoperative laboratory values, AANA Standards of Practice, and much more.

JOHN J. NAGELHOUT
KAREN L. ZAGLANICZNY
VALDOR L. HAGLUND, JR

ACKNOWLEDGMENTS

The production and success of this book required the collaborative efforts of many contributors. We wish to recognize each of the following contributors for his or her knowledge and expertise in the field of anesthesia and extensive review and research in each topic area:

Janet Baskin, CRNA, MS
Carol Bernicke, CRNA, MS
Michael D. Duronio, CRNA, MS
Geri Evon-Gabourie, CRNA, MS
Curt Feldhak, CRNA, MS
Nancy Fisher, CRNA, MS
Donna Funke, CRNA, MS
Carrie Hajjar, CRNA, MS
Jennifer Hourigan, CRNA, MS
Mary Jennett, CRNA, MS
Kendra Kayser, CRNA, MS
Patti S. Leupp, CRNA, MS
Cynthia Lynn, CRNA, MS

Ronald Manningham, CRNA, MS
Kellie Martin, CRNA, MS
Louise Minore, CRNA, MS
Lisa Mueller, CRNA, MS
Colette Neenan, CRNA, MS
Oscar Ong, CRNA, MS
Sally Range, CRNA, MS
Alan R. Roberts, CRNA, MS
Roxanna Robinson, CRNA, MS
Susan Vander Laan, CRNA, MS
Richard VanTuyl, CRNA, MS
Ruth I. Watts, CRNA, MS

We are also indebted to others who have facilitated the development and realization of this book. These include the staff at W.B. Saunders Company, Maura Connor, Editor, Stephanie Klein, Editorial Assistant, Frank Messina, Senior Copy Editor, Frank Polizzano, Production Manager, and Thomas Eoyang, Vice President and Editor-in-Chief of Nursing Books. We acknowledge the support of the staff at Henry Ford Hospital, Detroit Receiving Hospital, University of Detroit Mercy, and Wayne State University during our worthwhile endeavors. Finally, we would also like to thank our professional colleagues, friends, and especially our families for their patient endurance and endless encouragement.

JOHN J. NAGELHOUT
KAREN L. ZAGLANICZNY
VALDOR L. HAGLUND, JR

NOTICE

Anesthesia is an ever-changing field. Standard safety precautions must be followed, but as new research and clinical experience broaden our knowledge, changes in treatment and drug therapy become necessary or appropriate. The editors of this work have carefully checked the generic and trade drug names and verified drug dosages to ensure that the dosage information in this work is accurate and in accord with the standards accepted at the time of publication. Readers are advised, however, to check the product information currently provided by the manufacturer of each drug to be administered to be certain that changes have not been made in the recommended dose or in the contraindications for administration. This is of particular importance in regard to new or infrequently used drugs. It is the responsibility of the treating physician, relying on experience and knowledge of the patient, to determine dosages and the best treatment for the patient. The editors cannot be responsible for misuse or misapplication of the material in this work.

THE PUBLISHER

CONTENTS

PART I

COMMON DISEASES

PART II

COMMON PROCEDURES

PART III

DRUGS

APPENDIX 1

PART 1

COMMON
DISEASES

CARDIOVASCULAR SYSTEM

A. Ischemic Heart Disease

* * *

DEFINITION

Ischemic heart disease (IHD) reflects the presence of atherosclerosis in the coronary arteries (coronary artery disease).

INCIDENCE

Ten million adults in the United States have IHD. It is the leading cause of morbidity and mortality in the United States, causing 500,000 deaths each year. The first manifestation of IHD often is an acute myocardial infarction resulting in sudden death.

The prognosis for patients with IHD is related to the development and severity of cardiac dysrhythmias, myocardial infarctions, and left ventricular (LV) dysfunction. About 25 million patients in the United States undergo surgery each year—of these, 7 million are considered to be at high risk for IHD.

ETIOLOGY

IHD is due to atherosclerosis in the coronary arteries. Dyspnea after onset of angina indicates acute LV dysfunction, which can lead to congestive heart failure (CHF) from myocardial ischemia. Risk factors are many; the most important are male gender and advanced age. Others include hypercholesterolemia, hypertension, cigarette smoking, diabetes, obesity, sedentary life style, family history of premature development of IHD, and psychosocial characteristics. There are three types of angina: stable, unstable, and variant (Prinzmetal's). *Stable angina* is predictable—chest pain occurs predictably at the same amount of cardiac work or stimulation, often with a heart rate of 125 beats per minute. *Variant angina* is due to coronary artery spasm of unknown cause that leads to ischemia and causes chest pain. *Unstable angina* is a combination of stable and variant angina. Plaque is present and decreases lumen size and spasm.

DIAGNOSTIC AND LABORATORY FINDINGS

Cardiac Evaluation

History and physical examination, chest radiography, and electrocardiography (ECG) should be performed in the patient with known or suspected

IHD. If the initial evaluation suggests IHD, stress testing is indicated: exercise ECG, radionucleotide tests (exercise thallium or dipyridamole thallium). If stress tests suggest IHD, proceed with cardiac catheterization.

History

Elicit the severity of, progression of, and function limitation imposed by the IHD. One must analyze symptoms of exercise tolerance, dyspnea, angina, and peripheral edema to detect functional impairment due to coronary disease. Symptoms may not be present at rest; the patient's response to physical activity must be evaluated (i.e., Can the patient climb two flights of stairs?). One must recognize the patient with borderline CHF—the added stress of anesthesia, surgery, and fluid administration may cause overt failure.

Evaluation of LV Function	
Good	Impaired
By History and Physical Examination	
Angina	Prior myocardial infarction
Essential hypertension	Evidence of CHF
No evidence of CHF	
By Cardiac Catheterization	
Ejection fraction > 0.55	Ejection fraction < 0.40
LV end-diastolic pressure < 12	LV end-diastolic pressure > 18
Cardiac index > 2.5 L/min per m²	Cardiac index < 21 L/min per m²
No area of ventricular dyskinesia	Multiple areas of ventricular dyskinesia

CLINICAL MANIFESTATIONS

Angina

Substernal chest pain with occasional radiation to the neck, jaw, left shoulder, or left arm that is often precipitated by exertion and may be relieved with rest or sublingual nitroglycerin.

	Exercise-Induced	Occurs at Rest	Night Pain	ST Segment
Stable	Yes	No (yes with emotion)	Occasionally with dreams	Depressed
Unstable	Yes	Yes	Yes	Depressed or elevated
Variant	Rarely	Yes	Early in AM	Elevated usually—can also be depressed

TREATMENT

The goal is to decrease myocardial oxygen demand and increase coronary blood flow. This can be achieved by various ways.

General Medical Means

1. Control related pathology—CHF, hypertension
2. Smoking cessation
3. Weight loss
4. Exercise
5. Stress modification
6. Antithrombotic medications—low-dose aspirin prevents reinfarct
7. Avoidance of heavy meals or cold prior to exertion

Drug Therapy

1. Nitrates
2. Beta-blockers
3. Calcium channel blockers
4. Combined therapy

Revascularization—When Patient's Condition Is Refractory to Drug Therapy

1. Coronary artery bypass graft
2. Angioplasty

ANESTHETIC CONSIDERATIONS

Preoperative

Decrease anxiety—sympathetic activation may increase myocardial oxygen demands and cause ischemia. Midazolam (Versed) can be used for sedation and amnesia. Nitroglycerin also may be used prophylactically.

Intraoperative

Prevent intraoperative events that adversely affect the balance between oxygen delivery and demand at the myocardium. Factors that can cause decreased oxygen delivery and increased oxygen requirements are listed below.

Decreased Oxygen Delivery	Increased Oxygen Requirements
1. Decreased coronary blood flow: increased heart rate, increased diastolic blood pressure (BP), hypocapnia	1. Sympathetic stimulation
2. Coronary artery spasm	2. Increased heart rate
3. Decreased oxygen content: anemia, arterial hypoxemia	3. Increased systolic BP
4. Increased preload	4. Increased myocardial contractility
	5. Increased afterload

The goal is to maintain heart rate and BP within 20% of normal values. Note that a heart rate above 100 beats per minute is more likely to cause signs and symptoms of ischemia on ECG.

Induction

Most induction drugs are acceptable. Keep laryngoscopy as short as possible to decrease sympathetic stimulation. The following drugs can be used if intubation or hypertension already exists:

1. Lidocaine 1 to 2 mg/kg intravenous (IV) 90 seconds prior to intubation
2. Nitroprusside (Nipride) 1 to 2 μg/kg IV 15 seconds prior to intubation
3. Esmolol 100 to 300 μg/kg per minute IV before and during intubation
4. Fentanyl 0.25 to 1 μg/kg per minute IV to decrease pressor response

Maintenance

Maintain normal or optimal LV function. Volatile anesthetics minimize the increased sympathetic activity and increased oxygen demand. Volatile anesthetics with or without nitrous oxide are acceptable, or a nitrous oxide/opioid combination with the addition of volatile anesthetics can be used to treat an undesired increase in BP.

Muscle Relaxation

Choice is determined by the effect on the heart. Vecuronium, doxacurium, cisatracurium, rocuronium, and pipecuronium have no cardiac effect. Pancuronium causes an increase in heart rate and therefore may cause an increased oxygen demand.

Reversal Agents

Anticholinesterase and anticholinergics are considered safe for these patients. Glycopyrrolate is preferred.

EMERGENCE

Same considerations apply here as for induction (i.e., prevent increased oxygen demand and decreased coronary blood flow). Patients with severe IHD may need treatment for hypertension episodes during emergence.

POSTOPERATIVE CARE

Adequate pain relief is essential to prevent sympathetic stimulation.

TABLE 1/I/B-1 Drugs of Choice for Common Arrhythmias

Arrhythmia	Drug of Choice	Alternatives	Remarks
Atrial fibrillation or flutter[1] *	Verapamil, diltiazem or a beta-blocker to slow ventricular response[1]	Digoxin to slow ventricular response Quinidine, procainamide, disopyramide, flecainide, propafenone or sotalol for long-term prevention Ibutilide for termination of the arrhythmia	Digoxin, verapamil, diltiazem and possibly beta-blockers may be dangerous for patients with Wolff-Parkinson-White syndrome. Amiodarone in low doses has also been effective for prevention. Radiofrequency catheter ablation has been used in selected patients.
Other supraventricular tachycardias[2]	Adenosine, verapamil[3] or diltiazem[3] for termination	Esmolol, another beta-blocker or digoxin for termination	DC cardioversion or atrial pacing may be effective for some patients. Radiofrequency catheter ablation can cure many patients. Quinidine, procainamide, disopyramide, diltiazem, beta-blockers, verapamil, flecainide, propafenone or digoxin may be effective for long-term suppression.
Ventricular premature complexes (VPCs) or nonsustained ventricular tachycardia	No drug therapy indicated for asymptomatic patients	For symptomatic patients, a beta-blocker	There is no evidence that prolonged suppression with drugs prevents sudden cardiac death. For post-MI patients, treatment with a beta-blocker has decreased mortality, and treatment with flecainide or moricizine has increased it.

6

Sustained ventricular tachycardia[4,5]	Lidocaine for acute treatment[4,5]	Procainamide, bretylium, amiodarone[4,5]	Sotalol, other beta-blockers, procainamide, quinidine, amiodarone, disopyramide, flecainide, propafenone or mexiletine may be effective for long-term prevention.[6] See footnote 6.
Ventricular fibrillation[7]	Lidocaine[7]	Amiodarone, procainamide, bretylium[7]	Self-limited if digoxin is stopped. Phenytoin can also be effective. Avoid DC cardioversion and bretylium, except for ventricular fibrillation or sustained ventricular tachycardia. A beta-blocker or procainamide can make heart block worse.
Cardiac glycoside–induced ventricular tachyarrhythmias[5,8]	Digoxin-immune Fab (digoxin antibody fragments—Digibind)	Lidocaine, phenytoin	
Torsades de pointes (acquired)	Magnesium sulfate	Cardiac pacing, isoproterenol	Causative agents (e.g., quinidine) should be discontinued. Magnesium sulfate in a dose of 1 g IV, repeated once if necessary, may be effective even in absence of hypomagnesemia. Potassium should be used to raise serum K to between 4 and 5.5 mEq/L[8]

* Superscript numbers refer to the numbered list in Table 1/I/B–2.
From *Drugs for cardiac arrhythmias*. Med Lett. 1996;38:75–76.

PROGNOSIS

IHD is a chronic condition that requires continuous management before and after surgery.

B. Arrhythmias

• • •

The current drugs of choice for common arrhythmias are listed in Table 1/I/B–1. The dosages and adverse effects of each drug are given in Table 1/I/B–2. Several reports have indicated that when given to asymptomatic or mildly symptomatic patients, at least some antiarrhythmic agents may increase rather than decrease mortality.

TABLE 1/I/B–2   Notes to Table 1/I/B–1

1. DC cardioversion is the safest and most effective treatment. For patients with atrial flutter, atrial pacing can also be effective. Patients with Wolff-Parkinson-White syndrome and atrial fibrillation should be treated with IV procainamide if hemodynamically stable and, if not, with DC cardioversion.

2. Vagotonic maneuvers (such as carotid sinus massage, gagging, the Valsalva maneuver, or increasing venous return by straight leg raising) may be tried first.

3. Verapamil and diltiazem are contraindicated for patients receiving intravenous beta-blockers or those with congestive heart failure and should be used with caution in patients taking oral quinidine.

4. DC cardioversion is the safest and most effective treatment. It is preferred by most cardiologists for sustained ventricular tachycardia causing hemodynamic compromise, but some first try a chest thump, IV lidocaine or both.

5. Some ventricular tachycardias can be caused or exacerbated by bradycardia or heart block. In the presence of high-grade heart block, antiarrhythmic drugs can cause cardiac standstill. When high-grade heart block is present, therefore, a temporary pacemaker should be inserted before using antiarrhythmic drugs; pacing may abolish the arrhythmia. When a drug must be used in the presence of heart block, lidocaine is least likely to increase the block.

6. Specialized techniques such as programmed stimulation of the heart may be required to select long-term therapy, and some patients may be candidates for implanted cardioverter/defibrillators (see *Med Lett.* 1994;36:86) or radiofrequency catheter ablation (see *Med Lett.* 1996;38:40).

7. Defibrillation is the treatment of choice; drugs are for prevention of recurrence.

8. KCl can be given carefully, 10–20 mEq/hr IV, to patients with low or normal serum potassium concentrations. Extreme care must be taken to keep serum potassium below 5.5 mEq/L. In the presence of heart block not associated with paroxysmal atrial tachycardia, potassium should be withheld if the serum concentration is greater than 4.5 mEq/L because high serum potassium may increase atrioventricular block.

C. Myocardial Infarction

◆　◆　◆

DEFINITION

Myocardial infarction (MI) occurs when heart muscle dies as a result of inadequate blood supply due to blockages, acute thrombosis, and spasm.

INCIDENCE AND PREVALENCE

It is important to ascertain whether a patient has a history of prior MI. The incidence of perioperative myocardial reinfarction strongly correlates with time elapsed since prior MI. The average reinfarction rate is about 6% if the time elapsed is 6 months. Thus, elective surgery, especially thoracic or abdominal, *should be delayed for 6 months following MI*. Even with a 6-month delay, these patients are still at greater risk than patients who have not suffered an MI. In high-risk patients, hemodynamic monitoring and aggressive treatment of fluids and cardiac alterations have reduced the risk of reinfarction.

The incidence of reinfarction is increased in patients undergoing intrathoracic or intra-abdominal operations lasting more than 3 hours. Other factors increasing the potential for reinfarction include hypotension lasting longer than 10 minutes, hypertension and tachycardia, diabetes, smoking, high cholesterol, and poor overall condition.

ETIOLOGY

When supply (blood flow) does not meet demand (oxygen consumption), ischemia or infarction occurs. Once a patient experiences an MI, his or her risk for perioperative MI increases.

LABORATORY TESTS

Laboratory tests as indicated by the history and physical examination may include electrolytes, complete blood count, blood urea nitrogen, creatinine, cardiac enzymes, Holter monitoring for ST and arrhythmia analysis, echocardiography for evaluation of valve function and left ventricular function, stress testing for evaluation of ischemia, dipyridamole or dobutamine stress testing for those patients who cannot tolerate exercise testing, radionuclide ejection fraction, and the gold standard of cardiac catheterization. The approach must be individualized to the needs and risks of the patient.

CLINICAL MANIFESTATIONS

Many patients are asymptomatic following an MI. Commonly seen manifestations of angina and coronary artery disease include poor exercise tolerance, chest pain (stable or unstable), dyspnea, congestive heart failure, and arrhythmias. These patients need to be risk-stratified according to the New York Heart Association Functional Classification and the American Society of Anesthesiologists classification.

TREATMENT AND ANESTHETIC CONSIDERATIONS

Basic anesthesia care starts with a thorough history and physical examination. The history reveals risk factors, activity tolerance, a determination of angina (stable or unstable), and any use of nitroglycerin. The physical examination reveals to the astute clinician any extra heart sounds, rates, rhonchi, edema, and other physical findings that may signify underlying cardiac problems. These data allow the clinician to better assess left ventricular function. The anesthesia provider must communicate with the primary physician and surgeon to weigh the risks and benefits for the patient.

The importance of minimizing stress and maximizing myocardial perfusion intraoperatively cannot be emphasized enough. Reduction of stress begins in the preoperative area with the use of individualized sedation. Stress and an increase in metabolic work during the perioperative period increases myocardial oxygen demand. The heart may not be able to handle the increased demand related to the underlying pathology of coronary artery disease, resulting in myocardial ischemia or MI. Supply and demand of oxygen must be balanced for optimal outcome.

Four questions must be answered before the patient goes into the operating room. These questions are answered largely by a careful history. The questions are: What is the extent of coronary artery disease? Is an additional diagnosis needed? Is additional therapy indicated (e.g., catheterization, percutaneous transluminal coronary angioplasty, or coronary artery bypass graft)? What is the extent of ventricular compromise? This is important in that the extent of ventricular compromise affects the anesthetic and titration of anesthetics. And finally, Will the patient tolerate surgery?

Standard monitoring is utilized with these patients. Electrocardiographic monitoring of lead II (for inferior ischemia) and lead V5 (for anterior ischemia) is essential in identifying ischemia. Other monitoring modalities to consider: ST-segment trend monitoring, esophageal lead (to identify P waves or if lead placement is a problem), transesophageal echocardiography (e.g., for evaluating left ventricular function or ischemic valve problems), Swan-Ganz catheter (to evaluate right-sided heart pressure, wedge pressure, fluid status, and a reflection of left ventricular function), and arterial line to evaluate hemodynamics. Options can be utilized to maximize the delivery of the anesthetic care based on the patient and the type of surgical procedure.

Aggressive treatment of ischemia is imperative. The reason for cognizant monitoring is to allow rapid assessment of patient changes and swift intervention in the patient at risk for perioperative cardiac complications. Appropriate interpretation of the data and aggressive treatment have been demonstrated to improve outcome.

Fluid management must be individualized and titrated appropriately for the type of surgery and degree of left ventricular function. A central venous pressure or Swan-Ganz catheter can offer guidance in fluid management in the high-risk patient. In the cardiac-compromised patient, fluid balance and fluid overload often are separated by a fine line. Thus, appropriate fluid management cannot be regarded lightly in cardiac patients. Intraoperative overhydration may lead to postoperative hypertension and, in patients with myocardial disease, may exacerbate congestive heart failure.

Urine output must be closely monitored in cardiac and high-risk patients. Urine output reflects cardiac output (in a patient with normal kidneys). Urine output also is an indicator of volume status.

The anesthetic plan of care must be tailored for the individual patient with coronary artery disease. General, regional, and local anesthetic techniques can be selected.

General anesthesia and spinal anesthesia parallel each other when risks of postoperative MI and cardiac death are compared. The combination of general anesthesia and postoperative epidural anesthesia for vascular surgery has been suggested to lower cardiac complications. The incidence and risk of congestive heart failure are higher with general anesthesia in patients with severe coronary artery disease.

It is important to note that patient outcome is based on *how* the agents and technique are administered and individualized for each patient.

Emergence should be slow and smooth. Avoid hypertension and prevent conditions that do not provide optimal cardiovascular stability. It is best to keep the patient from shivering, because it increases myocardial oxygen demand and stresses the heart. Extubation may need to be delayed until cardiovascular status and stability are evaluated.

Ongoing postoperative observation of high-risk patients is essential to identify and aggressively treat cardiac complications. These complications include congestive heart failure, extremes of blood pressure, arrhythmias, cardiac ischemia, and MI. Identification and control of tachycardia, fever, pain, extremes in blood pressure, and fluid management may minimize the potential for postoperative ischemic events and improve outcome.

Recognizing the importance of preoperative assessment of the complications and mortality related to anesthesia and surgery is the first step toward prevention. Patients at risk for perioperative cardiac complications can be risk-stratified, and the information can be used to plan the safest anesthesia and intraoperative monitoring.

D. Hypertension

◆   ◆   ◆

DEFINITION

Systolic blood pressure (SBP) greater than 160 mm Hg or diastolic blood pressure (DBP) greater than 90 mm Hg or both. Mortality and morbidity increase with increasing levels of either SBP or DBP.

INCIDENCE

Hypertension (HTN) is the most common circulatory derangement, affecting 60 million Americans. Prevalence of HTN increases with age. Approximately half of those over 65 years of age have systolic or diastolic HTN.

ETIOLOGY

Blood pressure (BP) is regulated by baroreceptors (feedback loops) and secretion of vasoactive hormones (renin, angiotensin, aldosterone, and catecholamines). Any abnormality in this system can lead to HTN. Essential HTN has no identifiable cause and accounts for more than 90% of patients with HTN. Secondary HTN does have a demonstrable cause, such as renal disease, coarctation, Cushing's syndrome, pheochromocytoma, primary aldosteronism, and pharmacologic agents.

DIAGNOSTIC AND LABORATORY FINDINGS

Usually, persistent elevation of SBP is greater than 160 mm Hg and that of DBP is greater than 90 mm Hg. Renal disease, coarctation, hyperadrenocorticism, and pheochromocytoma are common secondary causes. Organ system involvement is determined through diagnostic testing.

TREATMENT

When DBP is greater than 90 mm Hg, drug treatment is usually employed, although isolated systolic HTN may respond to diet modification and weight loss. Patients with borderline HTN can decrease their BP with exercise and weight loss. If DBP exceeds 105 mm Hg, aggressive treatment is needed to decrease morbidity and mortality from myocardial infarction, congestive heart failure, cerebrovascular accident, and renal failure.

Drugs used to treat HTN include diuretics, angiotensin converting enzyme inhibitors, calcium channel blockers, beta-blockers, and vasodilators. Initial treatment often is with a diuretic, angiotensin converting enzyme inhibitor, or beta antagonist. Potassium levels should be monitored, as hypokalemia or hyperkalemia may be a side effect. Combination treatment is frequently used because treatment with a single drug may evoke undesirable physiologic responses. (Diuretics often cause a compensatory increase in renin activity, which reflects a decrease in intravascular volume.)

ANESTHETIC CONSIDERATIONS

Preoperative

Determine adequacy of BP control and review patient medications and associated pharmacology. Evaluate associated organ dysfunction (orthostatic hypotension, ischemic heart disease, cerebrovascular disease, peripheral vascular disease, renal dysfunction). Continue anti-HTN medications preoperatively. Management of emergency surgery in a patient with uncontrolled HTN includes maintaining a BP of 140/90, provided no evidence of cerebral ischemia or renal dysfunction is present.

Ideally, patients should be normotensive prior to surgery to decrease the incidence of cardiac ischemia. Also, BP is likely to decrease more during anesthesia in the hypertensive patient. It must be noted that chronic HTN is frequently associated with hypovolemia and ischemic heart disease; therefore, a decrease in BP is more likely to result in cardiac ischemia.

Induction

Expect exaggerated changes in BP and hypotension due to drug-induced vasodilation in the presence of decreased intravascular fluid volume. Laryngoscopy and intubation may cause HTN and should be performed as quickly as possible. One may need to deepen anesthesia by increasing the inhalation of volatile anesthetic or by utilizing opioids prior to intubation. Lidocaine can also attenuate the pressor response. Doses of labetalol or esmolol just prior to laryngoscopy may help to attenuate the BP response.

Maintenance

The goal during this period is to adjust the level of anesthesia so as to minimize the wide changes in BP. A volatile anesthetic is ideal for permitting a rapid adjustment in the depth of anesthesia in response to a change in BP. HTN in response to pain is the most common intraoperative change. All anesthetic gases produce a dose-dependent decrease in BP, with no drug preferable over another. Anesthesia can also be maintained using nitrous oxide/opioid technique. A volatile anesthetic may be needed at times to control undesirable increases in BP during periods of surgical stimulation.

The anesthesia provider needs to select the vasoactive agents to treat HTN, hypotension, or both if needed.

Monitors include routine use of electrocardiographic monitoring leads II and V_5 to best detect cardiac ischemia. Direct arterial pressure monitoring may be warranted.

Postoperative

HTN in the early postoperative period is common because of an exaggerated sympathetic response with or without relative hypovolemia related to intraoperative fluid replacement. Postoperative HTN requires prompt assessment and treatment to decrease risk of cardiac ischemia, dysrhythmia, congestive heart failure, cerebrovascular accident, and bleeding. If HTN continues despite adequate analgesia, hydralazine (2.5 to 10 mg IV every 10 to 20 minutes) or labetalol (0.1 to 0.25 mg/kg IV every 10 minutes) or esmolol (0.5 to 1.0 mg/kg, as needed) may be used.

E. Congestive Heart Failure

◆ ◆ ◆

DEFINITION

Congestive heart failure (CHF) is, as the name suggests, failure of the myocardium to function properly; this improper function causes pulmonary congestion, which can lead to pulmonary edema. CHF may involve one or both sides of the heart.

COMMON DISEASES

ETIOLOGY

CHF is usually due to: (1) cardiac valve abnormalities, (2) impaired myocardial contractility secondary to ischemic heart disease or cardiomyopathy, (3) systemic hypertension, or (4) pulmonary hypertension (cor pulmonale). CHF in the preoperative period is the most important contributor to postoperative cardiac morbidity and mortality. The heart has adaptive mechanisms that allow it to maintain its cardiac output (CO). These include: (1) Frank-Starling relation (increase in stroke volume that accompanies an increase in end-diastolic pressure), (2) inotropic state, (3) afterload, (4) heart rate, (5) myocardial hypertrophy and dilation, (6) sympathetic nervous system activity, and (7) humoral-mediated responses.

DIAGNOSTIC AND LABORATORY FINDINGS

1. Cardiac index is less than 2.5 L/min per kg with severe CHF.
2. Ejection fraction is often less than 0.50.
3. End-diastolic pressure parallels the end-diastolic volume and is increased in the presence of CHF. Left ventricular end-diastolic pressure is normally less than 12 mm Hg, and right ventricular end-diastolic pressure is normally less than 5 mm Hg.

CLINICAL MANIFESTATIONS

Left Ventricular Failure

1. Fatigue
2. Dyspnea due to interstitial pulmonary edema
3. Orthopnea
4. Paroxysmal nocturnal dyspnea
5. Acute pulmonary edema
6. Tachypnea and rales
7. Tachycardia and peripheral vasoconstriction
8. Oliguria
9. Pleural effusion

Right Ventricular Failure

1. Systemic venous congestion—jugular venous distention
2. Hepatomegaly
3. Ascites
4. Peripheral edema—dependent and pitting edema

TREATMENT

Treatment of CHF includes use of digitalis preparations, vasodilators, and inotropes.

Digitalis

Digitalis is the only orally effective positive inotropic agent currently in use. Digoxin is excreted mainly by the kidneys, and its elimination parallels creatinine clearance. During the perioperative period, sensitivity to digoxin can be increased if there are decreases in renal function or hypokalemia. Prophylactic treatment with digitalis is controversial in the patient with CHF who is undergoing elective surgery. Elderly patients undergoing thoracic surgery, however, may benefit. Digitalis may be continued in the preoperative period, especially if it is used to control heart rate. Digitalis toxicity should be suspected during the preoperative period if the patient complains of nausea and vomiting, cardiac dysrhythmia is present, and the digitalis level is greater than 3 mg/mL. Treatment of digitalis toxicity includes correction of hypokalemia, treatment of dysrhythmias, and insertion of a temporary pacemaker if complete heart block is present. If surgery cannot be delayed and the patient has digitalis toxicity, it is important to avoid sympathomimetics (ketamine) and hyperventilation (can cause hypokalemia).

Diuretics

Monitor plasma potassium, especially if the patient is treated with digitalis preparations. Chronic administration of loop diuretics can lead to hypovolemia, orthostatic hypotension, and hypokalemia.

Vasodilators

CO can be maintained by manipulating the peripheral circulation with vasodilators. The CO is increased by decreasing impedance to the forward ejection of the left ventricle. Hypotension can result, however, and is a limiting factor in treating CHF with vasodilators. An arterial line and pulmonary arterial catheter are useful in monitoring cardiac filling pressures, CO, systemic vascular resistance, and peripheral vascular resistance. Commonly used vasodilators include the following:

1. Nitroglycerin 0.5 to 5 μg/kg per minute IV
2. Hydralazine 25 to 100 mg PO
3. Nitroprusside 0.5 to 5 μg/kg per minute IV
4. Prazosin 1 to 5 mg PO
5. Captopril 25 to 75 mg PO
6. Enalapril 5 to 40 mg PO

Inotropes

Dopamine, intravenous dobutamine, or both are often used perioperatively to improve cardiac contractility. This combination provides the beneficial renal effects of dopamine and the beta effects of dobutamine at doses that are unlikely to increase afterload. A pulmonary arterial catheter should be used to monitor the effects of these drugs on CO and filling pressures.

ANESTHETIC CONSIDERATIONS

If surgery cannot be delayed, the goal is to optimize CO. Ketamine is a good choice for induction of anesthesia in the patient with CHF. Volatile anesthetics must be used with caution because they produce dose-dependent cardiac depression. Severe CHF requires the careful titration of all anesthetic agents for maintenance of anesthesia. Positive-pressure ventilation of the lungs may help by decreasing pulmonary congestion and improving arterial oxygenation. Invasive monitoring, including an arterial line, should be considered in the patient with CHF. CO is to be supported with dopamine, dobutamine, or both as necessary. Regional anesthesia may be used for peripheral surgery in the patient with CHF. Selection of the anesthetic technique and agents is individualized for each patient, with consideration of the medical history and surgical procedure.

F. Shock

•   •   •

HEMORRHAGIC SHOCK

DEFINITION

A potential complication of acute blood loss. Decreased intravascular fluid volume leading to decreased venous return and inadequate tissue perfusion.

ETIOLOGY

Hemorrhagic shock is a result of acute blood loss, frequently owing to trauma. There is decreased intravascular fluid volume, venous return, and cardiac output (CO) with inadequate tissue perfusion. Sympathetic nervous system activity is increased during acute hemorrhage, redirecting blood flow to the brain and heart. If this is prolonged, a detrimental decrease in renal and hepatic flow can occur. Anaerobic metabolism is increased and is seen as metabolic acidosis.

TREATMENT

Blood replacement therapy includes administration of whole blood or packed red cells. Crystalloids are also used because fluid shifts accompany hemorrhage. Treatment requires continuous monitoring of arterial pressure, cardiac filling pressures, and urine output to guide volume replacement. A pulmonary arterial catheter is helpful to determine CO and systemic vascular resistance. Dopamine is useful in some patients, especially if the goal is to cause a mild inotropic effect and increase the renal blood flow. Vasopressors, however, may be necessary to preserve cerebral and cardiac perfusion until intravascular fluid volume can be replaced. Fresh-frozen plasma and platelets are administered as needed.

ANESTHETIC CONSIDERATIONS

Induction and maintenance requires invasive monitoring of blood pressure. Ketamine is used to induce anesthesia because it stimulates the sympathetic nervous system. Additional anesthetic agents are carefully titrated according to the patient's hemodynamic status. Treatment of hemorrhagic shock aims to stop the bleeding and replace the volume lost, ideally with whole blood or packed red blood cells while maintaining adequate perfusion pressures to the vital organs.

SEPTIC SHOCK

DEFINITION

Shock due to the presence of pathogenic organisms or their toxins in the blood.

ETIOLOGY

Early Phase

This is characterized by hypotension with decreased systemic vascular resistance and increased CO, fever, and hyperventilation. Vasodilation may be due to endotoxins derived from cell walls of bacteria that cause the release of vasoactive substances (histamine phase can last up to 24 hours).

Late Phase

CO is increased in this phase. Lactic acidosis develops, which reflects impaired tissue oxygen CO as well as dilation of peripheral vessels that allows shunting of blood across tissues. Intravascular fluid volume may fall because of damaged muscle. Oliguria is often present. Coagulation defects are common.

DIAGNOSTIC AND LABORATORY FINDINGS

Septic shock is suggested by the development of hypotension in the presence of perioperative oliguria.

TREATMENT

Treatment includes intravenous antibiotics and restoration of intravascular fluid volume. Antibiotics should be started immediately. Typically, two antibiotics are used to cover both gram-positive and gram-negative bacteria (clindamycin for gram-positive and gentamicin for gram-negative). Fluid replacement may be guided by measurement of right-sided or left-sided heart filling pressures and urine output. Dopamine is effective when supportive function is needed.

ANESTHETIC CONSIDERATIONS

No specific anesthetic drug has been proven to be ideal in the presence of septic shock. The anesthetic management is individualized to each patient.

G. Valvular Heart Disease

◆ ◆ ◆

DEFINITION

Valvular heart disease is characterized by anatomic abnormalities that initially alter cardiac loading conditions. The most frequently encountered cardiac valve lesions produce pressure overload (mitral stenosis, aortic stenosis) or volume overload (mitral regurgitation, aortic regurgitation) on the left atrium or left ventricle.

AORTIC STENOSIS

INCIDENCE AND PREVALENCE

Isolated aortic stenosis is the most common cardiac valvular abnormality. Valvular aortic stenosis without accompanying mitral valve disease is more common in men and is usually congenital or degenerative in origin.

ETIOLOGY AND PATHOLOGY

Congenital

Isolated nonrheumatic aortic stenosis usually results from progressive calcification and stenosis of a congenitally abnormal bicuspid valve. Congenitally stenotic aortic valves may be either unicuspid, bicuspid, or tricuspid, but the bicuspid variety is the most common, occurring in more than 50% of patients. Aortic stenosis due to rheumatic fever almost always occurs in association with mitral valve disease, accounting for less than 3% of aortic stenosis cases.

Acquired

The most common form of acquired valvular aortic stenosis is calcific aortic stenosis in which degeneration increases with age. Calcium deposits build up on normal cusps, preventing them from opening completely.

The anatomic obstruction to left ventricular ejection of blood into the aorta produces an increase in left ventricular pressure in order to maintain forward stroke volume. Left ventricular output is maintained by the presence of the left ventricular hypertrophy, which may sustain a large pressure gradient across the aortic valve for many years without a reduction in cardiac output, left ventricular dilation, or the development of symptoms.

Significant aortic stenosis is associated with a peak systolic transvalvular pressure gradient exceeding 50 mm Hg and an aortic valve orifice area of less than 1 cm^2. Atrial contraction is important to filling of the left ventricle. The atrial contribution to ventricular filling may be as high as 40% in patients with aortic stenosis (about 20% normally). Left ventricle enddiastolic pressures are often elevated, causing symptoms of pulmonary congestion despite normal left ventricular contractility. Increased intraventricular pressure stimulates the parallel replication of sarcomeres, resulting in concentric ventricular hypertrophy. Muscle mass is increased, but cavity size remains the same because there is not volume overload.

DIAGNOSIS

A long latent period exists during which obstruction increases gradually and the pressure load on the myocardium increases while the patient remains asymptomatic. Patients with advanced aortic stenosis have dyspnea on exertion, angina, and orthostatic or exertional syncope.

Aortic stenosis has a characteristic systolic murmur, best heard in the second right intercostal space with transmission into the neck. Echocardiography shows thickening and calcification of the aortic valve and decreased mobility of the valve leaflets in almost all patients with calcific aortic stenosis. The incidence of arrhythmias leading to severe hypoperfusion accounts for syncope and the increased incidence of sudden death in patients with aortic stenosis.

TREATMENT

When significant symptoms develop, most patients die without surgical treatment within 2 to 5 years. Percutaneous transluminal valvuloplasty may be an alternative to surgery, but restenosis usually occurs within 6 to 12 months.

ANESTHETIC CONSIDERATIONS

Maintain normal sinus rhythm
Avoid bradycardia
Avoid sudden increases or decreases in systemic vascular resistance
Optimize intravascular fluid volume to maintain venous return and left ventricular filling

Spinal and epidural anesthesia are contraindicated in patients with severe aortic stenosis and employed cautiously in patients with mild to moderate aortic stenosis, because such anesthesia can produce an undesirable decrease in systemic vascular resistance. Prophylactic antibiotics are recommended.

PROGNOSIS

The 5-year survival rate for adults with valve replacement is approximately 85%.

AORTIC REGURGITATION

INCIDENCE AND PREVALENCE

Rheumatic fever is a common cause of primary disease of the valve leading to regurgitation. Other causes include infective endocarditis, trauma, congenital bicuspid valve, and diseases of connective tissue.

ETIOLOGY AND PATHOLOGY

Aortic regurgitation may be caused by primary disease of the aortic valve leaflets, the wall of the aortic root, or both.

The basic hemodynamic problem in aortic regurgitation is a decrease in forward left ventricular stroke volume because of regurgitation of part of the ejected stroke volume from the aorta back into the left ventricle.

In *chronic* aortic regurgitation, the left ventricle progressively dilates and undergoes eccentric hypertrophy. This increases end-diastolic volume, which maintains an effective stroke volume because end-systolic volume is unchanged. Because ventricular compliance initially increases, left ventricular end-diastolic pressure is usually normal or only slightly elevated.

In *acute* aortic regurgitation, the regurgitant blood fills a ventricle of normal size that cannot accommodate the combined large regurgitant volume and inflow from the left atrium. The sudden rise in left ventricular end-diastolic pressure is transmitted back to the pulmonary circulation and causes acute pulmonary congestion.

DIAGNOSIS

Most patients with chronic aortic regurgitation remain asymptomatic for 10 to 20 years. When symptoms do develop, exertional dyspnea, orthopnea, and paroxysmal nocturnal dyspnea are the principal complaints.

In acute aortic regurgitation, patients develop sudden clinical manifestations of cardiovascular collapse, with weakness, severe dyspnea, and hypotension. Chronic aortic regurgitation is recognized by its characteristic diastolic murmur (best heard in the second right intercostal space), widened pulse pressure, decreased diastolic pressure, and bounding peripheral pulses.

TREATMENT

Arterial blood pressure is decreased to reduce the diastolic gradient for regurgitation using afterload reduction via arterial vasodilators and angiotensin converting enzyme inhibitors. Early surgery is indicated for patients with acute aortic regurgitation because medical management is associated with a high mortality rate. Patients with chronic aortic regurgitation should undergo surgery before irreversible ventricular dysfunction occurs.

ANESTHETIC CONSIDERATIONS

Avoid sudden decreases in heart rate
Avoid sudden increases in systemic vascular resistance
Minimize drug-induced myocardial depression

Most patients tolerate spinal and epidural anesthesia provided intravascular volume is maintained. Prophylactic antibiotics are recommended.

PROGNOSIS

Favorable clinical responses to valve replacement have been reported in patients with evidence of relatively severe preoperative ventricular dysfunction. Aortic valve replacement significantly improves left ventricular performance in most patients with chronic aortic regurgitation.

MITRAL STENOSIS

INCIDENCE AND PREVALENCE

Pure mitral stenosis occurs in 25% of patients; mitral stenosis and mitral regurgitation occur in 40%.

ETIOLOGY AND PATHOLOGY

The predominant cause is rheumatic fever, which occurs about four times as frequently in women as in men. Less common etiologies include congenital mitral stenosis in infants and children and complications in association with the carcinoid syndrome, systemic lupus erythematosus, and rheumatic arthritis.

After the episode of acute rheumatic fever, stenosis of the mitral valve takes about 2 years to develop. Symptoms generally develop after 20 to 30 years, when the mitral valve orifice is reduced from its normal 4 to 6 cm^2 opening to one of less than 2 cm^2. Characteristically, mitral valve cusps fuse at their edge, and fusion of the chordae results in thickening and shortening of these structures. This valvular obstruction produces an increase in left atrial volume and pressure. Left ventricular filling and stroke volume in the presence of mild mitral stenosis are usually maintained at rest by the increased left atrial pressure. Stroke volume may decrease when effective atrial contraction is lost or with stress-induced tachycardia. Acute elevations in left atrial pressure occur and are rapidly transmitted back to the pulmonary capillaries.

Pulmonary hypertension results from passive backward transmission of the elevated left atrial pressure and irreversible increases in pulmonary vascular resistance. Chronic elevations in pulmonary capillary pressure are partially compensated by increases in pulmonary lymph flow, but an acute rise results in pulmonary edema. Transudation of fluid into the pulmonary interstitial space, decreased pulmonary compliance, and increased work of breathing lead to dyspnea on exertion.

DIAGNOSIS

About 50% of patients present with acute onset of congestive heart failure, often in association with paroxysmal attacks of atrial fibrillation. This arrhythmia occurs in about 40% of all patients with mitral stenosis. Stasis of blood in the distended left atrium predisposes to the formation of thrombi, which can be displaced as systemic emboli. The principal symptom of mitral stenosis is dyspnea due to reduced compliance of the lungs. Rupture of pulmonary-bronchial venous communications causes hemoptysis.

Mitral stenosis is recognized by the opening snap that occurs early in diastole and by a rumbling diastolic heart murmur best heard at the cardiac apex. The chest radiograph may show left atrial enlargement and evidence of pulmonary edema.

COMMON DISEASES

TREATMENT

Medical management is primarily supportive and includes limitation of physical activity, diuretics, and sodium restriction. Digoxin is useful in patients with atrial fibrillation, and beta-adrenergic blockers may control heart rate in some patients. Anticoagulation therapy is used in patients with a history of emboli and in those at high risk (over 40 years old and large atrium with chronic atrial fibrillation).

Surgical correction is undertaken once significant symptoms develop. Recurrent mitral stenosis following valvuloplasty is usually managed with valve replacement. Catheter balloon valvuloplasty using a percutaneous venous introduction and a trans-septal approach to the mitral valve may be used to decrease the degree of mitral stenosis in selected patients.

ANESTHETIC CONSIDERATIONS

Avoid sinus tachycardia or rapid ventricular response rate during atrial fibrillation

Avoid marked increases in central blood volume associated with overtransfusion or the head-down position

Avoid drug-induced decreases in systemic vascular resistance

Avoid events that may exacerbate pulmonary hypertension and evoke right ventricular failure, such as arterial hypoxemia and hypoventilation

Prophylactic antibiotics are recommended

Epidural is preferable to spinal anesthesia if regional anesthesia is planned because of the more gradual onset of sympathetic blockade.

PROGNOSIS

When mitral stenosis produces total incapacity, 20% of patients die within 6 months without surgical correction.

MITRAL REGURGITATION

INCIDENCE AND PREVALENCE

Severe mitral regurgitation requiring surgery occurs in about 5% of men and less than 1.5% of women.

ETIOLOGY AND PATHOLOGY

Abnormalities of the mitral annulus, mitral leaflets, chordae tendineae, and papillary muscles may cause mitral regurgitation. Chronic mitral regurgitation is usually the result of rheumatic fever, congenital or developmental abnormalities of the valve apparatus, or dilatation, destruction, or calcification of the mitral annulus. Acute mitral regurgitation is usually due to myocardial ischemia or infarctions, infective endocarditis, or chest trauma.

Because the regurgitant mitral orifice parallels the aortic valve, the impedance to ventricular emptying is reduced in mitral regurgitation. Almost half of the regurgitant volume is ejected into the left atrium before the aortic valve opens. The volume of mitral regurgitant flow depends on the systemic vascular resistance and forward stroke volume. Effective forward cardiac output is usually depressed in seriously symptomatic patients, whereas total left ventricular output (forward and regurgitant) is usually elevated.

There is little enlargement of the left atrium, but marked elevation of the mean left atrial pressure and pulmonary congestion are prominent symptoms. Atrial compliance determines the predominant clinical manifestations. Patients with normal or reduced atrial compliance (acute mitral regurgitation) have mainly pulmonary vascular congestion and edema. Patients with increased atrial compliance (chronic mitral regurgitation with a large dilated left atrium) primarily show signs of low cardiac output. Most patients are between the two extremes and exhibit symptoms of both pulmonary congestion and low cardiac output.

DIAGNOSIS

Symptoms usually take over 20 years to develop. Chronic weakness and fatigue secondary to low cardiac output are prominent features. The cardinal feature of mitral regurgitation is a blowing pansystolic murmur, best heard at the cardiac apex and often radiating to the left axilla. The regurgitant flow is responsible for the v wave present on the recording of the pulmonary artery occlusion pressure. The size of the v wave correlates with the magnitude of the regurgitant flow.

TREATMENT

Medical treatment includes digoxin, diuretics, and vasodilators. Afterload reduction increases forward stroke volume and decreases the regurgitant volume. Surgical treatment is usually reserved for patients with moderate to severe symptoms.

ANESTHETIC CONSIDERATIONS

Avoid sudden decreases in heart rate
Avoid sudden increases in systemic vascular resistance
Minimize drug-induced myocardial depression
Monitor the size of the v wave as a reflection of regurgitant flow

Prophylactic antibiotics are recommended. Spinal and epidural anesthesia are well tolerated, provided bradycardia is avoided.

PROGNOSIS

In most patients with mitral regurgitation, the clinical state and the quality of life improve following valve replacement. The cause of the mitral regurgitation also is important in the outcome following surgical treatment. In patients in whom mitral dysfunction is secondary to ischemic heart disease, the 5-year survival rate is about 30%; in rheumatic mitral regurgitation, the 5-year survival rate is approximately 70%.

TRICUSPID REGURGITATION

INCIDENCE AND PREVALENCE

Functional tricuspid regurgitation occurs in patients with right ventricular hypertension secondary to any form of cardiac and pulmonary vascular disease.

ETIOLOGY AND PATHOLOGY

Tricuspid regurgitation is generally due to dilatation of the right ventricle from the pulmonary hypertension that usually results from chronic left ventricular failure. Tricuspid regurgitation can be secondary to infective endocarditis (associated with intravenous drug abusers), rheumatic fever, or chest trauma.

Chronic left ventricular failure often leads to sustained increases in pulmonary vascular pressures. This chronic afterload increase causes the right ventricle to dilate progressively, and excessive dilatation of the tricuspid annulus eventually results in regurgitation. The right atrium and the vena cava are compliant and accommodate the volume overload with a minimal increase in right atrial pressure.

DIAGNOSIS

Patients with isolated tricuspid regurgitation are often totally asymptomatic for many years. Certain physical signs may be present immediately (pulsatile neck veins, pansystolic murmurs). Early fatigability and generalized weakness or a vague sensation of fullness in the right upper quadrant (congestive hepatomegaly) may also be described.

TREATMENT

Tricuspid regurgitation is generally well tolerated by most patients. Even surgical removal of the tricuspid valve is usually well tolerated. Treatment of the underlying disease process is more important than the tricuspid regurgitation itself.

ANESTHETIC CONSIDERATIONS

Maintain intravascular fluid volume and central venous pressure in high-normal range

Avoid any increase in pulmonary vascular resistance

Avoid positive end-expiratory pressure and high mean airway pressures because they reduce venous return and increase right ventricular afterload

Most patients tolerate spinal and epidural anesthesia well

Prophylactic antibiotics are recommended

PROGNOSIS

Excellent results have been reported with the use of tricuspid annuloplasty in patients with moderate tricuspid regurgitation. Management of severe tricuspid regurgitation entails annuloplasty or valve replacement. Durability of more than 10 years has been established with valvular prostheses.

H. Cardiomyopathy

♦ ♦ ♦

DEFINITION

Cardiomyopathies are characterized by myocardial dysfunction unrelated to the usual causes of coronary disease (atherosclerosis, valvular abnormalities, or hypertension). Progressive and life-threatening congestive heart failure (CHF) is common to all cardiomyopathies.

ETIOLOGY

Cardiomyopathies can be classified according to their associated hemodynamics and morphologies: (1) dilated, (2) restrictive, (3) hypertrophic, and (4) obliterative.

DILATED CARDIOMYOPATHY

This is characterized by a decreased myocardial contractility, often involving both ventricles and seen as decreased cardiac output (CO) and increased ventricular filling pressures. Functional mitral or tricuspid insufficiency may occur if dilation is severe. Electrocardiography may reveal left ventricular hypertrophy, ST and T-wave abnormalities, first-degree heart block, or a bundle branch block. Common dysrhythmias include premature ventricular contractions and atrial fibrillation. Chest radiographs may show cardiac enlargement and interstitial pulmonary edema. Diagnosis by echocardiography requires an ejection fraction of less than 0.40, a dilated and hyperkinetic left ventricle, and mild to moderate regurgitation. Mural thrombi often form, and systemic embolization is common.

The most common cause of dilated cardiomyopathy is multiple myocardial infarctions due to diffuse coronary artery disease. Risk factors include alcohol abuse and peripartum patients who manifest signs and symptoms 1 to 6 weeks after delivery. In some patients in whom febrile illness occurs frequently prior to the onset of cardiac dysfunction, a virus may be the cause.

TREATMENT

Patients with dilated cardiomyopathy must avoid unnecessary physical activity and exhibit total abstinence from alcohol. CHF is treated with digoxin and diuretics. Vasodilator treatment or an inotrope with vasodilator properties (amrinone or milrinone) may also be helpful. Ventricular dysrhythmias are treated with procainamide or quinidine. Because of the increased risk of pulmonary embolism, these patients are also treated with anticoagulants. Patients with associated collagen vascular disease, sarcoidosis, or inflammation on endocardial biopsy are treated with corticosteroids preoperatively. Tachydysrhythmias can be treated with beta-blockers. Patients with coronary artery disease and dilated cardiomyopathy may benefit from coronary revascularization to improve left ventricular (LV) function. With advanced CHF, these patients may be candidates for heart transplant, provided pulmonary hypertension does not exist.

ANESTHETIC CONSIDERATIONS

1. Avoid drug-induced myocardial depression
2. Maintain normovolemia
3. Prevent increases in afterload

Excess cardiovascular depression on induction in patients with a history of alcohol abuse may reflect undiagnosed dilated cardiomyopathy; however, failure of this expected sedative response to intravenous induction agents may reflect a slow circulation time. During maintenance, myocardial depression produced by volatile agents must be considered. Opiates exhibit benign effects on cardiac contractility but may not produce unconsciousness. Also, an opioid, nitrous, benzodiazepine technique may cause unexpected cardiac depression. Increases in heart rate associated with surgical stimulation may be treated with beta-blockers. Nondepolarizing muscle relaxants that exhibit few cardiovascular effects (vecuronium) are advised. Intravenous fluids should be guided by cardiac filling pressures; therefore a pulmonary artery catheter aids early recognition of the need for inotropes or vasodilators. Prominent a waves reflect mitral or tricuspid regurgitation. Intraoperative hypotension is treated with ephedrine. Phenylephrine, which has predominantly alpha stimulation, could cause adverse increases in afterload due to increased systemic vascular resistance (SVR).

Regional anesthesia may be used in selected patients, although caution is indicated in avoiding abrupt sympathetic blockade.

PROGNOSIS

Prognosis of dilated cardiomyopathy is poor, with a 5-year survival rate of 25% to 40%. The cause of death in 75% of these patients is CHF, and sudden death due to cardiac dysrhythmia is common. Pulmonary embolism or sudden death from dysrhythmia is found in over 50% of these patients on autopsy.

RESTRICTIVE CARDIOMYOPATHY

This condition manifests itself as impaired diastolic filling that produces increased filling pressures and decreased CO and mimics constrictive pericarditis. Restrictive cardiomyopathy causes a greater impairment of LV than right ventricular (RV) filling. LV filling pressures are usually greater than

RV filling pressures, and the left ventricle becomes less compliant. There is no effective treatment for this disease, and death is often the result of cardiac dysrhythmia or intractable CHF. Anesthetic management follows the same principles used in cardiac tamponade.

HYPERTROPHIC CARDIOMYOPATHY

This disease is an autosomal dominant hereditary condition. The peak incidence is in patients in their early fifties or seventies. Most of the elderly patients diagnosed with this condition are female.

The genetic defect involves an increased density of calcium channels, thus affecting the contractile process of the heart. The disease manifests itself as unexplained myocardial hypertrophy, often with greater thickening of the interventricular septum compared with the wall of the left ventricle. Echocardiography reveals a large variation in the location and extent of the hypertrophy. The disease is therefore often referred to as *hypertrophic cardiomyopathy with or without LV outflow obstruction*. These patients should not participate in sports because of the risk of sudden death. There is hypertrophy of the left ventricle, which becomes slitlike and elongated. The ejection fraction is often greater than 0.80, reflecting the hypercontractile condition of the heart even with severe LV outflow obstruction. Mitral regurgitation may be present and indicates interference with movement of the septal leaflet by the hypertrophied septum. The degree of ventricular outflow obstruction is influenced by contractility, preload, and afterload.

CLINICAL MANIFESTATIONS

The major symptoms include angina, syncope, tachydysrhythmias, and CHF. Angina that is relieved by placing the patient in the recumbent position is pathognomonic for this disease, because the increase in LV size in recumbency decreases the outflow obstruction. These patients are especially susceptible to coronary ischemia due to the marked LV hypertrophy, particularly when subendocardial blood flow is decreased from excessive pressure in the left ventricle.

In order to maintain CO, these patients depend on the atrial kick; therefore, atrial fibrillation is poorly tolerated. In addition, tachydysrhythmias impair diastolic filling time, which also decreases CO. These patients are prone to systemic embolization, and even asymptomatic patients are at risk for sudden unexpected death from LV outflow obstruction or ventricular tachycardia.

Cardiac murmurs may indicate LV outflow obstruction or mitral regurgitation in patients with hypertrophic cardiomyopathy. These murmurs are characterized by their marked variation with different maneuvers. Valsalva's maneuver decreases LV size, which increases the outflow obstruction; LV systolic pressures increase, causing the murmur of mitral regurgitation to intensify as well. Nitroglycerin and the standing position also intensify the murmur. Chest radiography and electrocardiography reveal LV hypertrophy, which may be the only sign in an asymptomatic patient. Abnormal Q waves may be seen because of the hypertrophied septum. This diagnosis should be considered in any young patient with an electrocardiogram suggestive of myocardial infarction. Cardiac catheterization may suggest mitral regurgitation or increased LV end-diastolic pressure. Decreased LV compliance causes increases in the height of the a wave to over 30 mm Hg. If LV outflow obstruction exists, there will be a pressure gradient across the aortic valve.

TREATMENT

The goal of treatment in these patients is to relieve the obstruction to LV outflow. This is often achieved with beta-blockers to lower the heart rate and contractility. Calcium channel blockers may help also. Caution should be taken to prevent drug-induced hypotension and negative inotropic effects; therefore, nitroglycerin should be avoided in these patients who present with angina. Should CHF exist also, the treatment is difficult. Diuretics can lead to hypovolemia and digoxin can increase cardiac contractility, both of which may worsen the obstruction. Cardioversion may be needed to maintain normal sinus rhythm. Patients with atrial fibrillation require anticoagulant treatment to prevent embolization. These patients are at risk for infective endocarditis and should receive prophylactic antibiotic treatment for dental or surgical procedures. Myotomy or myomectomy under bypass may be needed in 10% to 15% of these patients. Mitral valve replacement may also be needed.

ANESTHETIC CONSIDERATIONS

Anesthetic management is directed at minimizing LV outflow obstruction. Any drug or event that decreases cardiac contractility or increases preload or afterload will decrease the LV outflow obstruction.

Preoperative

Preoperative medications should decrease anxiety and activation of the sympathetic nervous system. Preoperative expansion of intravascular fluid volume will help to maintain intraoperative stroke volume and to lessen the adverse effects of positive-pressure ventilation.

Induction

Intravenous induction is acceptable with care to avoid sudden decreases in SVR. Slight myocardial depression can be tolerated. Ketamine is not a good choice because the associated increased myocardial contractility will enhance LV outflow obstruction and decrease the stroke volume. Laryngoscopy should be brief, and responses may be blunted by using a volatile anesthetic, opioid, or beta antagonist before laryngoscopy.

Maintenance

During maintenance, mild cardiac depression while maintaining intravascular fluid volume and SVR is desirable. Opiates alone are not the best choice because they do not provide cardiac depression and can decrease SVR. Opiates combined with nitrous oxide, however, may be helpful in providing myocardial depression and a slight increase in SVR. Regional anesthesia may increase the LV outflow obstruction because of the hemodynamic changes that result. Nondepolarizing muscle relaxants with little effect on the circulation are best for skeletal muscle paralysis. Tachycardia associated with pancuronium is not desirable in these patients, nor are the drug-induced histamine release and hypotension that can result from atracurium.

Invasive monitors, such as a pulmonary artery catheter, as well as transesophageal echocardiography and Doppler color flow imaging, may be useful. Intraoperative hypotension in response to decreased preload or afterload can be treated with an alpha agonist (phenylephrine, 50 to 100 μg IV). Beta agonists, such as ephedrine, dopamine, or dobutamine, are to be avoided because the associated increase in cardiac contractility and heart rate can worsen the outflow obstruction. A key factor in maintaining the blood pressure is the prompt replacement of blood loss and titration of fluids to the cardiac filling pressures. Persistent hypertension can be treated by titration of the volatile anesthetic. Vasodilators (sodium nitroprusside or nitroglycerin) are not used for this because they decrease SVR and worsen the problem. Maintenance of normal sinus rhythm is vital because ventricular filling depends on atrial contraction. Functional rhythm is treated with a decrease in the delivered concentration of volatile anesthetic. If this is not effective, atropine may be helpful. Beta-blockers may be needed to slow a persistently increased heart rate.

OBLITERATIVE CARDIOMYOPATHY

Obliterative cardiomyopathy is considered a variant of restrictive cardiomyopathy and is characterized by a marked decrease in ventricular compliance. This condition may occur in association with hypereosinophilic syndromes. Cardiac dysrhythmia, conduction disturbances, systemic embolization, and valvular inefficiency are common. Treatment may include steroids.

I. Peripheral Vascular Disease

◆   ◆   ◆

DEFINITION

Inflammation or disease of the peripheral vasculature.

ETIOLOGY

Peripheral vascular disease (PVD) may manifest as systemic vasculitis or arterial occlusive disease; there are many types of PVD.

TAKAYASU'S ARTERITIS

Takayasu's arteritis is a chronic inflammation of the aorta and its major branches and causes multiple organ dysfunction.

MANAGEMENT OF ANESTHESIA

Corticosteroid supplementation may be needed in patients already treated with these drugs. These patients may be taking anticoagulants; therefore, regional anesthesia may be controversial. Blood pressure may be difficult to measure noninvasively in the upper extremities, and a radial arterial line may be needed. Hyperextension of the head during laryngoscopy may compromise blood flow through the carotid arteries that are shortened because of the vascular inflammatory process. Preoperatively, it is useful to evaluate the range of motion of the cervical spine and any associated problems. Finally, the major goal of anesthesia in these patients is to maintain adequate perfusion pressure intraoperatively.

THROMBOANGIITIS OBLITERANS

DEFINITION

An inflammatory and occlusive disease that involves arteries and veins of the extremities, causing intermittent claudication. It often affects Jewish males aged 20 to 40 years.

MANAGEMENT OF ANESTHESIA

Prevention of cold-induced vasospasm is a major concern. This can be done by raising the ambient room temperature and trying to maintain body temperature. Blood pressure monitoring is best done noninvasively because placing an arterial line in the artery that supplies a potentially ischemic extremity may be questionable. Regional anesthesia is acceptable; however, avoid the use of epinephrine or other vasoconstrictors.

PROGNOSIS

The prognosis depends on the progression of the associated underlying disease. Raynaud's phenomenon is often associated with a period of "remission."

CHRONIC PERIPHERAL ARTERIAL OCCLUSIVE DISEASE

DEFINITION

This disease is usually due to peripheral atherosclerosis and often occurs in association with coronary or cerebral atherosclerosis.

ETIOLOGY AND CLINICAL MANIFESTATIONS

Occlusion of the distal abdominal aorta or the iliac arteries frequently occurs as claudication of the hips and buttocks. Elderly patients often present with occlusion of the common femoral or superficial femoral arteries. This produces a syndrome of claudication in or below the calf.

TREATMENT

Treatment includes revascularization, such as femoral-femoral bypass or any femoral-distal bypass procedure.

ANESTHETIC CONSIDERATIONS

The major risk for revascularization procedures lies in the associated ischemic heart disease. These procedures are done under general anesthesia; however, regional (epidural) anesthesia prior to anticoagulant therapy has not been associated with untoward events. Infrarenal clamping and unclamping in the presence of PVD is associated with minimal hemodynamic derangements; therefore, only a central venous pressure monitor usually is required. Thromboembolic complications, particularly in the kidneys, usually reflect dislodgement of atheroembolic debris. Spinal cord damage is unlikely, and special monitoring is not necessary.

SUBCLAVIAN STEAL SYNDROME

Occlusion of the subclavian or innominate artery by an atherosclerotic plaque proximal to the origin of the vertebral artery may result in reversal of blood flow from the brain, resulting in syncope. The pulse in the ipsilateral arm is usually absent or diminished (10 mm Hg lower).

CORONARY-SUBCLAVIAN STEAL SYNDROME

This syndrome occurs when incomplete stenosis of the left subclavian artery leads to a reversal of blood flow. The patient may present with angina and a decreased systolic blood pressure of at least 20 mm Hg in the ipsilateral arm. Bilateral brachial artery blood pressure measurement may be helpful in the preoperative assessment in patients with an internal mammary to coronary artery bypass.

ANEURYSMS OF THE THORACIC AND ABDOMINAL AORTA

DEFINITION

Diseases of the aorta are frequently aneurysmal, whereas occlusive disease is most likely to affect the peripheral arteries.

ETIOLOGY

The primary event in aortic dissection is a tear in the intima through which blood surges into a false lumen, separating the adventitia for various distances. Associated conditions include hypertension (present in 70% to 90% of patients with aneurysm), Marfan's syndrome, decelerations, blunt chest trauma, pregnancy, and iatrogenic injury (due to site or aortic cannulation or where the aorta has been cross-clamped). Aortic dissections that involve the ascending aorta are considered type A, and those that involve the descending aorta (distal to the left subclavian artery) are considered type B. Aneurysms can also be classified as saccular, fusiform, or dissecting.

CLINICAL MANIFESTATIONS

Signs and symptoms include (1) excruciating chest pain, (2) diminution or absence of peripheral pulses, stroke, paraplegia, and ischemia of extremities, (3) vasoconstriction and hypertension, (4) myocardial infarction, and (5) cardiac tamponade.

TREATMENT

Treatment is most effective with early recognition of the problem. Early short-term treatment includes pharmacologic measures to decrease systolic blood pressure to about 100 mm Hg and utilizing beta-blockers or other cardioactive agents to decrease contractility and vascular resistance. Definitive treatment requires surgical repair.

ANESTHETIC CONSIDERATIONS

Abdominal Aortic Aneurysm

History-taking and physical examination, with a focus on cardiac function, are essential. Hypertension and diabetes should be checked for. Hemoglobin and hematocrit, electrolytes, prothrombin time, partial thromboplastin time, urinalysis, and glucose testing also are indicated. Glucose should be kept below 200 mg/dL.

Monitors

These patients receive the routine monitors, which include an electrocardiogram with leads II and V5 and an arterial catheter; intraoperative laboratory tests include activated coagulation time, potassium ion, arterial blood gases, glucose, and hemoglobin and hematocrit. Transesophageal echocardrography and pulmonary artery catheter monitoring may be used for hemodynamic monitoring.

Induction

Most intravenous induction agents are acceptable in conjunction with a nondepolarizing muscle relaxant. A nasogastric tube and Foley catheter can be placed. Positioning is supine or lateral, depending on the location of the incision.

Maintenance

General anesthesia or a combined general and spinal/epidural technique is acceptable. Selection of the anesthetic agents depends on the medical history and physical condition of the patient.

Intravenous Fluids

A midline abdominal incision requires 10 to 15 mL/kg per hour, and a retroperitoneal approach requires 10 mL/kg per hour. NOTE: *Adequate fluid replacement is the major factor in preventing renal failure.* It is important to monitor the hemodynamic parameters and urine output. Keep blood pressure up by 10 to 15 mm Hg during cross-clamping, and keep it 3 to 5 mm Hg higher than preoperative values before removal. Mannitol may be given (25 g) prior to cross-clamping. Heparin (5000 to 10,000 units) also is used prior to cross-clamping. Activated coagulation times are monitored (normal value and at the beginning of and 5 minutes after heparin administration). The goal is to reach an activated coagulation time that is two to three times above normal. Protamine may be given to reverse this effect.

Hemodynamics

If narcotics are insufficient to establish control, nitroprusside or nitroglycerin may be used. Blood pressure should be below baseline prior to cross-clamping. The level of the clamp affects blood pressure changes: (1) Inferior—no increase in blood pressure, (2) suprarenal—shows a greater increase in blood pressure, (3) supraceliac—shows the greatest increase in blood pressure. Also, when the patient has aortic occlusive disease as opposed to aneurysmal disease, blood pressure will not rise as much.

Blood Loss

Blood loss may be replaced with autologous blood, packed red blood cells, and colloid therapy such as hetastarch. Administration of fresh-frozen plasma and platelets depends on coagulation values and total units of packed red blood cells transfused.

Unclamping

1. Lighten depth of anesthesia prior to unclamping (allow blood pressure to be 30 to 40 mm Hg above normal).
2. Be prepared to transfuse 1 unit of blood.
3. The surgeon can reclamp until anesthesia can restore blood pressure.
4. Use vasopressor as needed.

Emergence

Assess preoperative fluid status, current fluid status, length of procedure, and adequacy of pain control. If the patient requires postoperative ventilation, sedation may be required.

Complications

Complications include renal failure, distal ischemia, coagulation defects, hemorrhage, visceral ischemia, spinal cord ischemia, and graft infection.

Thoracic Aortic Aneurysm

Note: Blood pressure should be monitored above the aneurysm (right radial artery or left radial artery if the aneurysm involves the innominate artery). This allows assessment of cerebral perfusion pressure as well as the perfusion pressure to the kidneys. During aortic resection maintain the mean arterial pressure at about 100 mm Hg in the upper body and above 50 mm Hg distal to the aneurysm. Depending on the site of the aneurysm, an endobronchial tube may be required.

These procedures are usually done with profound hypothermia and total circulatory arrest or bypass with moderate hypothermia and sometimes with perfusion. One must be able to replace large volumes of blood rapidly. Have at least 8 to 10 units of blood available. Keep heart rate and blood pressure below normal. The most common approach is through a thoracotomy incision. Cross-clamping is applied just below the level of the left subclavian artery and distal to the aortic lesion, producing a large increasing or mechanical decompression with the oxygenator. If cross-clamping is done without shunt, vasodilator therapy is needed to control left ventricular afterload. Pulmonary artery catheters are utilized. The risk of ischemic cord damage increases as the cross-clamp period extends beyond 30 minutes. Postoperative complications are similar to those for abdominal aortic aneurysm. These patients are at a higher risk of renal failure and visceral, distal, and spinal cord ischemia.

J. Pericardial Processes/Tamponade

◆   ◆   ◆

PERICARDITIS

DEFINITION

Inflammatory process of the pericardium.

ETIOLOGY

This condition is often due to a viral infection.

CLINICAL MANIFESTATIONS

There is a sudden onset of severe chest pain.

Auscultation reveals a friction rub, leathery in quality, increasing in intensity on exhalation. Sinus tachycardia and low-grade fever are common.

TREATMENT

Treatment is symptomatic with analgesics and corticosteroids. Acute pericarditis in the absence of pericardial effusion does not alter cardiac function.

PERICARDIAL EFFUSION

DEFINITION

Accumulation of fluid in the pericardial space, often associated with pericarditis.

ETIOLOGY

The pericardial space normally contains 20 to 25 mL of pericardial fluid; intrapericardial pressure is subatmospheric and decreases on inspiration and increases on exhalation. Clinical effects depend on whether the fluid is creating a tamponade effect. If the fluid evolves gradually, the pericardium can stretch to accommodate the increased fluid volume without a large increase in pressure. Should this stretching be acute, tamponade is possible.

DIAGNOSTIC AND LABORATORY FINDINGS

Echocardiography is best at detecting pericardial effusion. Computed tomography can also be beneficial.

CHRONIC CONSTRICTIVE PERICARDITIS

DEFINITION

This condition resembles cardiac tamponade in that venous pressure is increased and stroke volume is decreased. Chronic constrictive pericarditis can interfere with diastolic filling of the heart.

ETIOLOGY

Most cases are idiopathic; however, chronic renal failure, radiation, rheumatoid arthritis, and cardiac surgery are all risk factors. There is a characteristic fibrous scarring and adhesion of both pericardial layers, similar to a rigid shell around the heart.

DIAGNOSTIC AND LABORATORY FINDINGS

Diagnosis depends on recognizing the increased venous pressure in a patient with no other signs of cardiac disease. This disease involves both sides of the heart; however, the prevalent manifestations are often those of right ventricular failure with venous congestion, hepatosplenomegaly, and ascites. Atrial dysrhythmia is common. Kussmaul's sign (exaggerated distention of neck veins on inspiration) is also common, whereas pulsus paradoxus is more typical of cardiac tamponade. Chest radiography reveals a normal to small heart with calcium evident in the pericardium. Electrocardiography reveals a low-voltage QRS complex, inverted t waves, and notched p waves. Computed tomography is best in revealing pericardial thickening.

TREATMENT

Treatment involves removal of the constricting pericardium, which can result in massive bleeding from the epicardium. Cardiopulmonary bypass may be needed, especially if bleeding is difficult to control. Surgical correction is not immediately followed by decreases in right atrial·pressure or increased cardiac output. Right atrial pressure normalizes within 3 months after surgery. Generally, myocardial function is normal.

ANESTHETIC CONSIDERATIONS

Provided there is no hypotension due to increased intrapericardial pressure, the selected anesthetic agents should not excessively (1) depress myocardial contractility, (2) cause hypotension, (3) lower the heart rate, or (4) impede venous return. Maintenance is best provided by a combination of midazolam, opioids, and nitrous oxide, with or without a low concentration of volatile anesthetic. Nondepolarizing muscle relaxants with minimal circulatory effects are best; however, the modest increase in heart rate with pancuronium is tolerated. Preoperative optimization of fluid status is important. If hemodynamic changes from increased intrapericardial pressure occur, the principles of anesthetic management for cardiac tamponade apply.

A pulmonary artery catheter is helpful because removal of the constrictive pericardium can be a long process and associated with changes in blood pressure and cardiac output. Dysrhythmia is common in this procedure, and antidysrhythmic drugs and a defibrillator should be readily available. These patients may need postoperative ventilatory support; dysrhythmia and low cardiac output may also require treatment postoperatively.

CARDIAC TAMPONADE

DEFINITION

Accumulation of fluid in the pericardial space that elevates intrapericardial pressure.

INCIDENCE

The incidence varies. In addition, cardiac tamponade may be an acute or chronic disease state.

ETIOLOGY

Cardiac tamponade is most commonly caused by trauma, infection, or neoplastic disease states. It can be present following cardiac surgery.

DIAGNOSTIC AND LABORATORY FINDINGS

Echocardiography is the best method to detect pericardial fluid. Chest radiography does not reveal a change in cardiac silhouette until 250 mL of fluid has accumulated.

CLINICAL MANIFESTATIONS

As intrapericardial fluid pressure rises, central venous pressure also rises; therefore, right atrial pressure may be monitored to determine whether tamponade is present. Other signs and symptoms include activation of the sympathetic nervous system, equalization of atrial filling pressures and pulmonary artery end-diastolic pressure, decreased voltage and electrical alternans on electrocardiography, paradoxical pulse, hypotension, and muffled heart sounds.

TREATMENT

Pericardiocentesis via local anesthesia is commonly used to treat cardiac tamponade. A pericardiotomy in the operating room under local or general anesthesia is recommended when tamponade develops from trauma or cardiac surgery. Temporary measures to maintain stroke volume include expansion of intravascular fluid volume, administration of a catecholamine to increase contractility, and correction of metabolic acidosis if necessary.

ANESTHETIC CONSIDERATIONS

If the intrapericardial pressure causing the tamponade cannot be relieved before induction of anesthesia, the goal is to maintain cardiac output. Avoid any anesthetic-induced decreases in contractility, systemic vascular resistance, and heart rate. Ketamine is a good choice for induction and maintenance. Pancuronium is also a good choice for muscle relaxation. Avoid vigorous positive-pressure ventilation, which can decrease venous return. Continuous central venous pressure and blood pressure monitoring (arterial line) should be started before induction. Maintain central venous pressure with generous administration of intravenous fluids to help maintain venous return. All equipment needed for emergency pericardiocentesis should be present in case of circulatory collapse after induction of anesthesia.

COMMON DISEASES

RESPIRATORY SYSTEM

A. Chronic Obstructive Pulmonary Disease/Emphysema/ Obstructive Disease

◆ ◆ ◆

DEFINITION

Chronic obstructive pulmonary disease (COPD) is a term used to describe a variety of disease processes, most commonly including emphysema, asthma, chronic bronchitis, bronchiectasis, and cystic fibrosis. These conditions cause an increase in resistance to flow of gases in the airway and can result in acute and chronic disease and in reversible and irreversible episodes.

INCIDENCE AND PREVALENCE

In the United States, COPD is most common in men older than 50 years of age. It is the second most common cause of mortality.

ETIOLOGY

The primary predisposing factor is history of long-term smoking. COPD is a result of three major pathophysiologic occurrences: (1) chronic infection secondary to irritation of bronchi and bronchioli from inhaling smoke or other irritating substances, (2) chronic obstruction of small airways due to excess mucus production, infection, and airway edema, and (3) entrapment of air in alveoli, resulting in abnormal enlargement of alveolar airspaces. Exacerbations can be precipitated by infection, congestive heart failure, oxygen therapy that blunts hypoxic drive, and pulmonary thromboembolism.

LABORATORY RESULTS

Chest radiography commonly shows hyperinflation and diaphragmatic flattening, right ventricular hypertrophy, dilated proximal pulmonary artery, and attenuated pulmonary vasculature in the presence of associated pulmonary vascular disease. In pulmonary function tests, the primary finding is a decreased forced expiratory volume in 1 second/forced vital capacity (FEV_1/FVC) ratio. Emphysematous patients also have increased respiratory volume and total lung capacity and decreased diffusing capacity for carbon monoxide. Arterial oxygen pressure (PaO_2) and arterial carbon dioxide pressure ($PaCO_2$) generally are not altered until the later stages of COPD. With electrocardiography, right-sided heart failure may appear as right ventricular hypertrophy. With chronic respiratory acidosis, $PaCO_2$ is elevated, and pH is low or normal. Acute exacerbations may result in markedly elevated $PaCO_2$ and acidic pH. Hematocrit is elevated.

CLINICAL MANIFESTATIONS

Patient History

Chronic bronchitis is often manifested by chronic productive cough, exertional dyspnea, and sometimes wheezing. Emphysema is primarily manifested by progressive exertional dyspnea, usually without productive cough or wheezing.

Physical Examination

Often, COPD patients have increased anteroposterior diameter, hyperresonance to percussion of thorax, and wheezing or rhonchi heard on auscultation of the chest. COPD patients may use accessory muscles for breathing, have a prolonged expiratory phase of respiration, and use "pursed lip" breathing; clubbing of the fingers also may occur.

TREATMENT

Conservative management includes low-flow oxygen via nasal cannula or Venturi mask, bronchodilators, beta$_2$-adrenergic agonists, ipratropium bromide, theophylline, and anti-inflammatory agents—cromolyn sodium, adrenocortical steroids. Emergent/aggressive therapy includes subcutaneous injection of epinephrine or terbutaline sulfate, inhaled bronchodilators, intravenous aminophylline, adrenocortical steroids, and intubation and mechanical ventilation in cases not responsive to other therapies.

ANESTHETIC CONSIDERATIONS

General anesthesia and regional techniques are both acceptable. Patients are susceptible to postoperative respiratory failure. If regional technique is used, avoid sedative drugs that cause ventilatory depression because these patients are extremely sensitive to the depressant effects of sedative agents. With regional anesthesia, avoid sensory level above T-6 because this can lower expiratory reserve volume and cause ineffective cough and airway clearance of secretions. With general anesthesia, humidify inspired gases. Volatile agents may produce bronchodilation. Nitrous oxide can cause enlargement and rupture of pulmonary bullae, leading to pneumothorax. Opioids may be used but can be associated with preoperative ventilatory depression. Controlled ventilation with high tidal volume (10 to 15 mL/kg) and slow inspiratory flow rates optimizes PaO_2 levels, decreases incidence of airflow turbulence, and optimizes ventilation-perfusion matching. If spontaneous ventilation is allowed, volatile agents can cause greater respiratory depression in patients with COPD than in patients with normal lungs. Ventilation should be adjusted according to arterial blood gases and pH.

PROGNOSIS

The overall short-term and long-term prognosis is good, and it is similar for both hospitalized patients with acute exacerbations and those with a comparable degree of COPD who remain stable with outpatient therapy. Right-sided heart failure is a poor prognostic sign.

B. Asthma

• ◆ •

DEFINITION

A condition involving episodic attacks of bronchospasm with associated dyspnea, cough, and wheezing. Biochemical autonomic, immunologic, infectious, endocrine, and physiologic factors play a role in this complex disorder. Bronchospastic episodes are generally short-lived and reversible, with complete recovery between episodes.

INCIDENCE AND PREVALENCE

Asthma affects 3% to 5% of the population, with 65% of patients developing symptoms before age 5. Males are affected twice as often as females.

ETIOLOGY

With asthma, an over-reactive parasympathetic nervous system and release of chemical mediators cause episodes of bronchiolar hyperreactivity in response to various stimuli. Environmental or "extrinsic" factors such as dust, cold, fumes, animal danders, pollens, and chemicals, or intrinsic factors such as emotional or physical stress, can precipitate a bronchospastic episode. Vagal afferents in the bronchi are sensitive to these stimuli, and reflex vagal activation occurs, causing bronchoconstriction. Airway obstruction develops because of airway constriction, edema of the airways, and excess mucus secretion, causing resistance to inspiratory and expiratory air flow. Hyperinflation distal to obstruction, altered pulmonary mechanics, and increased work of breathing occur secondary to impaired expiration. Inspired air distribution varies with regional differences in airway resistance. Altered ventilation-perfusion relationships in different portions of the lung may result in hypoxemia without hypercapnia and hyperventilation with respiratory alkalosis. Worsening obstruction leads to hypercapnia and respiratory acidosis.

LABORATORY RESULTS

Chest radiographs may be normal or show hyperinflation of the lungs. They may also reveal other causes or complications of asthma, such as pulmonary edema, pneumonia, or pulmonary hypertension. Early in the asthma attack, arterial blood gases will reveal mild hypoxemia, hypocarbia, and respiratory alkalosis. When the asthma attack becomes severe, hypoxemia worsens, and hypercarbia and respiratory acidosis develop. In pulmonary function tests, forced expiratory volume in 1 second and forced vital capacity are decreased, and functional residual capacity and total lung capacity are increased. Electrocardiography may show premature ventricular contractions, right bundle branch block, or evidence of right atrial or ventricular compromise. The eosinophil count may be elevated.

CLINICAL MANIFESTATIONS

During full remission, patients are asymptomatic with normal pulmonary function. During attacks, patients become dyspneic and have inspiratory and expiratory wheezing, nonproductive cough, prolonged expiration, tachycardia, and tachypnea. Patients may complain of chest tightness and may be utilizing accessory muscles for respiration.

TREATMENT

Treatment includes bronchodilators, beta$_2$-adrenergic agonists, ipratropium bromide and theophylline, oxygen therapy, anti-inflammatory agents (cromolyn sodium or hydrocortisone, methylprednisolone or prednisone), and fluid therapy.

ANESTHETIC CONSIDERATIONS

Preoperative evaluation should include the patient's history of the disease and current status, including lung sounds and medications. Active wheezing may predispose the patient to a life-threatening event under anesthesia. Patients with frequent bronchospasm should be on therapeutic doses of theophylline, bronchodilating inhalers, and in some cases glucocorticoids. Check for compliance with effectiveness of treatment. Benzodiazepines should be administered gradually to avoid respiratory depression and apnea. Narcotics must also be carefully administered, and those associated with histamine release should be avoided. Regional anesthesia in appropriate cases can help avoid bronchospasm induced by airway manipulation. Intubation of the airway may trigger bronchospasm; the patient should be deeply anesthetized prior to attempting intubation. Lidocaine given intravenously before intubation may blunt airway response to intubation. Halothane, enflurane, isoflurane, and desflurane have bronchodilating properties, but isoflurane and desflurane can cause airway irritation. When muscle relaxation is required, curare and atracurium should be avoided because of their ability to cause histamine release. Inspired gases should be warmed and humidified. If intraoperative bronchospasm occurs, inhaled bronchodilators, subcutaneous terbutaline, aminophylline, or volatile anesthetic agents may be used to treat it. Intraoperative bronchospasm may be detected by noting changes in lung sounds, airway pressures, and ease of ventilation. Anticholinesterase agents used for reversal of nondepolarizing muscle relaxants may precipitate bronchospasm. Use of an anticholinergic agent prior to giving the anticholinesterase agent will prevent bronchospasm. In patients who are not at high risk for aspiration, deep extubation is recommended to decrease the risk of bronchospasm on extubation.

PROGNOSIS

Asthma, especially in the presence of an asthma attack, significantly increases intraoperative morbidity and mortality rates. Asthma results in approximately 5000 deaths in the United States each year.

C. Pneumonia

◆ ◆ ◆

DEFINITION

Pneumonia is an acute infection of the lung parenchyma caused by bacteria or viruses.

INCIDENCE AND PREVALENCE

More than 1 million cases of pneumonia are diagnosed each year. It most frequently occurs in the winter months but may occur in association with a number of risk factors: (1) recent upper respiratory infection, (2) age (infants and elderly persons are at increased risk), (3) immunosuppression, (4) chronic obstructive pulmonary disease, (5) sepsis, (6) smoking, (7) mechanical ventilation, (8) airway obstruction by tumors, secretions, or a foreign body, and (9) neurologic impairment.

ETIOLOGY

Microorganisms enter the lungs via several routes. Microorganisms exhaled by other persons or from aerosols delivered from contaminated respiratory equipment can be inspired. A commonly inhaled microorganism is the influenza virus. Aspiration of oropharyngeal secretions may contain gram-positive or gram-negative microorganisms. Usually, gram-negative bacteria and *Staphylococcus* are transmitted via the circulation; in susceptible persons, the pathogen multiplies, releasing toxins and stimulating inflammatory and immune responses. The antigen-antibody reaction and endotoxins from some microorganisms damage alveolocapillary and bronchial mucous membranes. Infectious debris and exudate secondary to inflammation and edema fill terminal bronchioli. Ventilation-perfusion alterations develop. *Staphylococcus* or gram-negative bacteria may cause necrosis of lung parenchyma.

LABORATORY RESULTS

Arterial blood gases may reveal hypoxemia secondary to shunting and respiratory alkalosis. In cases of severe lung impairment or impaired tissue oxygenation, arterial blood gases may show hypercarbia and metabolic acidosis. Blood and sputum cultures/Gram stains are used to identify the type of microorganism. Polymorphonuclear leukocytosis is common. In chest radiographs, dehydration may mask patterns of infiltration. Lobar, segmental, or diffuse patterns of infiltration may be present. Electrocardiography may reveal dysrhythmias such as tachycardia or premature ventricular contractions or patterns of myocardial ischemia.

CLINICAL MANIFESTATIONS

Fever, chills, productive or nonproductive cough, malaise, pleural pain, dyspnea, and hemoptysis may be present. Symptoms may be minimal or masked in the elderly, debilitated, or neutropenic patient.

TREATMENT

Bacterial pneumonia is treated with antibiotics chosen according to sputum culture and sensitivity results. Viral pneumonia is treated with supportive therapy alone. Important and beneficial treatments for all types of pneumonia include (1) adequate hydration, (2) good pulmonary hygiene, including deep breathing, coughing, and chest percussion, (3) rest, and (4) oxygen. In severe cases, mechanical ventilatory support with supplemental oxygen may be required to maintain adequate gas exchange.

ANESTHETIC CONSIDERATIONS

Ensure that the patient has been started on appropriate antibiotic therapy. Mobilization of secretions improves lung mechanics and ventilation-perfusion matching. Patients with significant coexisting cardiovascular or pulmonary disease are far less tolerant of hypoxemia and increased work of breathing associated with pneumonia. Preoperative, induction, and maintenance doses of intravenous agents are introduced gradually. Higher oxygen concentrations may be used with an intravenous-based anesthetic. Regional anesthesia is desirable when applicable because it greatly reduces the risk of postoperative pulmonary dysfunction. Because they decrease the normal ventilatory response to hypercarbia, halothane, isoflurane, and enflurane in residual concentrations may reduce respiratory drive, especially after a prolonged procedure. General anesthesia interferes with mucociliary clearance: (1) use warmed, humidified inspired gases and (2) suction the patient frequently during the operation. Patients with marginal pulmonary function or those with upper abdominal or chest incisions may require postoperative mechanical ventilation following general anesthesia.

PROGNOSIS

In most cases, full recovery is likely with early and adequate treatment.

COMMON DISEASES

D. Tuberculosis

. . .

DEFINITION

Tuberculosis is a chronic granulomatous disease that is spread primarily via aerosol transmission.

INCIDENCE AND PREVALENCE

Prior to specific antimicrobial therapy, tuberculosis was a significant cause of death and disability in North America. It now affects approximately 28,000 people in North America, with prevalence highest among the elderly, the debilitated, persons living in crowded conditions, the malnourished, and the immunosuppressed.

ETIOLOGY

Tuberculosis is caused by the acid-fast bacillus *Mycobacterium tuberculosis*. Once inspired, the bacilli multiply, causing nonspecific pneumonitis. Some bacilli migrate to lymph nodes, encounter lymphocytes, and precipitate the immune response. Phagocytes engulf colonies of bacilli in the lung, isolating them and forming granulomatous tubercules. Infected tissues inside the tubercles create caseation necrosis, a cheesecake-like material. Isolation of the bacilli is completed by formation of scar tissue around the tubercle. After approximately 10 days, the immune response is complete and further bacilli multiplication is prevented. After isolation of bacilli and development of immunity, tuberculosis can remain dormant for life. Reactivation may occur if live bacilli escape into bronchi or in states of decreased immunity. Patients with laryngeal tuberculosis or lung cavitation have the highest infectivity rate.

LABORATORY RESULTS

Diagnosis is made via positive tuberculin skin testing, chest radiography, and positive sputum culture. A positive skin test alone may indicate only exposure to the tuberculin bacteria and is not by itself evidence of active disease. Chest radiographic findings of tuberculosis in the presence of acquired immunodeficiency syndrome (AIDS) may be atypical.

CLINICAL MANIFESTATIONS

Many patients are asymptomatic. Common manifestations include low-grade fever, especially in the afternoon; fatigue; weight loss; anorexia; lethargy; and a gradually developing cough that produces purulent sputum. Occasionally, patients develop pleural effusions, meningitis, bone or joint disease, genitourinary abscesses, or peritonitis. Night sweats are common. Chest pain, dyspnea, and hemoptysis are uncommon.

TREATMENT

Pharmacotherapy, primarily with isoniazid, rifampin, streptomycin, or ethambutol, may be used.

ANESTHETIC CONSIDERATIONS

Respiratory isolation is indicated until the patient is verified as a nontransmitter of tuberculosis. Disposable equipment, including filters and anesthetic circuits, is advisable. Nondisposable anesthetic equipment must be thoroughly sterilized. Postpone elective surgery in actively infected individuals until adequate chemotherapy has been administered (usually 3 weeks of treatment) and verified by a negative sputum sample. Consider the implications of organ dysfunction that may be secondary to the disease or its treatment. Lungs are most commonly affected by the disease, and chemotherapeutic agents used for treatment may lead to toxicity of the liver, kidneys, or peripheral nervous system.

PROGNOSIS

Seventy-five per cent of patients generally have organism-free sputum after 10 weeks of appropriate therapy. Length of therapy ranges from 9 to 18 months. Bacilli are usually rendered inactive after 3 weeks of chemotherapy.

E. Pulmonary Embolism

♦   ♦   ♦

DEFINITION

Pulmonary embolism is an occlusion of the pulmonary vascular bed by an embolus. It may be due to blood clots, fats, tissue fragments, tumor cells, air, amniotic fluid, or foreign objects.

INCIDENCE AND PREVALENCE

Pulmonary embolism is a leading cause of morbidity and mortality in the United States and is responsible for 50,000 deaths per year. It is the most common cause of acute pulmonary disease in hospitalized patients.

ETIOLOGY

Pulmonary embolism is primarily due to venous stasis, alterations or abnormalities in the blood vessel wall, and hypercoagulation. Most pulmonary emboli arise from thromboses in the pelvis or a lower extremity. They may occur as (1) a massive occlusion or blockage of a major portion of the pulmonary circulation, (2) embolus with infarction of a portion of lung tissue, (3) embolus without infarction or one not severe enough to cause permanent lung injury, or (4) multiple pulmonary emboli, either chronic or recurrent. The pattern of occurrence and severity determine the degree

COMMON DISEASES

of hypoxic vasoconstriction, pulmonary edema, atelectasis, vagal stimulation, and release of neurohumoral substances such as histamine. Pulmonary emboli may also cause systemic hypotension, pulmonary hypertension, decreased cardiac output, and shock.

LABORATORY RESULTS

Pulmonary angiography is the most definitive diagnostic tool. Chest radiographs may be normal or show subtle changes. Ventilation-perfusion scans may reveal an embolus if a perfusion defect exists in an area of normal ventilation. Arterial blood gases may be normal but typically reveal hypoxemia, respiratory alkalosis, and hypocapnia. Electrocardiography may show tachycardia or signs of right-sided ventricular failure, including tall, peaked t waves, right-axis deviation, or right-sided bundle branch block.

CLINICAL MANIFESTATIONS

Clinical manifestations range from tachypnea, tachycardia, dyspnea, and anxiety to pleural pain, pleural friction rub, pleural effusion, hemoptysis, fever, leukocytosis, severe pulmonary hypertension, and shock. Physical examination may reveal wheezing, rales, or pleural friction rub on chest auscultation, and tachycardia, splitting of the second heart sound, or systolic ejection murmur over the pulmonic valve.

TREATMENT

Prevention is the best treatment. Low-dose heparin, coumadin, aspirin, dextran, pneumatic leg compression, elastic compression stockings, and early ambulation can help in pulmonary embolus prophylaxis. Heparin administration is the initial treatment once a pulmonary embolus has been diagnosed. Thrombolytic therapy is indicated in cases of massive pulmonary embolism or circulatory collapse.

ANESTHETIC CONSIDERATIONS

Patients undergoing surgery often are at risk for deep venous thrombosis and, thus, pulmonary embolus. Subcutaneous heparin, dextran, and pneumatic leg compression devices may help prevent perioperative deep venous thrombosis. Regional anesthesia may decrease the incidence of deep venous thrombosis, and therefore the risk of pulmonary embolism, for some surgical procedures. Patients with a history of pulmonary embolism or deep venous thrombosis may be on anticoagulant therapy, so one must check prothrombin time and partial thromboplastin time. Avoid regional anesthesia in the presence of a prolonged bleeding time or residual anticoagulation. Vena cava umbrella filters are most often placed under local anesthesia with sedation. Hypotension may occur during placement of the apparatus because of decreased venous return. Sudden unexplained hypotension, bronchospasm, decreased end-tidal carbon dioxide, elevated central venous pressure, and elevated pulmonary artery pressure may indicate intraoperative pulmonary embolism.

PROGNOSIS

Statistics on prognosis are unavailable.

F. Cor Pulmonale

* * *

DEFINITION

Right ventricular hypertrophy and eventual right-sided heart failure.

INCIDENCE AND PREVALENCE

Cor pulmonale is noted in 10% to 30% of patients admitted to the hospital with congestive heart failure. It occurs in males 5 times more often than in females.

ETIOLOGY

Cor pulmonale usually is caused by left-sided heart failure and often is due to pulmonary disease and elevated pulmonary vascular resistance.

LABORATORY RESULTS

Chest radiography generally shows evidence of chronic obstructive airway disease and right ventricular hypertrophy. Chest radiographs may show dilatation of the main pulmonary artery and primary branches and decreased markings of peripheral pulmonary vasculature. Electrocardiography may reveal right arterial and ventricular hypertrophy evidenced by peaked t waves in leads II and III, atrioventricular fibrillation, right-axis deviation, and right bundle branch block. In pulmonary function tests, changes are generally consistent with the primary pulmonary disease.

CLINICAL MANIFESTATIONS

In cor pulmonale, clinical manifestations are difficult to detect and may resemble those of a coexisting respiratory disorder. Fatigue, retrosternal chest discomfort, dyspnea, cough, and activity-induced weakness or syncope may occur. Physical assessment may reveal distended neck veins, right ventricular gallop, pulmonic and tricuspid valve murmurs, split-second heart sound, jugular venous distention, pulsus paradoxus, hepatosplenomegaly, and dependent peripheral edema.

TREATMENT

Treatment centers on treating the underlying left-sided heart failure or pulmonary disease. The goal is to reduce pulmonary hypertension and to normalize arterial oxygen and carbon dioxide partial pressures and pH if pulmonary vascular constriction is reversible. Rest, supplemental oxygen, antibiotics, digitalis, diuretics, and bronchodilators can provide effective treatment.

ANESTHETIC CONSIDERATIONS

Elective operations must be avoided until reversible components of pulmonary disease are corrected. Avoid administration of anesthetics in the presence of pulmonary infections. Bronchospasm should be absent or treated. The patient should be appropriately hydrated and electrolytes within normal limits. Sedatives and narcotics are potentiated in these patients and may easily cause respiratory depression—dose judiciously and carefully monitor patient response. Anticholinergics may increase the heart rate and physiologic dead space; their use should therefore be limited. Monitoring should include routine standard monitors as well as Foley, arterial line, and pulmonary artery catheterization. Regional anesthesia is appropriate when high sensory levels are not required. Intermittent positive-pressure ventilation may improve arterial oxygenation. Significant decreases in arterial carbon dioxide may lead to metabolic alkalosis and hypokalemia.

PROGNOSIS

The prognosis is best in patients with chronic obstructive pulmonary disease who have near-normal arterial oxygenation and is worst in patients with intrinsic vascular disease or pulmonary fibrosis.

G. Pulmonary Hypertension

◆   ◆   ◆

DEFINITION

High blood pressure in the pulmonary arteries, or an increase in pulmonary artery pressure of 5 to 10 mm Hg above normal (15 to 18 mm Hg).

INCIDENCE AND PREVALENCE

Primary pulmonary hypertension is rare and generally affects women 20 to 40 years old. Secondary hypertension is more common. It can occur secondary to any cardiovascular or respiratory disorders that (1) increase volume or pressure of blood entering the pulmonary arteries or (2) narrow or obstruct the pulmonary arteries.

ETIOLOGY

An increase in pulmonary vasculature resistance may have anatomic or vasomotor etiologies.

Primary Pulmonary Hypertension

Pulmonary arterioles become narrowed because of vascular smooth muscle hypertrophy and formation of fibrous lesions around the vessels. Vessel narrowing or obliteration increases resistance, causing pulmonary hypertension. High pulmonary pressures are generated back to the right ventricle, eventually leading to right ventricular failure or cor pulmonale. Death usually ensues within 5 years of diagnosis secondary to cor pulmonale.

Secondary Pulmonary Hypertension

There are four causes of secondary hypertension: (1) elevated left ventricular filling pressures, as in coronary artery disease and mitral valve disease (with elevation of left-sided heart pressures, pulmonary vascular pressures must increase to maintain flow), (2) increased pulmonary blood flow (left-to-right shunts), as in ventricular septal defects or patent ductus arteriosus, (3) obliteration or obstruction of the pulmonary vascular bed by chronic obstructive airway disease, pulmonary embolism, pulmonary vasculitis, or pulmonary fibrosis, and (4) pulmonary vascular vasoconstriction secondary to hypoxemia, acidosis, or both. Secondary hypertension is reversible if the underlying cause is resolved.

LABORATORY RESULTS

Diagnosis must be confirmed with right-sided heart catheterization and when all other possible causes have been ruled out. Chest radiographs may show an enlarged border of the right side of the heart. Electrocardiography may reveal right ventricular hypertrophy.

CLINICAL MANIFESTATIONS

Symptoms often are masked by primary pulmonary or cardiovascular disease. Pulmonary hypertension may not be evidenced until pulmonary artery pressure equals systemic pressure. Resting pulmonary artery pressure generally does not rise until the effective cross-sectional area of the vascular bed is decreased by 50% or more. Patients may complain of fatigue, chest discomfort, and dyspnea, especially with exertion and tachypnea.

TREATMENT

Primary Pulmonary Hypertension

No curative treatment is available. Oxygen, cardiotonic glycosides, diuretics, fluid control, and bronchodilators may be used as palliative treatments.

Secondary Pulmonary Hypertension

Treatment of the underlying disorder is most effective. Oxygen may reverse hypoxic vasoconstriction. Digitalis and diuretics may be used for right ventricular failure.

COMMON DISEASES

ANESTHETIC CONSIDERATIONS

Correct reversible coexisting disease processes preoperatively. Obtain baseline arterial blood gases and pH. Preoperative medications may depress ventilation. Anticholinergics may depress mucociliary activity and impair clearance of secretions. Bronchospasm and increases in pulmonary and systemic pressures may be avoided during intubation if the depth of anesthesia is adequate. Regional anesthesia may be appropriate for cases not requiring high secondary levels. Nitrous oxide may increase pulmonary vascular resistance when high doses of opioids are given. Monitoring requirements depend on the severity of disease and type of surgery.

PROGNOSIS

The prognosis with primary pulmonary hypertension is poor; most patients die within 5 years of diagnosis. The prognosis is better with secondary pulmonary hypertension and is best when the underlying cause is reversed.

H. Upper Respiratory Infection

◆   ◆   ◆

DEFINITION

Viral or bacterial infection of the upper respiratory tract.

INCIDENCE AND PREVALENCE

Statistics are unavailable.

ETIOLOGY

Bacterial upper respiratory tract infections often are secondary to impairment of normal host defense mechanisms, such as mucociliary transport and cough reflexes. Viral respiratory infections impair normal respiratory defense mechanisms.

Types of Upper Respiratory Infection

1. *Sinusitis:* frontal and maxillary sinusitis are more common in adults; ethmoid sinusitis is more common in children. May lead to intracranial infection.

2. *Otitis media:* results from spread of bacteria to the middle ear from the nasopharynx. Most frequently caused by pneumococci or *Haemophilus influenzae.*

3. *Pharyngitis:* pharyngitis is usually viral; 20% of all bacterial cases are caused by group A streptococci.

4. *Peritonsillar abscess:* secondary to streptococcal tonsilitis.

5. *Retropharyngeal infection:* caused by retropharyngeal spread of infection; most cases occur in children.

6. *Ludwig's angina:* cellulitis of the submandibular, sublingual, and submental areas. Usually caused by streptococci.

7. *Epiglottitis:* infection of the upper airway epiglottis. Usually due to H. *influenzae*, type B. Rapidly progressive and potentially lethal.

LABORATORY RESULTS

1. *Sinusitis:* based on signs and symptoms and chest radiographs (?)
2. *Otitis media:* based on evaluation of signs and symptoms concerning the tympanic membrane
3. *Pharyngitis:* throat culture determines causative organism
4. *Peritonsillar abscess:* signs and symptoms
5. *Retropharyngeal infections:* signs and symptoms
6. *Ludwig's angina:* signs and symptoms
7. *Epiglottitis:* signs and symptoms

CLINICAL MANIFESTATIONS

Sinusitis is manifested by pain and tenderness over the affected sinuses, nasal drainage, fever, and facial or forehead discomfort. Purulent otitis media results in bulging tympanic membranes and obscured bony landmarks. Serous otitis media results in retracted tympanic membranes and no alteration in bony landmarks. Chronic otitis media results in hearing loss and tympanic membrane perforation. Acute mastoiditis is a rare complication. Pharyngitis usually is manifested by throat pain, fever, and often dysphagia. Peritonsillar abscess is manifested by fever, chills, dysphagia with drooling, and a muffled voice. Trismus may also be present. The manifestations of retropharyngeal infections are similar to those of pharyngitis and peritonsillar abscess. Ludwig's angina manifests as edema of the anterior neck and floor of the mouth, fever, and dysphagia secondary to elevation of the tongue. Upper airway obstruction can occur. Epiglottitis is manifested by rapid progression of fever, inspiratory stridor, drooling and dysphagia, and severe respiratory distress.

TREATMENT

Sinusitis: decongestants and analgesics. If intracranial spread ensues, high-dose antibiotics and surgical drainage are required.

Otitis media: analgesics, antibiotics, decongestants, and, in case of progressive hearing loss, myringotomy.

Pharyngitis: analgesics; antibiotics for bacterial pharyngitis.

Peritonsillar abscess: surgical drainage and antibiotics.

Retropharyngeal infections: surgical drainage and antibiotics, usually as necessary.

Ludwig's angina: analgesics, antibiotics. Airway compromise may mandate intubation, and intubation of the trachea may be impossible, necessitating tracheostomy.

ANESTHETIC CONSIDERATIONS

Anesthetic considerations are based on the specific type and severity of an upper respiratory infection. In the presence of active upper airway infection, risks of delaying surgery must be weighed against risks of proceeding with anesthesia. If surgery is not an emergency, it is safest to delay the procedure in the presence of fever, with an elevated leukocyte count, when the surgery is on the thorax or abdomen, or when surgery is expected to last longer than 1 hour.

PROGNOSIS

Complete recovery is likely for most upper respiratory infections, especially with appropriate treatment. Some upper respiratory infections, such as epiglottitis, are associated with higher mortality.

I. Restrictive Pulmonary Diseases

• • •

DEFINITION

Pulmonary dysfunction secondary to decreased lung elasticity, resulting in poor lung compliance and increased work of breathing. May be of the extrinsic or of the acute or chronic intrinsic type.

INCIDENCE AND PREVALENCE

Statistics are unavailable.

ETIOLOGY

Acute Intrinsic Restrictive

Acute intrinsic restrictive pulmonary disease is usually a result of intravascular fluid leakage into the interstitium and alveoli secondary to capillary endothelial damage or increased pulmonary vascular pressures.

Acute intrinsic restrictive pulmonary disorders include adult respiratory distress syndrome, aspiration pneumonitis, neurogenic pulmonary edema, high-altitude pulmonary edema, and opiate-induced pulmonary edema.

Chronic Intrinsic Restrictive

Chronic intrinsic restrictive pulmonary disease is generally a progressive pulmonary fibrosis that causes vascular destruction and may lead to pulmonary hypertension, cor pulmonale, and pneumothorax.

Chronic intrinsic restrictive pulmonary disorders include hypersensitivity pneumonitis, sarcoidosis, eosinophilic granuloma, and alveolar proteinosis.

Chronic Extrinsic Restrictive

Chronic extrinsic restrictive pulmonary disease is due to extrinsic disorders that hamper expansion of the lungs and may be the result of pleural, thoracic cage, or diaphragmatic disorders. Lung compression leads to decreased lung volumes, causing increased airway resistance. Mechanical changes of the chest increase the work of breathing; increasing pulmonary vascular resistance is secondary to compression of the pulmonary vessels, and poor cough ability may cause recurrent pulmonary infections and eventually lead to obstructive pulmonary disease.

Chronic extrinsic restrictive pulmonary diseases include fibrosis, effusion, kyphoscoliosis, pectus excavatum, obesity, ascites, and pregnancy.

CLINICAL MANIFESTATIONS

Clinical manifestations depend on the particular restrictive disorder. They may include tachypnea, dyspnea, cough, bronchospasm, pulmonary vascular vasoconstriction, pulmonary hypertension, cor pulmonale, and arterial hypoxemia.

TREATMENT

Treatment also depends on the specific restrictive disorder and may include oxygen therapy, bronchodilators, corticosteroids, and mechanical ventilation with positive end-expiratory pressure.

ANESTHETIC CONSIDERATIONS

1. Restrictive pulmonary disease does not dictate drug choices for induction and maintenance of general anesthesia.
2. Select and administer drugs to avoid postoperative ventilatory depression.
3. Regional anesthesia may be acceptable, but levels above T-10 may impair respiratory muscle function.
4. Controlled ventilation may maximize oxygenation and ventilation.
5. Poorly compliant lungs may require high inflation pressures.
6. Postoperative mechanical ventilation may be necessary.

7. Extubation should be done only when patients clearly meet criteria.

8. Decreased lung volumes may impair cough and interfere with postoperative secretion removal.

J. Adult Respiratory Distress Syndrome

◆   ◆   ◆

DEFINITION

Adult respiratory distress syndrome (ARDS) is a term that refers to a variety of infiltrative lung lesions resulting from diffuse alveolocapillary injury and resulting in a significant increase in capillary alveolar permeability. This leads to increased lung water and high concentrations of proteins in the lung parenchyma and alveoli, often resulting in acute respiratory failure and death.

INCIDENCE AND PREVALENCE

Approximately 150,000 to 200,000 new cases of ARDS are diagnosed each year in the United States. ARDS is precipitated by a number of conditions and frequently affects young people who were previously in excellent health.

ETIOLOGY

1. Alveolocapillary damage may occur directly secondary to aspiration or inhalation injuries or indirectly from the activation and aggregation of formed elements such as neutrophils and release of inflammatory mediators (leukocytes and macrophages) in response to sepsis, trauma, shock, activation of complement, the coagulation cascade, and other causes.

2. Specific causative mechanisms are not known.

3. Initial alveolocapillary damage results in increased permeability, pulmonary edema, inactivation of surfactant, impaired gas exchange, and decreased lung compliance with decreased ventilation and shunting of pulmonary blood flow. If the syndrome does not begin to resolve following the initial phase, it leads to a fibrotic phase. This results in collagen formation with progressive obliteration of alveoli, respiratory bronchioli, and interstitium, a decrease in lung compliance, decreased ventilation-perfusion, and respiratory failure.

LABORATORY RESULTS

Chest radiographs may initially be clear to show bilateral diffuse infiltrates. Later, infiltrates become extensive and may progress to complete opacification. In early stages, arterial blood gases may show hyperventilation-induced respiratory alkalosis and mild hypoxemia that improves with administration of supplemental oxygen. In the later stages of ARDS, hypoxemia is not improved by oxygen administration, and hypercarbia develops because of increased dead space ventilation.

CLINICAL MANIFESTATIONS

Classically, ARDS patients have rapid shallow respirations, respiratory alkalosis, marked dyspnea, diffuse decreased chest wall compliance, and hypoxemia unresponsive to oxygen therapy. In later stages of the syndrome, metabolic acidosis, hypotension, decreased cardiac output, and death may occur.

TREATMENT

Early recognition and treatment with supportive therapy and prevention of complications afford the best chance of recovery from ARDS. Therapy may include fluid management, oxygen administration, mechanical ventilation with use of positive end-expiratory pressure, inspiratory hold or reverse inspiratory/expiratory ratio, steroid administration, and cardiac drugs. Extracorporeal membrane oxygenation is sometimes used in the most severe cases, but it is associated with complications and has not been proven to improve survival.

ANESTHETIC CONSIDERATIONS

1. The goal is to provide adequate anesthesia while maintaining a physiologic state that is often precarious.

2. Regional anesthesia may be acceptable if not contraindicated by hemodynamic instability, coagulopathy, or sepsis.

3. Ventilation with high fractional inspired oxygen and positive end-expiratory pressure are often requested and may make patient transport difficult.

4. High positive end-expiratory pressure levels may cause hemodynamic instability.

5. Arterial line, central venous pressure, and pulmonary artery catheters are required.

6. Altered volume of distribution and rate of drug metabolism, as well as altered liver and kidney function, require more gradual and decreased dosing of benzodiazepines, narcotics, muscle relaxants, induction agents, and inhalation agents.

7. Use of dinitrogen monoxide is rarely possible because of high fractional inspired oxygen requirements.

PROGNOSIS

Fifty-two per cent of ARDS patients die despite therapy.

K. Pneumothorax and Hemothorax

◆ ◆ ◆

DEFINITION

Pneumothorax is the presence of air or gas in the pleural space. Hemothorax is the presence of blood in the pleural space.

INCIDENCE AND PREVALENCE

Spontaneous pneumothorax occurs unexpectedly in healthy persons, mostly men 20 to 40 years of age. Secondary pneumothorax and hemopneumothorax are generally due to trauma.

ETIOLOGY

Spontaneous pneumothorax is caused by rupture of blebs on the visceral pleura. Cause of this bleb formation is unknown. Secondary pneumothorax is caused by rib fractures and by rupture of a bleb or bulla as with chronic obstructive pulmonary disease or secondary to mechanical ventilation, especially if positive end-expiratory pressure is used. Hemothorax is secondary to trauma.

LABORATORY RESULTS

Chest radiography usually shows subcutaneous emphysema, pneumomediastinum, and pneumopericardium. Free fluid, as with hemothorax, may be best seen on a cross-table lateral film.

CLINICAL MANIFESTATIONS

Pneumothorax

Onset is with sudden pleural pain, tachypnea, and mild dyspnea. With large or tension pneumothorax, mediastinal shift may occur. The chest may be asymmetric. Breath sounds are absent over the affected area. Hypoxemia, hypotension, and severe dyspnea may occur.

Hemothorax

Symptoms are similar to those of pneumothorax and may include signs of hypovolemia in the case of significant chest trauma.

TREATMENT

Unless the pneumothorax is small and not expanding, a chest tube must be placed to decompress the chest. If a chest tube is not immediately available in the presence of tension pneumothorax, a large-bore needle can be inserted into the anterior second intercostal space for immediate decompression.

Tension pneumothorax is a life-threatening emergency. Hemothorax is also treated with a chest tube on the affected side and may also require fluid or blood replacement if blood loss is significant.

ANESTHETIC CONSIDERATIONS

Pneumothorax or hemothorax can significantly interfere with oxygenation and ventilation. Decreased cardiac output, as with tension pneumothorax, can exacerbate intrapulmonary shunting. Cyanosis indicates both cardiac and pulmonary involvement. Nitrous oxide can quickly expand the size of a pneumothorax if a chest tube is not in place. In the case of a ventilator-related pneumothorax, mortality is significantly reduced if a chest tube is placed in less than 30 minutes. Development of tension pneumothorax during general anesthesia is manifested by sudden hypotension, loss of pulmonary compliance, or decreased ventilating volume. Patients with significant trauma may require fluid resuscitation and cardiovascular support. Agents chosen should have minimal cardiac depressant effects.

PROGNOSIS

Prognosis depends on the severity of chest trauma associated with pneumothorax or hemothorax. Specific statistics are unavailable.

COMMON DISEASES

CENTRAL NERVOUS SYSTEM

A. Seizures

• • •

DEFINITION

Results of abnormal electrical discharge in the brain.

INCIDENCE AND PREVALENCE

Seizures affect approximately 0.5% to 1% of the U.S. population. Numerous forms of seizures exist. Most common are generalized tonic-clonic seizures. The likelihood of a recurrent seizure after a single seizure is approximately 50% in the following 3 years, with the greatest incidence during the first 6 months.

ETIOLOGY

Most seizures are idiopathic. Idiopathic seizure disorders usually begin in childhood. Seizure onset in adults may indicate an expanding intracranial hematoma, tumor, intracranial hemorrhage, metabolic disturbance, infection, trauma, alcohol or addictive drug withdrawal, eclampsia (in pregnant women), previous trauma causing an irritative phenomenon in the brain, and local anesthesia toxicity.

DIAGNOSTIC AND LABORATORY FINDINGS

Seizures can be detected with electroencephalography (signals can be augmented with methohexital, etomidate, or ketamine), electrolyte abnormalities, and examination of cerebrospinal fluid for infection. Magnetic resonance imaging is better than computed tomography to detect focal intracranial lesion.

CLINICAL MANIFESTATIONS

Clinical manifestations include focal or generalized tonic-clonic seizure activity and an increase in the cerebral metabolic rate of oxygen.

TREATMENT

First priority is to protect and secure the airway, oxygenate, and ventilate. Supportive care and treatment of the underlying problem are needed.

Grand Mal Seizures

Medications used are diazepam (Valium) 2 mg/min IV until the seizure stops or a total of 20 mg. Dilantin with an intravenous load of 15 mg/kg over 20 minutes. Infuse no faster than 50 mg/min, followed by daily maintenance doses of 300 to 500 mg orally or IV for adults. Therapeutic serum level is 10 to 20 μg/mL. For phenobarbital, the dosage is 100 mg/min IV up to a total of 20 mg/kg. Therapeutic serum level is 20 to 40 μg/mL.

Eclamptic Seizures

Use magnesium sulfate (a mild central nervous system depressant and vasodilator). Initial load is 2 to 4 g IV over 15 minutes, then a continuous infusion of 1 to 3 g/h. Therapeutic serum level is 4 to 8 mEq/L.

Local Anesthesia Toxicity

Use thiopental 50 to 100 mg, midazolam 1 to 5 mg, or diazepam 5 to 20 mg IV push.

ANESTHETIC CONSIDERATIONS

Check electrolytes, cultures, and drug level preoperatively. Know the anticonvulsant medications being used and their possible cardiopulmonary effects and potential interactions with the anesthetic being used. With phenytoin (Dilantin), infuse and flush with normal saline; infuse no faster than 50 mg/min. Arrhythmias, hypotension, and arrest occur if administration is too fast. The requirement for nondepolarizing muscle relaxants (NDMRs) may be increased. Other seizure medications used are phenobarbital, primidone, carbamazepine (increases requirement for NDMRs), valproic acid, and ethosuximide. Metrizamide, a water-soluble contrast agent, can produce seizures if allowed to enter the intracranial compartment in high concentration.

Patients on antiepileptic drugs have resistance to the effects of neuromuscular blocking agents and opioids because of changes in the number of receptors, altered drug metabolism, and interaction with endogenous neurotransmitters. A paralyzing dose of muscle relaxant stops peripheral but not central nervous system manifestations of seizure activity.

Methohexital can activate epileptic foci. Ketamine potentially can lower seizure threshold. Atracurium (metabolite/laudanosine) is a central nervous system stimulant. Enflurane in concentrations greater than 2.5% and hypocarbia of less than 25 mm Hg may produce seizures. Magnesium sulfate increases sensitivity to both depolarizing and NDMR. Hyperventilation of the lungs decreases delivery of additional local anesthesia to the brain; respiratory alkalosis and hyperkalemia result in hyperpolarization of nerve membranes.

PROGNOSIS

Seizures are a chronic condition managed for life. Seizures secondary to eclampsia resolve after delivering of the baby. Some seizure patients undergo epilepsy surgery and electrophysiologic mapping. Awake craniotomy with local anesthesia and intravenous sedation requires a cooperative patient. Otherwise, general anesthesia is used for these procedures.

B. Cerebrovascular Disease

◆   ◆   ◆

DEFINITION

A collection of disorders that affect the vasculature of the brain. The two major subdivisions of stroke are hemorrhage and ischemia.

INCIDENCE AND PREVALENCE

Cerebrovascular disease is the third leading cause of death in the United States.

ETIOLOGY

The major risk factors for the development of cerebrovascular disease are hypertension and diabetes. Other risk factors include atherosclerosis, inflammatory processes, dissecting aneurysm, disorders affecting the heart wall, congestive heart failure, polycythemia, cigarette smoking, use of oral birth control pills, and postpartum infarction. The different classifications of cerebrovascular disease can manifest as follows:

1. *Transient ischemic attack*—a temporary and focal episode of neurologic dysfunction that develops suddenly and lasts a few minutes to hours, but never more than 24 hours; 25 of 60 of these patients eventually suffer strokes.

2. *Reversible ischemic neurologic deficit*—neurologic symptoms that persist up to 6 to 8 weeks before they resolve.

3. *Progressive stroke*—a stroke in progress. Neurologic symptoms and deficits develop slowly and are not reversible.

4. *Complete stroke*—neurologic deficits are predominant; *amaurosis fugax*—transient ischemic attack involving the retina.

DIAGNOSTIC AND LABORATORY FINDINGS

Computed tomography, magnetic resonance imaging, and clinical examination are useful.

CLINICAL MANIFESTATIONS

Clinical manifestations involve numerous neurologic deficits. See the classification of symptoms under "Etiology."

TREATMENT

Reduce risk factors: hypertension, high-fat diet, smoking, obesity. Prevent strokes and carotid surgery may be indicated (approximately 100,000 operations are performed each year).

ANESTHETIC CONSIDERATIONS

Anesthetic considerations through preoperative evaluation of cardiovascular, neurologic, and pulmonary systems along with laboratory results and current medications. If the patient is scheduled for carotid endarterectomy, consider the benefits and risks associated with regional versus general anesthesia. Selection of anesthetic agents is based on the individual patient's need. The goal is to ensure a smooth induction, maintenance, and emergence, with avoidance of wide swings in blood pressure. In addition, an awake and extubated patient is the expected outcome to facilitate neurologic assessment. Have cardioactive agents and drips of nitroprusside, nitroglycerin, and neosynephrine available.

PROGNOSIS

Mortality from acute stroke ranges from 15% to 30%. The leading cause of death in victims of stroke is another stroke. The risk of a recurrent stroke in a patient who has had a previous stroke is approximately 9% each year. A generally accepted 5-year repeat stroke rate is about 45%.

C. Hydrocephalus

◆ ◆ ◆

DEFINITION

An abnormal accumulation of cerebrospinal fluid (CSF) caused by an excessive production or decreased uptake that leads to an increase in intraventricular pressure, causing adjacent brain tissue compression and progressive enlargement of the cranium.

INCIDENCE AND PREVALENCE

Hydrocephalus occurs in 3 of every 1000 births, usually secondary to meningomyelocele. Hydrocephalus is common after subarachnoidal hemorrhage due to impaired CSF circulation through the basal cistern. It can be a complication of an aneurysm rupture. Hydrocephalus may occur in neonates because of obstruction of CSF circulation within the ventricular system or at the site of reabsorption.

ETIOLOGY

Hydrocephalus can be divided into two causes—obstructive and nonobstructive.

Obstructive	Results from obstruction to CSF flow; depending on the site, can be further divided into communicating and noncommunicating.
Communicating obstructive (Extraventricular hydrocephalus)	Results from obstruction to CSF absorption by the arachnoid villi, usually from remote inflammatory disease or traumatic subarachnoid hemorrhage.
Noncommunicating obstructive (Intraventricular hydrocephalus)	Secondary to obstruction along CSF pathway between the lateral and 4th ventricular outlet (ventricles dilate proximal but not distal to the obstruction).

Obstructive hydrocephalus results from congenital malformation scar tissue, fibrin deposits following intraventricular hemorrhage or infection, tumors, or cysts.

Nonobstructive hydrocephalus	Results from excessive CSF production by the choroid plexus. Choroid plexus papillomas or benign tumors of the glomus of the lateral ventricles are common etiologies.

DIAGNOSTIC AND LABORATORY FINDINGS

Hydrocephalus can be identified by computed tomography or magnetic resonance imaging and by elevated intracranial pressure.

CLINICAL MANIFESTATIONS

Early signs and symptoms	Apnea, bradycardia, vomiting, increasing head circumference, headaches, mentation changes
Late signs and symptoms	Bulging fontanelle, "setting sun" eyes—6th cranial nerve palsy, limb spasticity, decreased level of consciousness to nonresponsiveness

ANESTHETIC CONSIDERATIONS

Intracranial pressure is elevated; the stomach is full. Avoid hypoventilation, hypoxia, and hypertension. Intravenous induction should be rapid and smooth. There should be minimal to no premedication or cricoid pressure. Know the baseline neurologic status. Once the airway is secure, hyperventilate the patient until ventricles are decompressed. The patient is maintained on N_2O/O_2 and increments of thiopental if needed until intracranial pressure is reduced, then an inhalation agent or opioid can be added. Sudden removal of a large CSF volume may lead to bradycardia and hypotension; this can be prevented by rapid replacement with saline and gradual release of fluids. Heat is lost because of wide surgical exposure (cranium to abdomen). Narcotics are given in small dosages (or not given at all) to enable rapid neurologic assessment upon awakening from anesthesia.

TREATMENT

Shunt insertion. CSF is shunted from the lateral ventricle to the peritoneal cavity (ventriculoperitoneal shunt). This is the preferable shunt because of its lower rate of complications and less frequent need for revision with growth. Ventriculoatrial and ventriculopleural shunts are less popular because of the risk of infection, microemboli, and hydrothorax. The lumboperitoneal shunt (between the lumbar subarachnoid space and the peritoneal space) may be used.

PROGNOSIS

Hydrocephalus is a chronic condition. It requires continual monitoring of shunt patency, signs and symptoms of infection, changes in the level of consciousness, and neurologic changes. Shunts may require revisions.

D. Parkinson's Syndrome

◆   ◆   ◆

DEFINITION

Also known as paralysis agitans, Parkinson's syndrome is the adult onset of degenerative disease of the central nervous system (extrapyramidal system) characterized by the loss of dopamine cell bodies in the substantia nigra in the brain. The dopamine deficiency causes the clinical signs and symptoms.

INCIDENCE AND PREVALENCE

Parkinson's syndrome occurs generally between 60 and 80 years of age. Distribution in males and females is equal.

ETIOLOGY

The exact cause is unknown. There is no hereditary component. The syndrome has been observed to develop after encephalitis, intoxication with carbon monoxide, and chronic ingestion of antipsychotic drugs.

DIAGNOSTIC AND LABORATORY FINDINGS

None presently.

CLINICAL MANIFESTATIONS

Clinical manifestations include slow resting tremors (generally of the pill-rolling type), bradykinesia, rigidity, a slow shuffling gait, and an expressionless face. The patient may present with a unilateral tremor or rigidity.

TREATMENT

The goal is to increase the activity of the remaining dopaminergic cells in the substantia nigra. This can be accomplished in three ways:

1. Administer L-dopa orally (dopamine precursor, crosses blood-brain barrier), thereby increasing the concentration of dopamine in the substantia nigra.

2. Administer oral medication such as bromocriptine, which increases the dopamine receptor activity in the substantia nigra. Other similar medications used occasionally are trihexyphenidyl hydrochloride (Artane) and amantadine, but these are less effective.

3. Administer deprenyl (selegiline) orally, which works by inhibiting the enzymes that break down dopamine in the substantia nigra.

ANESTHETIC CONSIDERATIONS

L-Dopa therapy should be continued during the perioperative period, including the usual morning dose on the day of surgery. The half-life of L-dopa and dopamine is short. Interruption of therapy for more than 6 to 12 hours can result in abrupt loss of therapeutic benefit from the drug. Abrupt withdrawal of L-dopa can lead to skeletal muscle rigidity that interferes with ventilation. L-Dopa sensitizes the cardiovascular system and may increase the risk of perioperative arrhythmias. Long-term L-dopa therapy tends to cause autonomic instability and blood pressure fluctuations. Venous and arterial monitoring may be required. L-Dopa therapy causes increased renal blood flow, increased excretion of sodium, decreased renin release, decreased intravascular fluid volume, and decreased blood pressure with induction, which may require aggressive administration of crystalloid and colloids. Avoid phenothiazines and butyrophenones (block dopamine may exacerbate symptoms). Ketamine may provoke exaggerated sympathetic nervous system response; its use is questionable.

PROGNOSIS

Symptoms are treated with medication, but patients still have disability secondary to rigidity and bradykinesia in addition to ambulatory difficulty.

E. Guillain-Barré Syndrome

• • •

DEFINITION

Acute idiopathic polyneuritis characterized by a sudden onset of weakness or paralysis, typically exhibited in the legs, spreading cephalad over the next few days to involve skeletal muscles of the arms, trunk, and head.

INCIDENCE

Guillain-Barré syndrome occurs in 1 to 2 persons per 100,000.

ETIOLOGY

Bulbar involvement is most frequently manifested as bilateral facial paralysis. The most common symptoms are difficulty in swallowing due to pharyngeal muscle weakness and impaired ventilation due to intercostal muscle paralysis. Because of lower motor neuron involvement, paralysis is flaccid and corresponding tendon reflexes are diminished. Sensory disturbances occur as paresthesias, most prominently in the distal part of the extremity and generally preceding the onset of paralysis. Pain takes the form of headache, backache, or tenderness of skeletal muscle to deep pressure. Autonomic nervous system dysfunction is a prominent finding in patients with acute Guillain-Barré syndrome (wide fluctuation in blood pressure, sudden profuse diaphoresis, peripheral vasoconstriction, resting tachycardia, cardiac conduction abnormalities on electrocardiography, orthostatic hypotension, thromboembolism). Complete spontaneous recovery can occur within a few weeks when segmental demyelination is the predominant pathologic change. The mortality rate of 3% to 8% is due to sepsis, respiratory distress syndrome, and pulmonary embolism.

DIAGNOSIS

Diagnosis is based on clinical findings (progressive bilateral weakness in the legs and arms). The concentration of protein in cerebrospinal fluid is increased, although cell counts remain normal. A viral etiology is supported by the observation that this syndrome develops after a respiratory or gastrointestinal infection in about half of cases.

TREATMENT

Treatment is mainly symptomatic. Monitor vital capacity (if less than 15 mL/kg, consider ventilatory support). Steroids are not considered useful. Plasma exchange or infusion of gamma globulin may be of some benefit.

ANESTHETIC CONSIDERATIONS

The function of the autonomic nervous system is altered (noxious stimuli can exaggerate response). A lower motor neuron lesion is present. Rapid induction could lead to aspiration. There is a compensatory cardiovascular response to changes in posture, blood loss, or positive pressure. An arterial line is needed. Avoid succinylcholine; use a nondepolarizing muscle relaxant. Postoperative ventilation support may be needed. Document neurologic findings as a baseline preoperatively.

PROGNOSIS

The prognosis varies.

F. Multiple Sclerosis

♦ ♦ ♦

DEFINITION

Demyelinating, acquired disease of the central nervous system characterized by random and multiple sites of demyelination of the corticospinal-tract neurons in the brain and spinal cord.

ETIOLOGY

The exact cause is unknown. Pathologic changes consist of loss of myelin covering the axons in the form of demyelinative plaques. Multiple sclerosis (MS) does not affect the peripheral nervous system.

INCIDENCE AND PREVALENCE

There is a relationship between geographic latitude (northern temperate zone in North America, Europe, and southern portions of New Zealand and Australia) and increased risk of developing MS (1 in 1000). Incidence is greater among urban dwellers and affluent socioeconomic groups. Evidence for a genetic factor is demonstrated by a 12-fold to 15-fold increase among first-degree relatives. MS is a disease of young adults. Females have a 2 : 1 greater incidence than males, and females tend to develop MS at a younger age. The development of symptoms later in life (after 35) is associated with a slower progression of symptoms. There may be a viral or inflammatory component. A transmissable agent has not been identified.

DIAGNOSTIC AND LABORATORY TESTS

Visual, brain stem, auditory, and somatosensory evoked potentials can be used to show slow nerve conduction due to demyelination in specific areas. Computed tomography and magnetic resonance imaging may demonstrate demyelinative plaques.

CLINICAL MANIFESTATIONS

Clinical manifestations reflect the site of demyelination in the central nervous system and spinal cord. Ascending spastic paresis of skeletal muscle is often prominent. Presenting symptoms may include unilateral vision impairment. Ten to 15% of patients develop full MS. Symptoms may develop over the course of a few days, remain stable for a few weeks, then improve. The incidence of seizure disorders increases with MS patients. The course of MS is characterized by exacerbations and remissions of symptoms at unpredictable intervals over a period of several years. Residual symptoms persist during remission.

TREATMENT

No treatment cures MS. Medications used include steroids (shortens duration of attack). Skeletal muscle spasticity is treated with baclofen (Lioresal), dantrolene, and diazepam (Valium). Immunosuppressive therapy and plasmapheresis may benefit some patients. Patients should avoid stress and fatigue.

ANESTHETIC CONSIDERATIONS

Document the baseline neurologic examination. Consider the impact of surgical stress on the natural progression of MS. Any postoperative increase in body temperature may be more likely than drugs to be responsible for exacerbation of MS. Spinal anesthesia has been implicated in postoperative exacerbation of MS, whereas epidural or peripheral nerve block has not. General anesthesia is most often chosen. Avoid succinylcholine (possibly exaggerated release of potassium). The response to nondepolarizing muscle relaxants (NDMRs) may be prolonged because of coexisting muscle weakness and decreased muscle mass.

PROGNOSIS

The course of MS is unpredictable. Exacerbations and remissions of neurologic symptoms are common. In the late-onset type, the course is generally progressive.

G. Myasthenia Gravis

♦ ♦ ♦

DEFINITION

Chronic autoimmune disease involving the neuromuscular junction.

INCIDENCE AND PREVALENCE

Myasthenia gravis (MG) occurs in 1 of every 20,000 adults. Females between 20 and 30 years of age are most often affected. Males are often

COMMON DISEASES

older than 60 years when the disease manifests. Females are affected more often than males.

ETIOLOGY

The basic defect is a decrease in the number of available receptors for acetylcholine at the postsynaptic neuromuscular junction that results in skeletal muscle weakness and easy exhaustion. This decrease in available receptors is due to their inactivation or destruction by circulating antibodies. An estimated 70% to 80% of functional acetylcholine receptors are lost (this explains the easy exhaustion of patients and the marked sensitivity to nondepolarizing muscle relaxants). The origin of the autoimmune response is unknown but the thymus gland may play a role. Hyperplasia of the thymus gland is present in more than 70% of patients, and 10% to 15% have thymomas. About 75% of patients undergo remission after thymectomy.

LABORATORY RESULTS

Patients should undergo clinical evaluation, the Tensilon test, and electromyography.

CLINICAL MANIFESTATIONS

MG is classified on the basis of the skeletal muscles involved and severity of the symptoms.

Type I   Limited to extraocular muscles in 10% of patients.
Type IIA   Slowly progressive and mild form of skeletal muscle weakness. Spares respiratory muscles. Responds to anticholinesterase well.
Type IIB   More severe. Does not respond well to drugs. Respiratory muscles may be involved.
Type III   Acute onset, rapid deterioration of skeletal muscle strength (within 6 months).
Type IV   Severe form. Results from type I or II.

The hallmark symptom of MG is weakness and rapid exhaustion of voluntary skeletal muscles with repetitive use followed by partial recovery with rest. Skeletal muscles innervated by the cranial nerves are especially vulnerable, as reflected by ptosis and diplopia, which may be the initial symptoms of the disease.

Signs and Symptoms

The clinical course of MG is marked by periods of exacerbation and remission. Electromyography shows decreased voltage with repetitive stimulation. The most common initial complaints are ptosis and diplopia from weakness in extraocular movement. Weakness of pharyngeal and laryngeal muscles (bulbar muscles) results in dysphagia, dysarthria, and difficulty in eliminating oral secretions. Skeletal muscle strength may be normal in well-rested patients, but exercise leads to weakness. Arm, leg, or trunk weakness can occur in any combination and is usually distributed asymmetrically. These patients may be at an increased risk for pulmonary aspiration of gastric contents. MG may be associated with cardiomyopathy. Other autoimmune diseases may be present (thyroid, rheumatoid arthritis, systemic lupus erythematosus, pernicious anemia). Pregnancy, emotional stress, and surgery may precipitate skeletal muscle weakness.

TREATMENT

1. *Anticholinesterase drugs*—inhibit enzyme responsible for hydrolysis of acetylcholine, thereby increasing the neurotransmitter at the neuromuscular junction. Neostigmine can be used (15-mg oral dose, equal to 1.5-mg IM dose, equal to 0.5-mg IV dose). Pyridostigmine lasts longer (3 to 6 hours) and produces fewer muscarinic side effects (60 mg orally equals 2-mg IV or IM dose). Phospholine iodine is extremely potent and is reserved for severe MG. Excessive anticholinesterase drug effects may result in skeletal muscle weakness (cholinergic crisis).

2. *Corticosteroids*—predisone, 50 to 100 mg orally every day (interferes with the production of antibodies; responsible for degradation of cholinergic receptors).

3. *Plasmapheresis*—removes circulating antibodies to acetylcholine, resulting in improved skeletal muscle strength.

4. *Thymectomy*—recommended for patients with drug-resistant MG. About 75% of these patients demonstrate a marked improvement in skeletal muscle strength; drug therapy is no longer required or dosage can be decreased.

ANESTHETIC CONSIDERATIONS

Preoperative opioids should be used with caution if at all. Explain to the patient that he/she may remain intubated and ventilated postoperatively. Criteria correlated with likelihood for controlled postoperative ventilation following transsternal thymectomy include:

1. Duration of MG greater than 6 years
2. Chronic obstructive pulmonary disease related to MG
3. Dose of pyridostigmine greater than 750 mg/d during the 48 hours preceding surgery
4. Preoperative vital capacity of less than 2.9 L is less likely to require postoperative ventilatory support with the transcervical approach

The muscle relaxant response is difficult to predict—use peripheral nerve stimulation. Sensitivity to NDMR, and to succinylcholine may increase. For induction, use short-acting intravenous anesthetics, short-acting NDMRs, or succinylcholine to facilitate intubation. For maintenance of anesthesia, use oxygen, nitrous oxide, and a volatile anesthetic agent. If an NDMR is used, the initial dose should be reduced by one half to one third. Assess with peripheral nerve stimulation. Narcotics may have a prolonged effect. The patient may require postoperative ventilatory support.

PROGNOSIS

MG is a chronic, lifelong disease.

H. Myasthenic Syndrome

• • •

DEFINITION

Also called Lambert-Eaton syndrome, myasthenic syndrome is a rare disorder of neuromuscular transmission resembling myasthenia gravis.

CLINICAL MANIFESTATIONS

Clinical manifestations include skeletal muscle weakness in patients with small cell carcinoma of the lung.

ETIOLOGY

Myasthenic syndrome is an autoimmune disease in which immunoglobulin G antibodies to presynaptic calcium channels are produced.

TREATMENT

Anticholinesterase drugs effective in treating myasthenia gravis are not effective with this syndrome. 4-Aminopyridine, which stimulates the presynaptic release of acetylcholine, may improve skeletal muscle strength.

ANESTHETIC CONSIDERATIONS

Patients are sensitive to depolarizing and NDMR. (Decrease dose.)

I. Intracranial Hypertension

• • •

DEFINITION

The cranial cavity has three intracranial constituents: blood volume, tissue volume, and cerebrospinal fluid volume. Intracranial elastance is hindered when one of these areas has been disrupted. Intracranial pressure (ICP) levels are increased when intracranial elastance is defective, so an ICP of

20 to 25 mm Hg is a threshold for intracranial hypertension and intervention should be implemented. The rigid skull allows little room for the brain, cerebrospinal fluid, or the cerebral blood volume to expand. Because these contents are practically incompressible, a volume change in any compartment requires a reciprocal change in one or both of the other compartments if the ICP is to remain normal.

ETIOLOGY

Head injury, stroke, intracranial hemorrhage, infection, tumor formation, postischemia or posthypoxic states, hydrocephalus, osmolar imbalances, and pulmonary disease can all cause increased ICP. As the ICP progressively increases, cerebral perfusion pressure is reduced, and focal ischemia occurs. If the ICP is already high, even small increases in intracranial volumes result in marked intracranial hypertension and global ischemia. When a space-occupying lesion is present, intracranial tissue shifts and localized pressure gradients develop, causing vascular compression and regional ischemia.

LABORATORY RESULTS

Magnetic resonance imaging and computed tomography are the two most prominent tests to evaluate tumors, hemorrhage, stroke, and areas of ischemia. Lumbar puncture is used to diagnose infections and hydrocephalus.

CLINICAL MANIFESTATIONS

Symptoms of increased ICP include headache, nausea and vomiting, mental changes, and disturbances in consciousness and vision. During early stages of intracranial hypertension, symptoms are most common in the early morning hours. Increases in arterial carbon dioxide pressure ($PaCO_2$) and the associated cerebral vasodilation that accompanies sleep produce an increase in intracranial contents that exceeds the limits of compensation, and the ICP increases. Progressive increases in ICP eventually result in unexplained fatigue and drowsiness. Papilledema may be seen, which is accompanied by visual disturbances. A first-time seizure in an adult with no apparent cause should arouse suspicion of increased ICP. Systemic blood pressure may be elevated in order to maintain cerebral perfusion pressure in the presence of intracranial hypertension.

TREATMENT

Patients with intracranial hypertension or reduced intracranial elastance can be managed using various interventions. All are based on the concept that ICP can be reduced or intracranial elastance can be improved by reducing one of the three intracranial constituents: blood volume, tissue volume, or cerebrospinal fluid volume. See specific interventions in the Anesthetic Considerations section that follows.

COMMON DISEASES

ANESTHETIC CONSIDERATIONS

Cerebral blood volume can be reduced in various ways. Endotracheal intubation limits the chances of increased cerebral blood flow (CBF) related to hypoxemia and hypercarbia. Neuromuscular blockade prevents increases in cerebral venous volume from coughing, straining, or actively exhaling. Cerebral venous drainage is facilitated by head elevation, but by reducing venous return, cardiac output, and mean arterial pressure, may actually reduce cerebral perfusion pressure. Appropriate analgesia and sedation prevent increases in the cerebral metabolic rate of oxygen and the accompanying increases in CBF. Hyperventilation acutely reduces CBF, although CBF usually returns to its original level even with prolonged hyperventilation. Barbiturates in sufficient doses suppress both the cerebral metabolic rate of oxygen and CBF in association with profound electrophysiologic suppression. Caution should be used when barbiturate therapy is implemented because of the vasodilator and myocardial depressive effects. Brain tissue volume is usually reduced by diuresis. Osmotic diuresis, using mannitol, reduces brain water. Mannitol can be used as a continuous infusion or as treatment for acute episodes of increased ICP. Maximum reduction of ICP is accomplished with large doses of mannitol administered rapidly, then followed by furosemide. When a patient emerges from anesthesia, increased ICP caused by coughing on the oral endotracheal tube should be considered. Both extubation while the patient is still anesthetized and lidocaine can be used if they are not contraindicated.

PROGNOSIS

Quick and appropriate management to reduce ICP leads to a full recovery for most patients.

J. Autonomic Dysreflexia

♦ ♦ ♦

DEFINITION

A disorder that appears after resolution of spinal shock. The differentiated spinal cord may produce a group of deleterious reflexes.

INCIDENCE AND PREVALENCE

The incidence and prevalence depend on the level of spinal cord transection. About 85% of patients with spinal cord transection above T-6 exhibit this reflex. Autonomic dysreflexia is unlikely to be associated with a transection below T-10. Surgery, however, is a potent trigger of autonomic dysreflexia, even in patients with no previous history of this response.

ETIOLOGY

Autonomic dysreflexia can be initiated by cutaneous or visceral stimulation below the level of spinal cord transection. Distention of a hollow viscus (bladder or rectum) is a common stimulus. This stimulus initiates afferent impulses that enter the spinal cord below that level. These impulses elicit reflex sympathetic activity over the splanchnic outflow tract. This outflow is isolated from inhibitory impulses such that generalized vasoconstriction persists below the level of injury. Vasoconstriction results in increased blood pressure, which is then perceived by the carotid sinus. Subsequent activation of the carotid sinus results in decreased efferent outflow from the sympathetic nervous system. Activity from the central nervous system is manifested as a predominance of parasympathetic nervous system activity at the heart and peripheral vasculature. This predominance cannot be produced below the level of spinal cord transection (this part of the body remains neurologically isolated). Therefore, vasoconstriction persists below the level of spinal cord transection. If spinal cord transection is above the level of splanchnic outflow (T4-T6), vasodilation in the neurologically intact portion of the body is insufficient to offset the effects of vasoconstriction (reflected by persistent hypertension).

LABORATORY RESULTS

None.

CLINICAL MANIFESTATIONS

The hallmark symptoms are hypertension and bradycardia. These result from stimulation of the carotid sinus and cutaneous vasodilation above the level of spinal cord transection. Hypertension persists because vasodilation cannot occur below the level of injury. Nasal stuffiness reflects vasodilation. Other symptoms may include headache, blurred vision (due to hypertension), increased operative blood loss, loss of consciousness, seizures, cardiac arrhythmias, and pulmonary edema.

TREATMENT

Treatment includes ganglionic blockers (trimethaphan, pentolinium), alpha-adrenergic antagonists (phentolamine, phenoxybenzamine), and direct-acting vasodilators (nitroprusside). General or regional anesthesia is used. Drugs that lower blood pressure by central action alone are not predictably effective.

ANESTHETIC CONSIDERATIONS

Control of airway and ventilation with large tidal volumes (10 to 15 mL/kg) are needed to avoid hypercarbia and atelectasis. Take special care in moving patients with chronic spinal cord injury—avoid fractures of weakened bones and pad pressure areas. Preoperative hydration helps prevent hypotension during induction and aids maintenance of anesthesia. Prevent autonomic hyperreflexia. NDMR should be used to facilitate intubation and prevent reflex skeletal muscle spasms. Avoid succinylcholine. Have nitroprusside and other cardioactive agents readily available to treat precipitous hypertension.

PROGNOSIS

Autonomic dysreflexia is a chronic, lifelong potential condition of spinal cord transection patients.

K. Spinal Cord Injury

◆ ◆ ◆

DEFINITION

The spinal cord is vulnerable to trauma, compression by intradural or extradural tumors, and vascular injuries.

INCIDENCE AND PREVALENCE

Approximately 10,000 persons suffer acute spinal cord injuries each year that result in paraplegia and quadriplegia. Two thirds are male, and 70% to 80% are ages 11 to 30. The mortality rate before reaching the hospital is 30% to 40%; the mortality rate during the first year decreases to 10%.

ETIOLOGY

Spinal cord injuries result from motor vehicle accidents, falls, sport injuries (especially from diving), and penetrating injuries from guns. The spinal cord itself is not usually severed but is injured by compression from bone, foreign body, hematoma, edema, and ischemia.

DIAGNOSTIC AND LABORATORY RESULTS

A clinical examination is needed.

CLINICAL MANIFESTATIONS

Clinical manifestations include changes in cardiopulmonary responses, fluid, and electrolytes, temperature control dysfunction, and abnormal response to drugs. Injuries at levels T2-T12 cause paraplegia but leave the upper extremities and diaphragm intact. Injuries at levels C5-T1 cause varying degrees of upper-extremity paralysis as well.

TREATMENT

For acute injury, the ABCs of resuscitation are used: A is airway, B is breathing, and C is circulation. Avoid neck motion and further cord damage. Maintain spinal cord perfusion with volume and vasoactive drugs. If the cord is compressed by bone or hematoma, decompression is necessary.

ANESTHETIC CONSIDERATIONS

Halo traction may be necessary for any fundamental change in airway management of cervical spine injury. A surgeon may be needed to help maintain neck immobility during intubation. Fiberoptic intubation may be needed. Nasal intubation is contraindicated in the presence of basilar skull fracture. Preparations should be made for immediate cricothyroidotomy, if necessary. Use anticholinergic agents to reduce secretions. Ventilate the patient with large tidal volumes (10 to 15 mL/kg) to avoid hypercarbia and atelectasis. Move the patient carefully to prevent injury to the limbs and trunk. Check pressure areas to prevent breakdown. Some cardioacceleration and vasoconstrictor tone is lost as a result of cord injuries that involve levels T1-T4. Spinal cord shock is present. Respiratory compromise is possible, depending on the level of spinal injury. Maintain spinal cord perfusion with volume and vasoactive agents.

PROGNOSIS

Spinal cord injury is a chronic condition that will require management for life.

SECTION IV

MUSCULOSKELETAL SYSTEM

A. Muscular Dystrophy

$\bullet\quad\bullet\quad\bullet$

DEFINITION

Muscular dystrophy is a hereditary disease characterized by painless degeneration and atrophy of skeletal muscles. There is progressive and symmetric skeletal muscle weakness and wasting but no evidence of muscle denervation, with reflexes and sensations remaining intact. Mental retardation is often present. Increased permeability of skeletal muscle membranes precedes clinical evidence of the disease. The most common and severe form of the disease is categorized as pseudohypertrophic (Duchenne's) muscular dystrophy. Other less common forms include limb-girdle, facioscapulohumeral (Landouzy-Dejerine), nemaline rod myopathy, and oculopharyngeal dystrophy.

ETIOLOGY

Pseudohypertrophic muscular dystrophy occurs in 3 of 10,000 births. It is caused by an X-linked recessive gene and becomes apparent in males aged 2 to 5 years.

CLINICAL MANIFESTATIONS

Initially symptoms such as waddling gait, frequent falling, and difficulty climbing stairs reflect involvement of the proximal skeletal groups of the pelvis. Affected skeletal muscle may become larger as a result of fatty infiltration, accounting for the designation of this disorder as pseudohypertrophic. Steady deterioration of skeletal muscle strength results in confinement to a wheelchair by 8 to 11 years of age. Kyphoscoliosis may develop, which reflects the unopposed actions of the antagonists of the dystrophic muscles. Skeletal muscle atrophy can predispose to long bone fractures. Degeneration of cardiac muscle invariably accompanies muscular dystrophy. Congestive heart failure is common. Characteristic electrocardiographic findings include a tall R wave in lead V1, a deep Q wave in limb leads, a short P-R interval, and sinus tachycardia. Mitral regurgitation may be due to papillary muscle dysfunction and decreased myocardial contractility.

Chronic weakness of inspiratory respiratory muscles and a decreased ability to cough can result in loss of pulmonary reserve and an accumulation of secretions, thus predisposing to recurrent pneumonias. Respiratory insufficiency often remains covert because impaired skeletal muscle function prevents patients from exceeding their limited breathing capacity. With further progression of the disease, kyphoscoliosis can contribute further to a restrictive pattern of lung disease. Sleep apnea is possible and may contribute to pulmonary hypertension.

LABORATORY RESULTS

Laboratory findings include a plasma creatine kinase concentration that is 30 to 300 times normal, even early in the disease, reflecting skeletal muscle necrosis and the increased permeability of skeletal muscle membranes. Plasma creatine kinase concentration is elevated in approximately 70% of female carriers. Skeletal muscle biopsy early in the course of the disease may demonstrate necrosis and phagocytosis of muscle fibers.

ANESTHETIC CONSIDERATIONS

Anesthetic considerations for the patient with pseudohypertrophic muscular dystrophy must account for the increased permeability of skeletal muscle membranes and decreased cardiopulmonary reserve. Succinylcholine may be associated with exaggerated potassium release, leading to life-threatening cardiac arrhythmias. Ventricular fibrillation upon induction of anesthesia that includes succinylcholine has been observed in patients later discovered to have pseudohypertrophic muscular dystrophy. Responses to nondepolarizing muscle relaxants usually are normal, but the possibility of a prolonged response should be considered when coexisting skeletal muscle weakness is prominent. Dantrolene should be available because of the increased incidence of malignant hyperthermia in these patients. Malignant hyperthermia has been observed after only a brief period of halothane administration alone, although most cases have been triggered by succinylcholine or with prolonged inhalation of halothane. Hypomotility of the gastrointestinal tract may delay gastric emptying, which in the presence of weak laryngeal reflexes increases the risk of pulmonary aspiration. Depressant effects of volatile anesthetics on myocardial contractility can be exaggerated. Cardiac arrest after induction of anesthesia has been reported in afflicted patients. Monitoring should be directed at early detection of malignant hyperthermia (capnography temperature) and cardiac depression. Postoperative pulmonary dysfunction must be anticipated, and clearance of secretions must be facilitated. Delayed pulmonary insufficiency may occur up to 36 hours postoperatively, despite apparent recovery to the preoperative level of skeletal muscle strength.

TREATMENT

Regional anesthesia avoids many of the unique risks of general anesthesia in these patients; during the postoperative period it provides analgesia, which may facilitate chest physiotherapy. Prognosis for these patients is poor: death usually occurs by 15 to 25 years of age because of congestive heart failure, pneumonia, or both.

PROGNOSIS

Muscular dystrophy requires chronic life-long management.

B. Kyphoscoliosis

• • •

DEFINITION

Kyphoscoliosis is a deformity of the costovertebral skeletal structures characterized by anterior flexion (kyphosis) and lateral curvature (scoliosis) of the vertebral column.

ETIOLOGY

The incidence of idiopathic kyphoscoliosis is about 4 per 1000 persons. This disease seems to have a familial predisposition, with females affected about 4 times more often than males.

A curve greater than 40° is considered severe and most likely to be associated with physiologic alterations in cardiac and pulmonary function. Restrictive lung disease and pulmonary hypertension progressing to cor pulmonale are the principal causes of mortality in patients with kyphoscoliosis. As the scoliotic curve worsens, more lung tissue is compressed, resulting in decreased vital capacity and dyspnea with mild exertion. Work of breathing is increased by abnormal mechanical properties of the thorax and by increased airway resistance resulting from small lung volumes. The alveolar to arteriolar difference for oxygen is increased. The arterial carbon dioxide pressure ($PaCO_2$) is usually normal, but relatively minor insults such as bacterial or viral upper respiratory tract infections may result in acute respiratory failure. A poor cough reflex contributes to frequent pulmonary infections. Pulmonary hypertension reflects increased pulmonary vascular resistance due to compression of lung vasculature by the curve in the spine and the pulmonary vascular response to arterial hypoxemia.

ANESTHETIC CONSIDERATIONS

Anesthetic management of these patients should begin with a thorough preoperative assessment of the physiologic derangements produced by the skeletal deformity. Pulmonary function tests, with special attention to the vital capacity and forced expiratory volume in 1 second, will reflect the magnitude of restrictive lung disease. Arterial blood gases and pH are helpful in detecting unrecognized arterial hypoxemia or acidosis that could be contributing to pulmonary hypertension. These patients may enter the preoperative period with pneumonia due to chronic aspiration of acidic gastric fluid. Any reversible components of pulmonary dysfunction, such as infections or bronchospasm, should be corrected before elective surgery is performed. Preoperative medication with depressant drugs should be administered cautiously if at all because of the narrow margin of ventilatory reserve in these patients, as well as the adverse effects on the pulmonary vascular resistance that would occur with respiratory acidosis from hypoventilation. Intraoperatively, ventilation of the lungs should be controlled to facilitate adequate arterial oxygenation and elimination of carbon dioxide. Nitrous oxide should be used with caution because it may increase pulmonary vascular resistance. Arterial oxygen saturation should be monitored continuously to ensure adequacy of oxygenation. Central venous pressure measurements may provide an early warning of increased pulmonary vascular resistance produced by nitrous oxide. It has been suggested that these patients have an increased incidence of malignant hyperthermia, so vigilant monitoring of end-tidal carbon dioxide and temperature is recommended.

COMMON DISEASES

C. Malignant Hyperthermia

◆ ◆ ◆

DEFINITION

Malignant hyperthermia is a hypermetabolic disorder of skeletal muscle triggered by anesthetic agents.

INCIDENCE AND PREVALENCE

This disorder is relatively rare, affecting approximately 1 of 50,000 anesthetics administered in adults and 1 of 15,000 anesthetics administered in children. A genetic component seems to be related to the incidence of malignant hyperthermia. The incidence increases when succinylcholine is used with other triggering agents. Triggering agents include succinylcholine, all inhalational anesthetic agents (except nitrous oxide), and potassium salts. Additional agents that may trigger malignant hyperthermia are curare and phenothiazine. Malignant hyperthermia has been found to be associated with other muscle disorders, such as Duchenne's muscular dystrophy.

ETIOLOGY

The precise etiology of malignant hyperthermia is not well understood; however, it is thought that a defect in calcium flux in the sarcoplasm leads to high concentrations of calcium. This high concentration of calcium allows for sustained muscle contraction. Accelerated metabolism associated with the sustained contractions is accompanied by acidosis and heat production. There is a depletion of adenosine triphosphate, acidosis, cell membrane destruction, and cell death.

LABORATORY RESULTS

The definitive diagnosis of malignant hyperthermia is made by muscle biopsy and in vitro isometric contracture testing in the presence of caffeine, halothane, or both. Although not definitive, creatinine kinase tests should be performed on patients considered susceptible to malignant hyperthermia. Elevated resting levels of creatine kinase are found in about 70% of malignant hyperthermia–susceptible patients. Other laboratory findings consistent with malignant hyperthermia crisis are carbon dioxide partial pressure (PCO_2) greater than 46 mm Hg; elevated lactate, potassium, and creatine phosphokinase levels; and pH less than 7.28.

CLINICAL MANIFESTATIONS

Clinical findings related to hypermetabolism may vary. Common are hypercarbia, tachycardia, hypoxemia, metabolic and respiratory acidosis, tachypnea, hyperkalemia, arrhythmias, hypotension, flushing, cyanosis, mottling, extreme increases in body temperature, sweating, tea-colored urine, and muscle rigidity. The earliest clinical sign is increased end-tidal carbon dioxide, followed by tachycardia. If untreated, malignant hyperthermia produces late signs of renal failure, disseminated intravascular coagulation, pulmonary edema, blindness, seizures, paralysis, and coma.

TREATMENT

A treatment protocol for malignant hyperthermia is outlined below:

1. Inform the surgeon and request termination of surgery, if possible.

2. Discontinue administration of all inhalation anesthetics and succinylcholine; hyperventilate the patient with 100% oxygen at a high flow rate; monitor end-tidal carbon dioxide.

3. Enlist the help of additional anesthesia staff; have a malignant hyperthermia cart brought to the operating room.

4. Reconstitute dantrolene with sterile water; administer intravenous dantrolene in 2.5-mg/kg boluses until signs of malignant hyperthermia abate.

5. Draw arterial blood gases; treat acidosis with sodium bicarbonate, with dose increases in 1- to 2-mEq/kg increments, or as guided by arterial blood gases. Draw blood samples for electrolyte, creatine kinase, myoglobin, glucose, and coagulation studies.

6. Treat hyperkalemia with an infusion of 10 U of regular insulin in 50 mL of 50% glucose.

7. Insert a three-way Foley catheter and obtain urine samples for myoglobin level determination; induce a urine output of greater than 2 mL/kg per hour by giving intravenous fluids, mannitol, and furosemide.

8. Initiate aggressive cooling as indicated by the patient's core temperature.

9. Treat persistent or life-threatening electrocardiographic arrhythmias with standard antiarrhythmic agents; Ca^{2+} channel blockers should not be used.

10. After the malignant hyperthermia event, the patient should be monitored for at least 24 hours in an intensive care unit.

The Malignant Hyperthermia Association of the United States (MHAUS) Malignant Hyperthermia Hotline consultant may be contacted for expert medical advice at (800) 644–9737. The malignant hyperthermia event should be reported to the North American Malignant Hyperthermia Registry at (717) 531–6936.

ANESTHETIC CONSIDERATIONS

A detailed anesthesia history is imperative. If the patient or family has a history of malignant hyperthermia, all triggering agents should be avoided. The anesthesia machine vaporizers should be removed, and the circuit and carbon dioxide absorber canisters should be changed. The machine should be flushed with oxygen (10 L/min) for 10 to 20 minutes prior to the operation. The patient should be well sedated. Consider administering dantrolene preoperatively (do not use phenothiazine). If malignant hyperthermia is diagnosed, patient and family counseling and education is necessary.

PROGNOSIS

The overall mortality rate is 10%. Without use of dantrolene, the mortality rate goes up to 70%. Early treatment may decrease the mortality rate to about 5%.

ENDOCRINE SYSTEM
A. Diabetes Mellitus

◆ ◆ ◆

DEFINITION

Diabetes mellitus is a chronic systemic disease characterized by a broad array of abnormalities, the most notable of which is disturbed glucose metabolism, resulting in inappropriate hyperglycemia.

ETIOLOGY

About 2.4% of the U.S. population (about 5.5 million persons) is diabetic. Diabetes is divided into two categories, insulin-dependent diabetes mellitus (IDDM) and non–insulin-dependent diabetes mellitus (NIDDM).

IDDM most often develops in childhood or adolescence (before 16 years of age), and evidence suggests a genetic predisposition to the disease. It probably results from destruction of pancreatic beta cells by an autoimmune process that may be precipitated by a viral infection. About 15% of patients with IDDM have other autoimmune diseases such as hypothyroidism, Graves' disease, Addison's disease, and myasthenia gravis. The genetic predisposition is more of a reflection of susceptibility to the disease, rather than its inheritance. These patients depend on exogenous insulin to prevent ketoacidosis.

NIDDM most often develops in middle or later life (after 35 years of age) and, again, evidence suggests a genetic predisposition. The prevalence increases steadily with age, particularly among black females. Many NIDDM patients may be on insulin therapy, but they are not usually prone to ketoacidosis. Nevertheless, NIDDM may progress to the extent that insulin is needed to prevent ketoacidosis. Patients with NIDDM, who are almost all overweight, constitute 90% of all diabetics. Obese nondiabetics require two to five times more insulin than do nonobese nondiabetics; thus, obesity may unmask latent diabetics.

Complications from diabetes are numerous. The most serious acute metabolic complication is ketoacidosis, defined as hyperglycemia in the presence of metabolic acidosis. The symptoms include nausea, vomiting, lethargy, and signs of hypovolemia due to dehydration, which is secondary to the osmotic effect of glucose. Causes of ketoacidosis include poor patient compliance with insulin regimen, insulin resistance because of infection, and silent myocardial infarction. Administration of a beta$_2$ agonist to inhibit labor in the presence of IDDM has been reported to abruptly precipitate ketoacidosis, even with prior subcutaneous insulin administration. Later complications of diabetes include macroangiopathies such as coronary artery disease, cerebrovascular disease, and peripheral vascular disease. These later complications are more common in the patient with NIDDM; sequelae such as premature myocardial infarction, angina pectoris, or peripheral vascular insufficiency often are the presenting symptoms in an undiagnosed diabetic. In the patient with IDDM, microvascular complications and disorders of the nervous system predominate. Retinopathy, nephropathy, and autonomic and peripheral nervous system neuropathies are common findings. Diabetic retinopathy occurs in 80% to 90% of people who have had IDDM for longer than 20 years. Autonomic nervous system dysfunction may affect more than 15% of diabetics. Delayed wound healing and postoperative infection are more likely in the diabetic. Stiff joint syndrome affects 30% to 40% of patients with IDDM, affecting all joints—most important to anesthesia, the atlanto-occipital joint may be involved, making laryngoscopy difficult.

TREATMENT

Treatment of diabetes includes diet, oral hypoglycemic drugs, and exogenous insulin. NIDDM is prevented primarily by avoidance or treatment of obesity. Transplantation of pancreatic tissue may be considered in selected patients.

ANESTHETIC CONSIDERATIONS

The goal of anesthetic management in the diabetic patient undergoing surgery is to mimic normal metabolism as closely as possible by avoiding hypoglycemia, excessive hyperglycemia, ketoacidosis, and electrolyte disturbances. Hypoglycemia is prevented by ensuring an adequate supply of exogenous glucose. Hyperglycemia and associated ketoacidosis, dehydration, and electrolyte abnormalities are prevented by the administration of exogenous insulin. The goal of blood glucose control is to maintain a level well above that considered to be hypoglycemic but below the level at which deleterious effects of hyperglycemia (hyperosmolarity, osmotic diuresis, electrolyte disturbances, impaired phagocyte function, impaired wound healing) become evident. Blood glucose concentration should be between 120 and 180 mg/dL^{-1}. Along with the careful preoperative, intraoperative, and postoperative monitoring of the blood glucose and electrolytes, a thorough preoperative evaluation should be done to determine whether other systems, such as cardiac, neurologic, and renal systems, are involved. Appropriate preoperative evaluations should be done, and intraoperative monitoring should be directed at these complications.

B. Diabetes Insipidus

♦   ♦   ♦

DEFINITION

Diabetes insipidus (DI) reflects the absence of antidiuretic hormone owing to the destruction of the posterior pituitary (neurogenic DI) or failure of the renal tubules to respond to antidiuretic hormone (nephrogenic DI).

ETIOLOGY

Neurogenic DI can be caused by intracranial trauma, hypophysectomy, neoplastic invasion, or sarcoidosis. Nephrogenic DI can be caused by hypokalemia, hypercalcemia, sickle cell anemia, obstructive uropathy, chronic renal insufficiency, or lithium.

CLINICAL MANIFESTATIONS

Clinical features include polydipsia and polyuria with poorly concentrated urine despite increased plasma osmolarity. Neurogenic and nephrogenic DI are differentiated on the basis of response to desmopressin, which produces concentration of the urine in neurogenic, but not nephrogenic, DI.

TREATMENT

Treatment includes careful monitoring of urine output, plasma volume, and plasma osmolarity. Isotonic fluids may be administered until osmolarity is greater than 290; then hypotonic fluids are necessary. Neurogenic DI may be treated with desmopressin at 3 mg/kg. Nephrogenic DI may be treated with chlorpropamide, an oral hypoglycemic drug that potentiates the effect of antidiuretic hormone on renal tubules.

ANESTHETIC CONSIDERATIONS

Anesthetic management for the patient with DI should include monitoring of urine output and plasma electrolyte concentrations during the perioperative period. If emergent surgery is needed, central venous pressure monitoring may aid evaluation of volume status.

C. Thyroid Disease

◆   ◆   ◆

DEFINITION

Thyroid hormone is one of major regulators of cellular metabolic activity, altering speed of reactions, total oxygen consumption, and heat production of the body.

ETIOLOGY

Thyroid-stimulating hormone (TSH) is released from the anterior pituitary, causing iodine to be taken up into the thyroid gland. The iodine is then incorporated into tyrosine residues, and the hormones triiodothyronine (T_3) and thyroxine (T_4) are formed and stored. Peripheral tissues convert

T_4 to T_3, which is three times more potent than T_4 and has a shorter half-life. Both T_4 and T_3 are partially bound to the plasma protein thyroid-binding globulin (TBG), although only the unbound forms are pharmacologically active. TBG levels can increase with acute liver disease, pregnancy, acute intermittent porphyria, and medications (oral hypoglycemics, exogenous estrogens, clofibrate, and opioids), and they can be decreased with chronic liver disease, nephrotic syndrome, anabolic steroids, and acromegaly. TBG has no direct role in cell metabolism, but its concentration can alter diagnostic test results when checking for thyroid disease.

HYPERTHYROIDISM

Hyperthyroidism is an increase in thyroid function resulting from an excess supply of thyroid hormones and is associated with Graves' disease, TSH overproduction, and pregnancy. In subacute thyroiditis, excess thyroid hormone leaks out of the gland owing to inflammation. Ovarian tumors or metastatic thyroid carcinoma may also produce extrathyroid gland hormone. Exogenous consumption of thyroid hormone can also lead to hyperthyroidism.

LABORATORY RESULTS

Laboratory findings in hyperthyroidism include elevated levels of T_3 and T_4. Because TBG concentration may affect the measured T_4, a resin T_3 uptake test may be performed to distinguish between protein-binding abnormalities and true metabolic changes associated with hyperthyroidism. TSH levels may be normal or decreased.

CLINICAL MANIFESTATIONS

Clinically, hyperthyroid patients present with nervousness, tachycardia, goiter, tremors, muscle weakness, heat intolerance, and weight loss despite high caloric intake. Exophthalmos occurs in approximately 7 of 10 cases of hyperthyroidism. Worsening of angina pectoris or unexpected onset of congestive heart failure or atrial fibrillation may reflect undiagnosed hyperthyroidism, especially in elderly patients in whom the increased amount of thyroid hormones is sufficient only to aggravate underlying heart disease.

Thyroid storm (thyrotoxicosis) is an abrupt exacerbation of hyperthyroidism caused by the sudden excessive release of thyroid gland hormones into the circulation. Hyperthermia, tachycardia, congestive heart failure, dehydration, and shock commonly occur. Thyroid storm may be precipitated by surgical stress but is usually seen 6 to 18 hours postoperatively. It may mimic malignant hyperthermia, sepsis, hemorrhage, or a transfusion/drug reaction.

TREATMENT

Treatments for hyperthyroidism include antithyroid drugs, subtotal thyroidectomy, or radioactive iodine. Thyroid storm therapy includes active cooling, hydrating beta-adrenergic blockade, use of steroids if there is any indication of adrenal insufficiency, and institution of long-term therapy with antithyroid drugs or iodine. Six weeks are required to become euthyroid. Only emergency surgery should be performed in thyrotoxic patients. Premedication, including beta-blockers, should be given generously. Sympathetic stimulation (pain, ketamine, pancuronium) should be avoided. Eyes should be protected well, especially if exophthalmos is present. Drug metabolism and anesthetic requirements are increased. Because of muscle weakness, muscle relaxants should be titrated carefully. Hypotension should be treated with direct-acting agents such as phenylephrine. Regional anesthesia may be beneficial in thyrotoxic patients, because it blocks the sympathetic response. Local anesthetics with epinephrine may lead to further arrhythmias.

HYPOTHYROIDISM

Hypothyroidism can be classified as either primary (because of destruction of the thyroid gland, where there is an adequate level of TSH), or secondary (because of central nervous system (CNS) dysfunction leading to decreased levels of TSH). Causes of primary hypothyroidism include chronic thyroiditis subtotal thyroidectomy, radioactive iodine therapy, or irradiation of the neck. Thyroid hormone deficiency may occur because of antithyroid drugs, excess iodide, or a dietary iodine deficiency. Causes of secondary hypothyroidism include hypothalamic dysfunction leading to thyrotropin-releasing hormone deficiency, or anterior pituitary dysfunction leading to TSH deficiency.

LABORATORY RESULTS

Laboratory findings in primary hypothyroidism include decreased levels of T_3 and T_4, with an increased concentration of TSH. Secondary hypothyroidism exhibits decreased levels of T_3, T_4, and TSH. Resin T_3 uptake is decreased in both incidences.

CLINICAL MANIFESTATIONS

Onset of clinical symptoms in the adult patient is insidious and may go unrecognized. Patients experience lethargy, constipation, cold intolerance, facial edema with an enlarged tongue, a reversible cardiomyopathy, pericardial effusion, ascites, anemia, and an adynamic ileus with delayed gastric emptying. There may be adrenal atrophy with decreased cortisol production, dilutional hyponatremia, and decreased water excretion. There is a decreased cardiac output, bradycardia, hypovolemia, and diminished baroreceptor reflexes. Myxedema coma (profound hypothyroidism) may be triggered by trauma, infection, and CNS depressants, leading to respiratory depression, congestive heart failure, and depressed consciousness.

TREATMENT

Treatment for hypothyroidism involves the exogenous supplementation of thyroid hormone. T_4 requires 10 days to have an effect. T_3 begins to have an effect in 6 hours. Treatment for myxedema coma includes intravenous administration of T_3, and, if adrenal insufficiency is suspected, cortisol. Digitalis may be used sparingly to treat congestive heart failure, because increases in myocardial contractility are not well tolerated by hypothyroid patients. Fluid replacement is important, keeping in mind that these patients may be vulnerable to water intoxication and hyponatremia.

Elective surgery must be postponed in any patient who is clinically hypothyroid. In hypothyroid patients who must undergo emergency procedures, anesthetic considerations should include avoidance of preoperative sedation because of profound CNS and respiratory sensitivity to depressants. Cortisol supplementation should be considered; intravascular volume should be optimized; and anemia should be corrected. Anesthetic techniques must take into consideration airway problems associated with a large tongue, poor gastric emptying, and increased sensitivity to all depressant medications.

COMMON DISEASES

D. Cushing's Disease

◆ ◆ ◆

DEFINITION

Cushing's disease (hyperadrenocorticism) may reflect (1) overproduction of adrenocorticotropic hormone by the anterior pituitary (about two thirds of cases), (2) ectopic production of adrenocorticotropic hormone by malignant tumors (especially carcinoma of the lung, kidney, and pancreas), (3) excess production of cortisol by a benign or malignant tumor of the adrenal cortex, or (4) exogenous (pharmacologic) administration of cortisol or related drugs.

LABORATORY RESULTS

Diagnosis is best made by measurement of plasma cortisol concentration in the morning after a midnight dose of dexamethasone. Dexamethasone suppresses plasma cortisol concentration in normal patients but not in Cushing's disease patients. Magnetic resonance imaging for pituitary tumors and computed tomography showing large adrenal glands are also used for diagnosis.

CLINICAL MANIFESTATIONS

Signs and symptoms include hypertension, hypokalemia, hyperglycemia, skeletal muscle weakness, osteoporosis, obesity, hirsutism, menstrual disturbances, poor wound healing, and susceptibility to infection.

TREATMENT

Trans-sphenoidal microadenomectomy is the preferred treatment for hyperadrenocorticism owing to excess secretion of adrenocorticotropic hormone by the anterior pituitary.

ANESTHETIC CONSIDERATIONS

Anesthetic management should account for the effects of excess cortisol secretion, especially as reflected in blood pressure, electrolyte balance, and blood glucose concentration. Osteoporosis is a consideration in positioning for the operative procedure. Plasma cortisol concentration decreases promptly after microadenomectomy or bilateral adrenalectomy. Intraoperative replacement therapy (cortisol, 100 mg IV) should be initiated.

E. Addison's Disease

◆   ◆   ◆

DEFINITION

Primary adrenal insufficiency (Addison's disease) reflects the absence of cortisol and aldosterone owing to the destruction of the adrenal cortex. The most common cause is adrenal hemorrhage in the patient in whom coagulation is hindered, but insufficiency can also develop as a result of sepsis or accidental or surgical trauma.

Diagnosis of hypoadrenocorticism requires measurement of the plasma cortisol concentration within 1 hour of administration of adrenocorticotropic hormone.

CLINICAL MANIFESTATIONS

Symptoms of primary adrenal insufficiency include weight loss, anorexia, nausea, vomiting, skeletal muscle weakness, abdominal pain, diarrhea or constipation, and hyperpigmentation over palmar surfaces and pressure points.

LABORATORY RESULTS

Laboratory findings include hyperkalemia and hypoglycemia. Lack of catecholamines may result in hypotension, which is often indistinguishable from shock due to loss of intravascular fluid volume.

TREATMENT

Treatment for primary adrenal insufficiency entails both glucocorticoid and mineralocorticoid replacement. Acute adrenal insufficiency (addisonian crisis) is a medical emergency, and treatment includes fluids, steroid replacement, inotropes as necessary, and electrolyte correction.

ANESTHETIC CONSIDERATIONS

Anesthetic management for patients with primary adrenal insufficiency should provide for exogenous corticosteroid supplementation. Etomidate should be avoided because it transiently inhibits synthesis of cortisol in normal patients. Doses of anesthetic drugs should be minimal because these patients may be sensitive to drug-induced myocardial depression. Invasive monitoring (arterial line and pulmonary artery catheter) is indicated. Because of skeletal muscle weakness, the initial dose of muscle relaxant should be reduced, and further doses should be governed by peripheral nerve stimulator response. Plasma concentrations of glucose and electrolytes should be measured frequently during the operation.

F. Acromegaly

♦   ♦   ♦

DEFINITION

Acromegaly is due to excess secretion of growth hormone in an adult, most often from an adenoma in the anterior pituitary gland. Failure of plasma growth hormone concentration to decrease 1 to 2 hours after the ingestion of 75 to 100 g of glucose is presumptive evidence of acromegaly, as is a growth hormone concentration greater than 3 mg/L^{-1}.

LABORATORY RESULTS

A skull radiograph and computed tomography are useful in detecting enlargement of the sella turcica, which is characteristic of an anterior pituitary adenoma.

CLINICAL MANIFESTATIONS

Clinical manifestations reflect parasellar extension of the anterior pituitary adenoma and peripheral effects produced by excess growth hormone.

An enlarged sella turcica, headaches, visual field defects, and rhinorrhea may occur with parasellar extension. Excess growth hormone is reflected by skeletal overgrowth (prognathism), soft tissue overgrowth (lips, tongue, epiglottis, vocal cords), connective tissue overgrowth (recurrent laryngeal nerve paralysis), peripheral neuropathy (carpal tunnel syndrome), visceromegaly, glucose intolerance, osteoarthritis, osteoporosis, hyperhidrosis, and skeletal muscle weakness.

TREATMENT

Treatment is trans-sphenoidal surgical excision of pituitary adenoma. If adenoma is extended beyond the sella turcica, surgery or irradiation is no longer feasible, and medical treatment with bromocriptine may be an option.

ANESTHETIC CONSIDERATIONS

Anesthetic management must account for potentially difficult upper air-way management and the possible need to insert a small-diameter tracheal tube. Awake intubation with or without a fiberoptic scope may be necessary. If diabetes mellitus is present, plasma glucose concentration should be monitored. Arterial line placement in the radial artery can lead to inadequate collateral circulation at the wrist, so Allen's test should be performed or an alternative site should be selected. Muscle relaxant use should be guided by peripheral nerve stimulation, especially in patients with a history of skeletal muscle weakness.

G. Pheochromocytoma

◆   ◆   ◆

DEFINITION

Pheochromocytoma is a catecholamine-secreting tumor that originates in the adrenal medulla or in chromaffin tissue along the paravertebral sympathetic chain, extending from the pelvis to the base of the skull.

ETIOLOGY

Pheochromocytoma typically occurs in patients 30 to 50 years of age, although one third of reported cases are in children, principally males. Pheochromocytoma may also be part of an autosomal dominant multiglandular neoplastic syndrome, a condition called multiple endocrine neoplasia. Less than 0.1% of patients with hypertension actually have pheochromocytoma; however, nearly 50% of deaths in patients with unsuspected pheochromocytoma occur during anesthesia and surgery or parturition. Pheochromocytoma and associated hypertension and hypermetabolism may mimic other diseases, including malignant hyperthermia.

LABORATORY RESULTS

Diagnosis requires chemical confirmation of excessive catecholamine release. Measurement of free norepinephrine from a 24-hour urine test is thought to be a more sensitive index of pheochromocytoma than measures of catecholamine metabolites (normetanephrine, metanephrine, vanillylmandelic acid). Normotension despite increased plasma concentration of catecholamines is thought to reflect a decrease in the number of alpha receptors (down-regulation) in response to increased circulating concentrations of the neurotransmitter. Clonidine (0.3 mg orally) suppresses the plasma concentration of catecholamines in hypertensive patients but not in patients with pheochromocytoma, reflecting the drug's ability to suppress increases in plasma catecholamine concentration resulting from neurogenic release but not from diffusion of excess catecholamine from a pheochromocytoma into the circulation. Computed tomography is the initial localizing procedure in the diagnosis of pheochromocytoma.

CLINICAL MANIFESTATIONS

The classic symptom of pheochromocytoma is paroxysmal hypertension. The triad of tachycardia, diaphoresis, and headache in a hypertensive patient is highly suggestive of pheochromocytoma. Conversely, absence of this triad virtually rules out the presence of pheochromocytoma. Tremulousness, palpitations, and weight loss are common, especially in young to middle-aged patients. Symptoms may last from minutes to several hours and are often followed by fatigue. Decreased intravascular fluid volume associated with sustained hypertension may manifest as orthostatic hypotension. A hematocrit greater than 45% may reflect hypovolemia caused by this mechanism. Death resulting from pheochromocytoma is often due to congestive heart failure, myocardial infarction, or intracerebral hemorrhage.

TREATMENT

Treatment consists of surgical excision of the catecholamine-secreting tumor only after medical control is optimized. Alpha blockade (phentolamine, prazosin) should be instituted and blood pressure normalized prior to surgery. Return to normotension facilitates an increase in intravascular fluid volume as reflected by a decrease in the hematocrit. If cardiac dysrhythmias or tachycardia persist after alpha blockade, beta blockade is indicated in the absence of congestive heart failure.

ANESTHETIC CONSIDERATIONS

Anesthetic management for the patient requiring excision of a pheochromocytoma is based on administration of drugs that do not stimulate the sympathetic nervous system. Alpha- and beta-antagonist therapy should be continued. Invasive monitors (arterial line and pulmonary artery catheter) should be inserted preoperatively. The depth of anesthesia should be adequate before laryngoscopy is begun. This is often accomplished by intravenous induction of anesthesia followed by establishment of a surgical level of anesthesia with a volatile agent; isoflurane is most commonly used. Halothane should be avoided because of its propensity to produce cardiac dysrhythmias in the presence of increased plasma catecholamine concentrations. Administration of lidocaine (1 to 2mg/kg IV) about 1 minute before initiation of laryngoscopy may attenuate the hypertensive response to intubation and decrease the likelihood of cardiac dysrhythmias. Furthermore, administration of short-acting opioid (fentanyl, 100 to 200 μg IV; sufentanil, 10 to 20 μg IV) just before starting laryngoscopy may attenuate pressor response. Nitroprusside and phentolamine should be readily available, should persistent hypertension accompany intubation of the trachea. Skeletal muscles should be paralyzed with a nondepolarizing muscle relaxant devoid of circulatory effects.

Anesthesia is maintained with an inhalation agent (isoflurane) and nitrous oxide; the isoflurane concentration is adjusted in response to any change in blood pressure. If hypertension persists despite delivery of the maximum concentration of isoflurane (1% to 2%), nitroprusside, esmolol, lidocaine, and phentolamine should be used as needed. A decrease in blood pressure may accompany surgical ligation of the venous drainage of pheochromocytoma, which may be treated by decreasing the isoflurane concentration along with rapid infusion of crystalloids, colloids, or both. Rarely, intravenous infusion of phenylephrine or norepinephrine is required until the peripheral vasculature adapts to decreased levels of endogenous catecholamine. Arterial blood gases, electrolytes, and blood glucose levels should be monitored intraoperatively. Postoperatively, invasive monitoring should be continued, and pain control should be maintained.

H. Hypoaldosteronism

◆ ◆ ◆

DEFINITION

Hypoaldosteronism is suggested by hyperkalemia in the absence of renal insufficiency. Isolated deficiency of aldosterone secretion may reflect (1) congenital deficiency of aldosterone synthetase or (2) hyporeninemia due to a defect in the juxtaglomerular apparatus or treatment with an angiotensin converting enzyme inhibitor leading to loss of angiotensin stimulation.

ETIOLOGY

Hyporeninemic hypoaldosteronism typically occurs in patients older than 45 years with chronic renal disease, diabetes mellitus, or both. Indomethacin-induced prostaglandin deficiency is a reversible cause of this syndrome.

CLINICAL MANIFESTATIONS

Symptoms include heart block secondary to hyperkalemia and postural hypotension with or without hyponatremia. Hyperchloremic metabolic acidosis is common.

TREATMENT

Treatment of hypoaldosteronism includes liberal sodium intake and daily administration of hydrocortisone.

ANESTHETIC CONSIDERATIONS

Anesthetic management begins with preoperative monitoring of the serum potassium level, which should be less than 5.5 mEq/L before elective surgery.

Electrocardiographic monitoring for effects of hyperkalemia (tall, tentlike T waves; heart block) is recommended. Avoid hypoventilation to prevent an additional increase in serum potassium. Succinylcholine should be avoided when possible to prevent potassium release. Intravenous fluids should be potassium-free. If hypovolemia is suspected, initiate fluid replacement, possibly governed by invasive (central venous pressure) monitoring.

I. Primary Hyperaldosteronism

♦ ♦ ♦

DEFINITION AND ETIOLOGY

Primary hyperaldosteronism (Conn's syndrome) is excess secretion of aldosterone from a functional tumor independent of a physiologic stimulus. Secondary hyperaldosteronism is when increased renin secretion is responsible for the excess secretion of aldosterone. Hyperaldosteronism should be suspected in a patient with diastolic hypertension (100 to 125 mm Hg) and a plasma potassium concentration of less than 3.5 mEq/L. Hypertension reflects aldosterone-induced sodium retention and the resultant increased extracellular fluid volume. Hypokalemic metabolic acidosis is present secondary to aldosterone-induced renal excretion of potassium. Skeletal muscle weakness is presumed to reflect hypokalemia. Hypokalemia nephropathy can result in polyuria and the inability to concentrate urine optionally.

LABORATORY RESULTS

Diagnosis of hyperaldosteronism is confirmed by increased plasma concentration of aldosterone and increased urinary potassium excretion (>30 mEq/L) despite coexisting hypokalemia. Measurement of plasma renin activity permits classification of the disease as primary (low renin activity) or secondary (increased renin activity).

TREATMENT

Treatment consists of supplemental potassium and administration of competitive aldosterone antagonists such as spironolactone. Hypertension may require treatment with antihypertensive drugs. Hypokalemia from drug-induced diuresis is decreased with a potassium-sparing diuretic such as triamterene. The definitive treatment for aldosterone-secreting tumor is surgical excision.

ANESTHETIC CONSIDERATIONS

Anesthetic management begins with preoperative correction of hypokalemia and treatment of hypertension. Unsuspected hypovolemia is evidenced by orthostatic hypotension during preoperative evaluation. Invasive monitoring (central venous pressure, pulmonary arterial catheter) may be necessary in these patients to monitor intraoperative filling pressures. Supplementation with exogenous cortisol is also a consideration.

COMMON DISEASES

HEPATIC SYSTEM
A. Hepatitis

* * *

DEFINITION

An inflammatory disease of hepatocytes that may be either acute or chronic (lasting >6 months) and can progress to cell necrosis and eventual hepatic failure.

ETIOLOGY

Some of the causes of both acute and chronic hepatitis include viral infections and drug-induced toxicity. The organisms responsible for viral hepatitis include (1) hepatitis A virus, (2) hepatitis B virus, (3) hepatitis C virus (formerly non-A, non-B virus), (4) Epstein-Barr virus, (5) cytomegalovirus, and (6) herpes simplex virus. Hepatitis A, or infectious hepatitis, is transmitted by the fecal-oral route or by ingestion of food contaminated with sewage. Hepatitis types B and C are transmitted percutaneously and by contact with body fluids. Hepatitis B, or serum hepatitis, is the most common type of viral hepatitis and may also be transmitted by nonparenteral routes (oral-to-oral and sexual). Drug-induced hepatitis may result from dose-dependent toxicity of a drug (or a metabolite), from an idiosyncratic drug reaction, or from a combination of both. Halothane has been associated with hepatic dysfunction with repeat administration at short intervals in adults.

DIAGNOSTIC AND LABORATORY RESULTS

Laboratory evaluation should include blood urea nitrogen, serum electrolytes, serum creatinine, glucose, transaminases, bilirubin, alkaline phosphatase, albumin, prothrombin time, platelet count, and hepatitis B surface antigen. Concentrations of plasma transaminase enzymes are elevated 7 to 14 days before the onset of jaundice and begin to decline shortly after jaundice is noticeable. Severe hepatitis is suggested by a plasma albumin concentration below 2.5 g/dL or a markedly prolonged prothrombin time unresponsive to vitamin K therapy. The presence of hepatitis B surface antigen in plasma indicates the potential for infectivity, and persistence for longer than 6 months in the absence of antibodies indicates that the patient is a chronic carrier and potentially infective to others.

CLINICAL MANIFESTATIONS

Symptoms of viral hepatitis include jaundice, dark urine, fatigue, anorexia, nausea, fever, and abdominal discomfort. Mild anemia and lymphocytosis occur. Hypomagnesemia may be present in chronic alcoholics and can predispose to arrhythmias.

TREATMENT

Correct dehydration and electrolyte abnormalities. Vitamin K or fresh-frozen plasma is used to correct coagulopathies. Treat bacterial infections and use neomycin, lactulose, or both to decrease plasma ammonia levels. Avoid factors that may aggravate hepatic encephalopathy. Orthotopic liver transplantation may be considered in selected patients.

ANESTHETIC CONSIDERATIONS

Correct coagulopathy with fresh-frozen plasma. Avoid premedication with sedatives. Barbiturates, opioids, and some muscle relaxants may have prolonged effects due to altered hepatic metabolism. Response to succinylcholine may also be prolonged because of depression of pseudocholinesterase. Factors known to reduce hepatic blood flow, such as hypotension, excessive sympathetic activation, and high mean airway pressures during controlled ventilation, should be avoided. Prevent hypoglycemia by administering exogenous glucose. Administer blood at a controlled rate to minimize the likelihood of citrate intoxication. Alcoholic patients may develop cross-tolerance to both intravenous and volatile anesthetics.

B. Cirrhosis/Portal Hypertension

♦ ♦ ♦

DEFINITION

A chronic disease process that destroys the hepatic parenchyma and replaces it with collagen. This distorts the liver's normal architecture, leading to obstruction of portal venous flow and subsequent portal hypertension as well as impairment of all the physiologic functions of the liver. Other complications include variceal hemorrhage secondary to the portal hypertension, intractable fluid retention in the form of ascites and the hepatorenal syndrome, and hepatic encephalopathy or coma.

ETIOLOGY

The most common cause of cirrhosis in the United States is alcohol (Laennec's cirrhosis). Other causes include chronic active hepatitis (postnecrotic cirrhosis), chronic biliary inflammation or obstruction (biliary cirrhosis), chronic right-sided congestive heart failure (cardiac cirrhosis), hemochromatosis, and Wilson's disease.

DIAGNOSTIC AND LABORATORY RESULTS

Laboratory changes in the presence of portal hypertension include a hematocrit of 30% to 35%, hyponatremia due to increased secretion of antidiuretic hormone, blood urea nitrogen greater than 20 mg/dL, and elevated plasma bilirubin, transaminases, and alkaline phosphatase concentrations.

CLINICAL MANIFESTATIONS

Gastrointestinal

Portal hypertension (>10 mm Hg) leads to the formation of ascites, esophageal varices, hemorrhoids, and gastrointestinal bleeding. Peptic ulcer disease is twice as common in patients with cirrhosis and may result in further hemorrhage. Patients develop anorexia and lose skeletal muscle mass. Gastric emptying is often slow, warranting premedication and a rapid sequence induction.

Circulatory

A hyperdynamic circulation characterized by an increased cardiac output is attributed to an increased vascular volume, decreased blood viscosity secondary to anemia, and generalized peripheral vasodilation. Cardiomyopathy can manifest as congestive heart failure. Palmar erythema and spider angiomas over the face, upper back, and arms are prominent. Hepatomegaly occurs with or without splenomegaly and ascites.

Pulmonary

Hyperventilation commonly results in primary respiratory alkalosis. Arterial hypoxemia develops because of right-to-left shunting (up to 40% of cardiac output). Elevation of the diaphragm from ascites reduces functional residual capacity, predisposing to atelectasis.

Renal

Decreased renal perfusion, enhanced proximal and distal sodium reabsorption, impaired free water clearance, hyponatremia, and hypokalemia are common. The hepatorenal syndrome may develop in these patients following gastrointestinal bleeding, aggressive diuresis, sepsis, or major surgery. This syndrome is characterized by progressive oliguria, azotemia, intractable ascites, and a high mortality rate unless liver transplantation is undertaken.

Hematologic

Anemia, thrombocytopenia, and leukopenia may be present. Coagulopathies result from decreased hepatic synthesis of coagulation factors (all except factor VIII and fibrinogen are affected) and reduced or impaired platelet function. Enhanced fibrinolysis due to decreased clearance of activators of the fibrinolytic system may also contribute to the coagulopathy.

Metabolic

Hypoalbuminemia, hyperaldosteronism, and hypoglycemia may be present.

Central Nervous System

Hepatic encephalopathy as well as coma may be manifested. Mental obtundation, asterixis (flapping motion of the hands), and fetor hepaticus (musty, sweet breath odor) are evident. Elevated intracranial pressure may require prompt treatment and continuous intraoperative monitoring.

TREATMENT

Treatment is supportive until liver transplantation can be undertaken. Variceal bleeding involves replacement of blood loss, vasopressin infusion (0.1 to 0.9 U/min IV), balloon tamponade (Sengstaken-Blakemore tube), or endoscopic sclerosis or the transjugular intrahepatic portosystemic shunt/ stent (TIPS) procedure to stop the bleeding. If bleeding does not stop or recurs, emergency surgical procedures such as shunts (portocaval or spleno- renal), esophageal transection, or gastric devascularization may be needed. Coagulopathies should be corrected by replacing clotting factors with fresh- frozen plasma or cryoprecipitate. Platelet transfusions should be performed prior to surgery for counts less than 100,000 mm^3. Preservation of renal function involves avoiding aggressive diuresis while correcting acute intra- vascular fluid deficits with colloid infusions.

ANESTHETIC CONSIDERATIONS

Reduce the dosage of muscle relaxants dependent on hepatic elimination (pancuronium and vecuronium) because of reduced plasma clearance. Atra- curium is the relaxant of choice. The duration of action of succinylcholine may be prolonged as a result of reduced levels of pseudocholinesterase. Half- lives of opioids may be prolonged, leading to prolonged respiratory depression. Avoid the use of halothane so as not to confuse the diagnosis if liver function test results deteriorate postoperatively. Regional anesthesia may be used in patients without thrombocytopenia or coagulopathy if hypotension is avoided (perfusion to the liver becomes highly dependent on hepatic arterial blood flow). Following removal of large amounts of ascitic fluid, colloid fluid replacement may be necessary to prevent hypotension. Whole blood may be preferable to packed red blood cells when replacing blood loss. Coagulation factors and platelet deficiencies should be corrected with fresh-frozen plasma and platelet transfusions, respectively. Citrate toxicity can occur in these patients because of impaired metabolism of the citrate

COMMON DISEASES

anticoagulant in blood products. Intravenous calcium should be given to reverse the negative inotropic effects of a reduction in serum ionized calcium levels.

C. Hepatic Failure

◆   ◆   ◆

DEFINITION

A massive necrosis of liver cells resulting in the development of a life-threatening loss of overall hepatic functional capacity exceeding 80% to 90%. Hepatic failure can result from acute or chronic liver disease.

INCIDENCE

The major causes of hepatic failure in the United States are related to the effects of viral hepatitis or drug-related liver injury. Each year, an estimated 2000 cases of hepatic failure in the United States are related to viral hepatitis. This accounts for 1% of all deaths and 6% of all liver-related deaths.

ETIOLOGY

Following is a categorical list of the potential causes of hepatic failure:

Viral
Hepatitis A, B, C, D, E viruses
Herpes simplex virus
Cytomegalovirus
Adenovirus
Epstein-Barr virus
Varicella zoster virus
Dengue fever virus
Rift Valley fever virus

Toxic Damage
Acetaminophen
Isoniazid
Phenytoin
Halothane
Methyldopa
Tetracycline
Valproic acid
Nicotinic acid
Carbon tetrachloride

Phosphorus
Pesticides
Ethyl alcohol

Metabolic
Wilson's disease
Acute fatty liver of pregnancy
Reye's syndrome
Sickle cell disease
Galactosemia

Other
Autoimmune hepatitis
Amanita phalloides (mushroom)
   poisoning
Budd-Chiari syndrome
Veno-occlusive disease
Hyperthermia
Partial hepatectomy
Jejunoileal bypass

DIAGNOSTIC AND LABORATORY FINDINGS

Most proteins associated with the promotion or inhibition of coagulation are synthesized in the liver. When one is reviewing laboratory data, special attention should be given to coagulation studies, liver function studies, complete blood count, electrolytes, glucose, blood urea nitrogen, and creatinine.

Lab Study	Normal	Liver Failure
WBC	3.5–10.6 cells/mm^3	Decreased
Hgb	11.5–15.1 g/dL	Decreased
Hct	34.4–44.2%	Decreased
Platelet count	150–450 mm^3	Decreased
PT	11–14 s	Increased
PTT	20–37 s	Increased
Bilirubin	Plasma: 0.3–1.1 mg/dL Indirect: 0.2–0.7 mg/dL Direct: <0.5 mg/dL	Increased. Jaundice is seen with plasma bilirubin levels >3 mg/dL.
SGOT (AST)	10–40 IU/L	Increased
SGPT (ALT*)	5–35 IU/L	Increased
LDH (LD-5*)	5.3–13.4%	Increased
ALP	87–250 U/L	Normal; used to differentiate biliary obstruction
Albumin	3.3–4.5 g/dL	Decreased levels <2.5 g/dL are precarious.
NH$_3$	<50 µg/dL	Increased NH$_3$ is converted to urea by the normal liver.
BUN	7–20 mg/dL	Normal or decreased due to impaired excretion of Na and retention of H$_2$O; increased in hepatorenal syndrome
Cr	0.6–1.3 mg/dl	Increased in hepatorenal syndrome
Na	135–145 mEq/L	Usually decreased. Increased Na may result after the administration of lactulose or if replacement of free H$_2$O is inadequate.
K	3.6–5.0 mEq/L	Decreased; related to the secondary effects of hyperaldosteronism, vomiting, diuretic use, or inadequate replacement. Increased K may result from the use of blood products.
Mg	1.6–3.0 mEq/L	Decreased
Ca	8.8–10.4 mg/dL	Decreased
P	2.5–4.5 mg/dL	Decreased
Glucose	70–110 mg/dL	Decreased; related to impaired gluconeogenesis and decreased insulin clearance.

* Specific of liver damage.

A 12-lead electrocardiogram should be performed to rule out any possible cardiac dysrhythmias related to acidemia, electrolyte abnormalities, or hypoxemia associated with hepatic failure. The liver failure patient is at risk for the development of acid-base derangements. Respiratory alkalosis may result from hyperventilation related to an abnormality of central regulation, or respiratory acidosis may be caused by endotoxins, increased intracranial pressure (ICP), or pulmonary sequelae, which depress respiratory centers. Metabolic acidosis is also possible, related to substantial tissue damage and decreased clearance of lactic acid by the failing liver.

The hypoxemia associated with liver failure can be attributed to aspiration, atelectasis, infection, hypoventilation, or any combination thereof. Results of radiographic examination of the patient's chest should be obtained to rule out evidence of pulmonary edema or adult respiratory distress syndrome. Arterial blood gases guide respiratory management and correction of acid-base abnormalities.

CLINICAL MANIFESTATIONS

No matter the exact cause of the patient's liver failure, it is important to remember that this malady affects the entire physiologic makeup. Physical examination is important for the approximation of liver and spleen size, evidence of bleeding abnormalities, identification of extravascular fluid shifts, and any other organ dysfunction.

Listed below are common clinical features of hepatic failure and their associated causes:

Clinical Feature	Cause
Jaundice	Increased circulating bilirubin
Spider angiomas "nevi"	Increased circulating estrogen
Testicular atrophy	Increased circulating estrogen
Gynecomastia	Increased circulating estrogen
Pectoral and axillary alopecia	Increased circulating estrogen
Palmar erythema	Increased circulating estrogen
Increased skin pigmentation	Increased activity of MSH
Anemia	Iron, B_{12}, or folate deficiency, hypersplenism, bone marrow suppression
Leukopenia	Hypersplenism; bone marrow suppression
Thrombocytopenia	Hypersplenism; bone marrow suppression
Increased bleeding tendencies, nosebleeds, gingival bleeding, menstrual bleeding, easy bruising	Anemia; thrombocytopenia; decreased production of clotting factors; decreased adherence of circulating platelets
Peripheral edema	Hypoalbuminemia; failure of the liver to inactivate aldosterone and ADH, with subsequent Na and H_2O retention
Ascites	Portal HTN; hypoalbuminemia; Na and H_2O retention

Clinical Feature	Cause
Increased risk of infection	ETT intubation with impaired cough reflex; IV catheters; central lines; urinary catheters; leukopenia; decreased neutrophil adherence; complement deficiencies
Weight loss and muscle wasting	Nausea and vomiting; anorexia; impaired gluconeogenesis; impaired insulin functioning; hypoproteinemia
Fetor hepaticus (pungent sour odor detected in exhaled breath)	Inability to metabolize methionine
Hepatic encephalopathy (hepatic coma)	Inability to metabolize ammonia; increased cerebral sensitivity to toxins; hypoglycemia
Hepatorenal syndrome	Decreased renal blood flow, particularly to the cortex; vasoconstriction; decreased GFR; renal retention of Na

COMMON DISEASES

TREATMENT

Management of the patient with liver failure should include admission to the intensive care unit. The health care team should be on constant guard for complications associated with liver failure, such as sepsis, cerebral edema, hypoglycemia, and electrolyte and bleeding abnormalities. Liver failure associated with acetaminophen poisoning or mushroom poisoning should be identified immediately, because antidotes are available for both. Patients not responsive to conventional treatment should be considered for transplantation as early as possible, before they are excluded by the development of infection or encephalopathic brain damage.

General treatment modalities for the patient with liver failure include the following:

1. Antibiotic prophylaxis
2. Urinary catheter
3. Central venous pulmonary catheter
4. Histamine$_2$ antagonist or sucralfate
5. Blood glucose checks every 1 to 2 hours
6. Aspiration precautions
7. Periodic assessment of neurologic status
   - Prevent sepsis
   - Monitor renal function and fluid status
   - Monitor fluid volume
   - Increase gastric pH and decrease risk of gastrointestinal bleeding
   - Prevent hypoglycemia and guide administration of intravenous dextrose
   - Prevent aspiration pneumonia and adult respiratory distress syndrome
   - Note that neurologic status may rapidly deteriorate because of increasing ammonia levels or increasing ICP
8. Early nutritional supplementation—prevent nutrition-related complications

ANESTHETIC CONSIDERATIONS

Only surgery to correct life-threatening conditions should be performed on the patient with liver failure. The patient's condition should be optimized prior to the surgical procedure. A normally "minor" procedure can become a major catastrophe when dealing with the patient with liver failure.

Premedication must be considered, taking into account the severity of the patient's disease process, the presence of altered consciousness, and the liver's diminished ability to metabolize pharmacologic agents. If the patient is thought to have a full stomach, antacids and histamine$_2$ antagonists may be administered.

Monitoring should conform to the established standards of care. The size and number of intravenous catheters should be individualized. Most cases involving liver failure require the use of an arterial line, a central venous pulmonary line, and a Foley catheter to enable monitoring of the patient's fluid status. Swan-Ganz or pulmonary arterial catheters may be used if the patient's condition so warrants.

For the patient with liver failure, the use of local anesthesia with sedation or regional anesthesia should be considered whenever possible. Coagulopathies must first be ruled out, and the surgical procedure itself must be considered. Patients may be considered to have a full stomach, especially in the presence of ascites. In this case a rapid-sequence induction is standard. The choice of induction agent and dosage administered should reflect the liver's diminished ability to metabolize pharmacologic agents and the patient's increased volume of distribution.

Both nondepolarizing and depolarizing muscle relaxants may be administered. Dosages may need to be individualized according to the patient's initial response. A peripheral nerve stimulator aids the practitioner in gauging the patient's response and adjusting subsequent doses. The breakdown of succinylcholine remains relatively normal despite advanced disease states. Vecuronium should be avoided because its primary site of metabolism is the liver. Indeed, atracurium should be the nondepolarizing muscle relaxant of choice because of its unique metabolic properties, which do not involve either the liver or the kidneys. If atracurium is unavailable, any other nondepolarizing muscle relaxant may be used, taking into account the patient's specific organ involvement and the drug's metabolic properties.

Isoflurane and desflurane are the inhalational agents of choice. Enflurane may also be considered, but the practitioner must consider the neurologic status of the patient. Halothane is contraindicated in patients with liver disease. Nitrous oxide may be safely instituted according to the nature of the surgery and as long as a high fraction of inspired oxygen is not required.

The use of opioids must take into account a prolonged half-life and decreased clearance. Because fentanyl does not decrease hepatic blood flow, it is often the opioid of choice for the liver failure patient.

The liver failure patient is at risk for major blood loss with any invasive procedure. Blood products should be available, and all losses should be replaced accordingly.

PROGNOSIS

In the United States, mortality rates due to liver disease have increased since the 1960s. Overall, the mortality rate from hepatic failure is 70% to 95%. Liver transplantation should be considered when conventional medical management fails; such consideration should take place early, before infection or encephalopathic brain damage renders the potential candidate ineligible. One-year patient survival rates after transplantation are 63% to 78%.

COMMON DISEASES

RENAL SYSTEM
A. Urolithiasis

. . .

DEFINITION

Urolithiasis, or kidney stones, is the presence of calculi typically composed of calcium oxalate. These are due to hypercalciuria or hyperoxaluria. Other types of stones include magnesium ammonium phosphate, calcium phosphate, and uric acid.

ETIOLOGY

Causes of hypercalcemia and hypercalciuria are primarily hyperparathyroidism, vitamin D intoxication, malignancies, and sarcoidosis. Small bowel bypass is associated with hyperoxaluria. Alterations in urine pH or the presence of metabolic disturbances can also result in formation of renal stones, which differ in composition from the typical oxalate variety.

TREATMENT

Extracorporeal shock wave lithotripsy is a noninvasive treatment of renal stones. It transmits shock waves through water, focusing them on the stone via biplanar fluoroscopy. The shock waves are triggered by the R wave of the electroencephalogram and delivered during the myocardial refractory period to avoid initiating any cardiac dysrhythmias. Patients with artificial cardiac pacemakers risk pacemaker dysfunction with this form of therapy.

ANESTHETIC CONSIDERATIONS

General anesthesia or regional anesthesia, including epidural and intercostal nerve blocks with local infiltration, may be used to provide analgesia during lithotripsy. The sitting position during anesthesia may be associated with peripheral pooling of blood, especially with the use of regional anesthesia and resultant vasodilatation. Immersion in water increases hydrostatic pressures on the abdomen and thorax, which can displace blood into the central circulation. This may result in acute congestive heart failure in patients with limited cardiac reserve. These hydrostatic forces on the thorax likewise result in decreases in chest wall compliance and functional residual capacity. This may produce ventilation-perfusion mismatches. Water in the immersion tub should be kept warm to avoid hypothermia. Extracorporeal shock wave lithotripsy is contraindicated in patients with abdominal aortic aneurysms, spinal cord tumors, or orthopedic implants in the lumbar region.

Parturients, obese patients, and patients with coagulopathies are also not likely candidates.

B. Acute Renal Failure

♦ ♦ ♦

DEFINITION

Acute renal failure is a rapid deterioration in renal function that results in retention of nitrogenous waste products (azotemia).

ETIOLOGY

Azotemia can be divided into prerenal, renal, and postrenal types, depending on its causes. Prerenal azotemia results from an acute decrease in renal perfusion. Renal azotemia is usually due to intrinsic renal disease, renal ischemia, or nephrotoxins. Postrenal azotemia is the result of urinary tract obstruction or disruption. Up to 50% of cases are due to ischemia and nephrotoxins following major trauma or surgery. This is also called *acute tubular necrosis*. Potential toxins include aminoglycosides, x-ray contrast dyes, and in some patients, nonsteroidal anti-inflammatory drugs. Other factors predisposing to acute renal failure include pre-existing renal impairment, advanced age, atherosclerotic vascular disease, diabetes, and dehydration.

LABORATORY RESULTS

Acute renal failure is thought of as either oliguric (urinary volume < 400 mL/d) or anuric (urinary volume < 100 mL/d). However, nonoliguric acute renal failure may now account for up to 50% of cases (urine volume > 400 mL/d). These patients have a lower urine sodium concentration than oliguric patients do. Moreover, they appear to have a lower complication rate and to require shorter hospitalization.

CLINICAL MANIFESTATIONS

Please refer to the chapter on chronic renal failure, which follows this chapter.

TREATMENT

Standard treatment includes restriction of fluids, sodium, potassium, and protein intake. Dialysis may be employed to treat or prevent uremic complications. Peritoneal dialysis and hemodialysis can be equally effective, yet elevation and immobilization of the diaphragm associated with continuous peritoneal dialysis may predispose to respiratory complications. Standard hemodialysis may also be replaced by continuous arteriovenous hemofiltration, which may be better tolerated in critically ill patients.

ANESTHETIC CONSIDERATIONS

Please refer to the chapter on chronic renal failure, which follows this chapter.

PROGNOSIS

Sepsis remains the most common cause of death in patients with acute renal failure. Urinary function improves over the course of several weeks but may not return to normal for up to 1 year.

C. Chronic Renal Failure

◆   ◆   ◆

DEFINITION

Chronic renal failure is characterized by a progressive decrease in the number of functioning nephrons, leading to an irreversible reduction in glomerular filtration rate.

ETIOLOGY

Common diseases leading to chronic renal failure are chronic glomerulonephritis, diabetic nephropathy, hypertensive nephrosclerosis, and polycystic renal disease.

LABORATORY RESULTS

Examine chest radiograph for possible fluid overload (be aware of when the patient was last dialyzed) or pulmonary edema. Check electrolytes, complete blood count, and coagulation factors, because all may be affected.

CLINICAL MANIFESTATIONS

Metabolic

Hyperkalemia, hyperphosphatemia, hypocalcemia, hypermagnesemia, hyperuricemia, and hypoalbuminemia are possible. Water and sodium retention results in extracellular fluid overload and hyponatremia. Failure to excrete nonvolatile acids causes a high anion gap and metabolic acidosis.

Hematologic

Anemia is present because of decreased erythropoietin production, decreased red cell production, and decreased cell survival. Anemia and metabolic acidosis result in a rightward shift of the oxyhemoglobin dissociation curve. Both platelet and white cell function are impaired in patients with renal failure. This is clinically manifested as a prolonged bleeding time and increased susceptibility to infection. Patients who have recently undergone hemodialysis may also have residual anticoagulant effects from heparin. Observe the prothrombin time and partial thromboplastin time, especially if regional anesthesia is being considered.

Cardiovascular

Cardiac output is increased to maintain oxygen delivery. Sodium retention and abnormalities in the renin-angiotensin system result in systemic arterial hypertension. Left ventricular hypertrophy is common. Extracellular fluid overload, along with the increased demands of anemia and hypertension, predispose these patients to cardiomegaly and congestive heart failure. Dysrhythmias may be due to metabolic abnormalities. Hypovolemia may develop if too much fluid is removed with dialysis.

Pulmonary

Chronic renal failure interferes with normal excretion of hydrogen ions by the kidneys, resulting in metabolic acidosis. Treatment of the acidosis may include hemodialysis or intravenous administration of sodium bicarbonate. Pulmonary edema may result from an increase in permeability of the alveolar-capillary membrane with the appearance of "butterfly wings" on chest radiographs.

Endocrine

Diabetes mellitus is common because of peripheral resistance to insulin. Secondary hyperparathyroidism due to chronic hypocalcemia leads to osteodystrophy and vulnerability to pathologic fractures.

Gastrointestinal

Anorexia, nausea, vomiting, and ileus are associated with azotemia. Gastric fluid volume and acidity are increased. These changes, combined with delayed gastric emptying related to autonomic neuropathy, predispose these patients to pulmonary aspiration.

Neurologic

Asterixis, lethargy, confusion, seizures, and coma are manifestations of uremic encephalopathy. Autonomic and peripheral neuropathies are common. Peripheral neuropathies are typically sensory and involve the distal lower extremities. The median and common peroneal nerves are most often affected.

TREATMENT

Treatment may include intermittent hemodialysis using an arteriovenous fistula or continuous peritoneal dialysis via an implanted catheter. Renal transplantation may become necessary.

ANESTHETIC CONSIDERATIONS

Monitoring

Avoid measuring blood pressure in an arm with an arteriovenous fistula. Consider invasive monitoring, especially for procedures involving major fluid shifts. Intra-arterial monitoring is indicated for patients with poorly controlled hypertension.

Premedication

Aspiration prophylaxis with a histamine$_2$ blocker and metoclopramide may be indicated.

Induction

Rapid-sequence induction with cricoid pressure is indicated for patients with nausea, vomiting, or gastrointestinal bleeding. Reduced protein binding of drugs results in more unbound drug to act at receptor sites. Succinylcholine should be avoided in patients with a serum potassium level greater than 5 mEq/L. Atracurium, mivacurium, and cisatracurium are the muscle relaxants of choice. Expect a prolonged response to the other nondepolarizing muscle relaxants.

Maintenance

Avoid agents that reduce cardiac output (principal compensatory mechanism for anemia). Isoflurane is the preferred volatile agent because it has the least effect on cardiac output. Enflurane should be avoided because of the potential adverse effects of fluoride on the diseased kidneys. Use of meperidine may result in accumulation of the metabolite normeperidine. Morphine and its effects may be prolonged. If regional anesthesia is considered, the adequacy of coagulation should be confirmed, and the presence of uremic neuropathies should be excluded. The duration of action of local anesthetics may be shortened because of elevated tissue blood flow secondary to increased cardiac output. Ventilation of the lungs should maintain normocapnia and reduce the effects of positive-pressure ventilation on cardiac output. Avoid hypoventilation, which results in respiratory acidosis. However, hyperventilation causing respiratory alkalosis shifts the oxyhemoglobin dissociation curve to the left and reduces tissue oxygen availability.

Fluid Management

Avoid lactated Ringer's injection in hyperkalemic patients when large volumes of fluid may be required because of the potassium concentration of 4 mEq/L.

HEMATOLOGIC SYSTEM
A. Anemia

◆ ◆ ◆

DEFINITION

A numeric deficiency of erythrocytes caused by either too-rapid loss or too-slow production of the cells. Therefore, numeric concentrations of hemoglobin are reduced, and the oxygen-carrying capacity of blood is decreased. This results in reduced oxygen delivery to peripheral tissues.

ETIOLOGY

Anemia may result from acute blood loss; however, iron-deficiency anemia due to persistent blood loss is the most frequent form of chronic anemia. Anemia is also associated with many chronic diseases, such as persistent infections, neoplastic processes, connective tissue disorders, and renal and hepatic disease. Other forms of anemia include aplastic anemia, which involves bone marrow depression, and megaloblastic anemias, which are related to deficiencies of vitamin B_{12} or folic acid. Lastly, various anemias can result from intravascular hemolysis of erythrocytes.

LABORATORY RESULTS

Erythrocyte production can be assessed from the reticulocyte count in peripheral blood. For instance, a low reticulocyte count in the presence of a low hematocrit suggests an erythrocyte production defect, rather than blood loss or hemolysis, as a cause of anemia. Decreases in hematocrit that exceed 1% per day are most likely related to acute blood loss or intravascular hemolysis.

CLINICAL MANIFESTATIONS

A history of decreased exercise tolerance characterized as exertional dyspnea is a frequent clinical sign of chronic anemia. A functional heart murmur and evidence of cardiomegaly may be detected upon physical examination. The decreased oxygen-carrying capacity of arterial blood is compensated for by a shift to the right of the oxyhemoglobin dissociation curve and an increase in the cardiac output. The decreased exercise tolerance reflects the inability of cardiac output to increase further and maintain tissue oxygenation when these patients become physically active.

TREATMENT

Packed erythrocytes can be transfused preoperatively to increase hemoglobin concentrations, but it should be remembered that about 24 hours are necessary to restore intravascular fluid volume and blood viscosity. Compared with a similar volume of whole blood, erythrocytes produce about twice the increase in hemoglobin concentration.

ANESTHETIC CONSIDERATIONS

Minimum acceptable hemoglobin concentrations that should be present before proceeding with elective surgery cannot be stated, although a concentration of 10 g/dL is frequently used as a guideline. If elective surgery is performed, the anesthetic should be geared toward preventing changes that may interfere with tissue oxygen delivery. For example, myocardial depression produced by the volatile anesthetics may reduce cardiac output and thus impair the patient's compensatory mechanisms. Likewise, shifts to the left of the oxyhemoglobin dissociation curve, as produced by hyperventilation of the lungs and resulting respiratory alkalosis, can impair release of oxygen from hemoglobin to the tissues. It is also important to maintain body temperature, because hypothermia causes a left shift in the oxyhemoglobin dissociation curve. Intraoperative blood loss should be promptly replaced and closely monitored. Finally, postoperatively, it is important to minimize shivering or increases in body temperature, because these changes can greatly increase total body oxygen requirements.

B. Sickle Cell Disease

◆ ◆ ◆

DEFINITION

Sickle cell disease represents an inherited group of disorders, ranging in severity from the usually benign sickle cell trait to the often fatal sickle cell anemia. All the variants of the disease have in common various quantities of hemoglobin S. Hemoglobin S differs from normal adult hemoglobin A by the substitution of valine for glutamic acid at the sixth position on the beta chain of hemoglobin molecules.

INCIDENCE AND PREVALENCE

The incidence of sickle cell trait among the black population of the United States is about 10%. Sickle cell anemia is present when patients are homozygous for hemoglobin S and affects approximately 0.3% to 1.0% of the Afro-American population in the United States. In the homozygous state, 70% to 98% of hemoglobin is the S type, resulting in severe hemolytic anemia.

ETIOLOGY

Sickle cell trait is the heterozygote manifestation of sickle cell disease containing the hemoglobin genotype AS. Erythrocytes of patients with the trait contain 20% to 40% hemoglobin S, with the remainder being hemoglobin A. Affected persons are usually asymptomatic. Sickle cell anemia occurs when deoxygenated forms of hemoglobin S result in deformation of erythrocytes into sickle shapes instead of their usual biconcave shape. This damages the erythrocyte membranes, leading to their rupture and chronic hemolytic anemia. Formation of sickle cells is exaggerated by low oxygen partial pressures (< 40 mm Hg). Formation tends to be greater in veins than in arteries, so maintenance of pH is important. Hypothermia also promotes formation of sickle cells because of vasoconstriction, which leads to stasis of blood flow and deoxygenation of hemoglobin.

CLINICAL MANIFESTATIONS

Most commonly, the clinical manifestations are infarctive events due to occlusion of blood vessels with sickle cells and anemia due to hemolysis. The cardiac output is generally increased to compensate for the chronic anemia. Furthermore, the oxyhemoglobin dissociation curve for hemoglobin S is shifted to the right (P-50 = 31 mm Hg). Patients are susceptible to bacterial infections because splenic function is lost secondary to repeated thrombosis. Multiple organ dysfunction produced by infarctive events is the major reason that survival beyond 30 years of age is unlikely.

LABORATORY RESULTS

In the steady state, hemoglobin concentrations are 5 to 10 g/dL. Observe arterial blood gases, electrolytes, liver function tests, and other tests depending on the patient's clinical symptoms and possible organ involvement.

TREATMENT

Treatment of a painful infarctive crisis is with hydration and mild alkalinization of blood. Partial exchange transfusions with erythrocytes containing hemoglobin A will reduce concentrations of hemoglobin S and decrease the incidence of further infarctive damage. The goal of exchange transfusions is to increase hemoglobin A concentrations to at least 40%.

ANESTHETIC CONSIDERATIONS

Avoid acidosis due to hypoventilation of the lungs, maintain oxygenation, prevent circulatory stasis due to improper body positioning or use of tourniquets, maintain intravascular fluid volume to prevent increased blood viscosity, and maintain normal body temperature. Administer preoperative medication judiciously to avoid depression of ventilation. Regional anesthesia may be preferred over general anesthesia, although with regional blocks, compensatory vasoconstriction and decreased arterial oxygen partial pressures in the unblocked area predispose the patients to infarction.

C. Polycythemia Vera

◆ ◆ ◆

DEFINITION AND ETIOLOGY

Polycythemia vera is a myeloproliferative disease that generally occurs in patients between 60 and 70 years of age. Hyperactivity of myeloid progenitor cells results in increased production of erythrocytes, leukocytes, and platelets.

LABORATORY RESULTS

Hemoglobin concentrations typically exceed 18 g/dL, and platelet counts can be greater than 400,000/mm^3.

CLINICAL MANIFESTATIONS

Clinical symptoms are due to hyperviscosity of the blood, which leads to stasis of blood flow and an increased incidence of vascular thrombosis, particularly in the cardiovascular and central nervous systems. Defective platelet function is the most likely mechanism for spontaneous hemorrhage, which may occur in these patients.

TREATMENT

Treatment entails reducing hemoglobin concentrations to near-normal levels by phlebotomy before elective surgery.

ANESTHETIC CONSIDERATIONS

Surgery in the presence of uncontrolled polycythemia vera is associated with a high incidence of perioperative hemorrhage and postoperative venous thrombosis. In emergency situations, viscosity of the blood can be reduced by intravenous infusions of cystalloid solutions or low-molecular-weight dextrans.

D. Leukemia

◆ ◆ ◆

DEFINITION

Leukemia is uncontrolled production of leukocytes due to cancerous mutation of lymphogenous cells or myelogenous cells. Lymphocytic leukemias begin in lymph nodes or other lymphogenous tissues and then spread to other areas of the body. Myeloid leukemias begin as cancerous production of myelogenous cells in bone marrow, with spread to extramedullary organs.

Cancerous cells usually do not resemble other leukocytes and lack the usual functional characteristics of white cells.

INCIDENCE, PREVALENCE, ETIOLOGY, CLINICAL MANIFESTATIONS, AND LABORATORY RESULTS

Acute lymphoblastic leukemia accounts for about 15% of all leukemias in adults. Central nervous system dysfunction is common. These patients are highly susceptible to life-threatening infections, including those produced by *Pneumocystis carinii* and cytomegalovirus.

Chronic lymphocytic leukemia accounts for about 25% of all leukemias and is most common in elderly males. Diagnosis is confirmed by the presence of lymphocytosis ($> 15,000/mm^3$) and lymphocytic infiltrates in bone marrow. There may be neutropenia, with an associated increased susceptibility to bacterial infections. Treatment is with cancer chemotherapeutic drugs classified as alkylating agents.

Acute myeloid leukemia can result in death in about 3 months if untreated. Patients present with fever, weakness, bleeding, and hepatosplenomegaly. Chemotherapy produces a temporary remission in about one half of patients.

Chronic myeloid leukemia presents with massive hepatosplenomegaly and white blood cell counts greater than $50,000/mm^3$. Fever and weight loss reflect hypermetabolism. Anemia may be severe. Splenectomy is routine in these patients.

TREATMENT

Cancer chemotherapy is the best available therapy for irradiation of cancerous cells anywhere in the body. Adverse clinical effects of these drugs include bone marrow suppression (susceptibility to infection, thrombocytopenia, and anemia), nausea, vomiting, diarrhea, ulceration of the gastrointestinal mucosa, and alopecia. Bone marrow transplantation is also becoming an increasingly successful treatment for leukemia.

ANESTHETIC MANAGEMENT

Management of anesthesia for the leukemia patient requires a clear understanding of the mechanisms of action, potential interactions, and likely toxicities associated with the use of cancer chemotherapeutic drugs. For instance, patients taking doxorubicin or daunorubicin (antibiotics) may develop cardiomyopathy leading to congestive heart failure, which is often refractory to cardiac inotropic drugs or mechanical cardiac assistance. Cardiomegaly and pleural effusions may be found on chest radiographs. Marked left ventricular dysfunction was found to persist for as long as 3 years after the drug was discontinued. Nonspecific and usually benign electrocardiographic changes have been observed in 10% of patients. Bleomycin is an antibiotic that can cause pulmonary toxicity in patients. Dyspnea and a nonproductive cough are typical initial manifestations. Pulmonary function tests demonstrate a restrictive pulmonary disease pattern. It is recommended that fractional inspired oxygen be maintained at less than 30% during surgery because patients are susceptible to the toxic pulmonary effects of oxygen while on bleomycin therapy. Strict aseptic technique is important because of immunosuppression. Look for signs of central nervous system depression, autonomic nervous system dysfunction, and peripheral neuropathies preoperatively. Renal or hepatic dysfunction should influence the choice of anesthesia and muscle relaxants. Volatile anesthetics may reduce myocardial contractility in patients with cardiotoxicity related to the chemotherapeutic drugs. Monitor arterial blood gases and consider replacing fluid losses with colloid rather than crystalloid solutions in patients with pulmonary fibrosis. Also consider possible postoperative ventilation, depending on the length of the procedure and the degree of fibrosis.

Avoid nitrous oxide in patients donating bone marrow or undergoing bone marrow transplantation because of potential drug-induced adverse effects on bone marrow. Donors may be given heparin before removal of bone marrow, which influences the use of spinal or epidural anesthesia for this procedure.

E. AIDS/HIV Infection

◆   ◆   ◆

DEFINITION

Acquired immunodeficiency syndrome (AIDS) is not a single disease but rather the appearance of various opportunistic infections due to generalized depression of the immune system. Immunodeficiency is caused by infection of helper T-lymphocytes with a retrovirus known as human immunodeficiency virus (HIV). This virus destroys T-lymphocytes, leaving the host susceptible to development of infection and neoplastic diseases.

INCIDENCE

Over 90% of adult patients with AIDS are men, and 70% of these persons are homosexual or bisexual males. Heterosexual intravenous drug users account for 15% of males with AIDS and 50% of affected females. Persons with hemophilia coagulation disorders account for 1% of all AIDS cases, and recipients of infected blood transfusions account for 2% of all cases.

ETIOLOGY

The virus is transmitted by sexual contact, inoculation by other body secretions, and transfusion of blood or blood products, especially factor VIII concentrates. Because HIV selectively infects lymphocytes, concentrations of the virus are probably highest in secretions containing lymphocytes, such as semen, vaginal secretions, and blood. There is no evidence of airborne transmission of AIDS.

COMMON DISEASES

CLINICAL MANIFESTATIONS

Patients develop severe immunosuppression due to destruction of T-lymphocytes, resulting in susceptibility to opportunistic infections. The most frequently encountered opportunistic, life-threatening infection is pneumonia due to the parasite *Pneumocystis carinii*. The most common malignant condition in AIDS patients is Kaposi's sarcoma. Fifty per cent of patients develop some element of central nervous system dysfunction. Weight loss, fatigue, idiopathic thrombocytopenia, chronic diarrhea, and anemia are nonspecific findings. Milder manifestations of AIDS include a transient mononucleosis-like syndrome and persistent generalized lymphadenopathy.

LABORATORY RESULTS AND DIAGNOSTIC FINDINGS

Laboratory findings include lymphopenia and reduction in the ratio of helper T-lymphocytes to suppressor T-lymphocytes. Detection of antibodies to HIV using an enzyme-linked immunoassay indicates that the patient has been infected with the virus. To increase reliability, a positive enzyme-linked immunoassay result is confirmed by a Western blot test. Persons infected with HIV usually develop antibody (seroconvert) against the virus within 6 to 12 weeks of being infected.

A positive antibody test result does not mean that the subject has AIDS or will develop the syndrome.

TREATMENT

Oral administration of zidovudine (formerly azidothymidine, or AZT) inhibits replication of some retroviruses, including HIV, and therefore may be useful in reducing the risk of developing opportunistic infections associated with AIDS. The drug is primarily eliminated by the kidneys following breakdown by the liver. Drugs such as probenecid, acetaminophen, aspirin, and indomethacin may competitively inhibit zidovudine's breakdown in the liver. Anemia and granulocytopenia are adverse effects of zidovudine therapy.

ANESTHETIC MANAGEMENT

Anesthetic management must assume that all patients are potentially infected with HIV or other bloodborne pathogens. Universal precautions must be followed. Disposable laryngoscope blades should be used if available, and bacterial filters should be placed in the anesthesia circuit. The choice of anesthetic drugs and techniques depends on accompanying systemic manifestations of AIDS and related opportunistic infections. For example, oxygenation may be impaired in patients with *P. carinii* infection. Frequently, patients are malnourished and dehydrated. Anemia due to chronic infection may require transfusion.

PROGNOSIS

The incubation period for AIDS may be 7 years or longer. The mortality rate approaches 70% within 2 years after diagnosis.

F. Coagulopathies

◆ ◆ ◆

HEMOPHILIA A

DEFINITION

Hemophilia A is a disorder of blood coagulation due to inadequate activity of factor VIII.

INCIDENCE AND PREVALENCE

It is estimated that hemophilia A is present in 1 of 10,000 males because the gene for factor VIII is carried on X chromosomes.

ETIOLOGY

Plasma concentrations of factor VIII and the severity of bleeding are directly related. For example, spontaneous hemorrhage is likely when factor VIII concentrations are less than 3% of the normal value.

LABORATORY RESULTS

Classically, patients present with a prolonged partial thromboplastin time but a normal prothrombin time and bleeding time.

CLINICAL MANIFESTATIONS

Deep tissue bleeding, hemarthrosis, and hematuria are common forms of clinical bleeding associated with hemophilia A. Central venous system bleeding is a major cause of death in these patients.

TREATMENT

Factor VIII levels should be increased to more than 50% prior to surgery. Fresh-frozen plasma is considered to have 1 U of factor VIII activity per milliliter. Cryoprecipitate has 5 to 10 U of activity per milliliter, whereas factor VIII concentrates have 40 U of activity per milliliter. Transfusions are given twice a day following surgery because of the short half-life of factor VIII (8 to 12 hours). If cryoprecipitate or factor VIII is administered, there is an increased risk of transmission of viral diseases, such as hepatitis or acquired immunodeficiency syndrome (AIDS).

ANESTHETIC CONSIDERATIONS

Avoid all intramuscular injections. Regional anesthesia is to be avoided because of the risk of bleeding. Consider the possibility of coexisting liver disease due to hepatitis from prior blood or factor VIII transfusions. Always follow universal precautions.

HEMOPHILIA B

DEFINITION

A disorder of blood coagulation due to absent or decreased activity of factor IX, also known as Christmas disease.

INCIDENCE AND PREVALENCE

Hemophilia B is similar to hemophilia A, but it is much less common (1 of 100,000 males).

ETIOLOGY

Measurement of factor IX levels establishes the diagnosis. Factor IX activity should be maintained at more than 30% of normal.

LABORATORY RESULTS

The partial thromboplastin time is prolonged in these patients.

CLINICAL MANIFESTATIONS

See under "Hemophilia A."

TREATMENT

Fresh-frozen plasma is no longer considered a therapy of choice for patients with hemophilia B. Specific procoagulant concentrates to raise plasma concentrations of factor IX are chosen.

VON WILLEBRAND'S DISEASE

DEFINITION AND ETIOLOGY

Von Willebrand's disease is a hematologic disease that is transmitted as an autosomal dominant characteristic affecting both sexes. It is most likely due to the deficiency of a protein (von Willebrand's factor) important for adequate activity of factor VIII and optimal function of platelets.

LABORATORY RESULTS

The classic expression is prolonged bleeding time, impaired aggregation of platelets, and decreased plasma concentrations of factor VIII.

CLINICAL MANIFESTATIONS

Epistaxis, bleeding from mucosal surfaces, and superficial bruising are common. Pregnancy produces an increase in factor VIII and von Willebrand's factor in parturients with mild to moderate forms of this disorder.

TREATMENT

Cryoprecipitate (40 μg/kg) provides von Willebrand's factor as well as factor VIII. Also, the synthetic analogue of antidiuretic hormone, desmopressin, effectively induces release of von Willebrand's factor.

ANESTHETIC CONSIDERATIONS

Avoid drugs that interfere with optimal aggregation of platelets. Properly position the patient to avoid bruising.

DISSEMINATED INTRAVASCULAR COAGULATION

DEFINITION

Disseminated intravascular coagulation is characterized by uncontrolled activation of the coagulation system, with consumption of platelets and procoagulants. Thrombi develop in the microcirculation, and bleeding results because of loss of coagulation factors into these thrombi.

ETIOLOGY

Normal mechanisms of controlling intravascular coagulation may be overwhelmed by extensive tissue damage in such cases as sepsis, burns, retained placenta after delivery, trauma to the central nervous system, and prolonged extracorporeal circulation. Large amounts of thromboplastic material are released into the circulation with subsequent activation of the extrinsic coagulation pathway. Consumption of platelets and procoagulants, including factors I, II, V, VIII, and XIII, reflects generalized activation of the entire coagulation system. Furthermore, impaired perfusion of the liver interferes with extraction of activated clotting factors.

LABORATORY RESULTS

Platelet counts are often less than 150,000/mm^3 because of consumption. Prothrombin time and partial thromboplastin time are prolonged. Decreased fibrinogen (< 150 mg/dL) reflects consumption of this procoagulant. Levels of fibrin degradation products are elevated.

CLINICAL MANIFESTATIONS

Clinically, patients demonstrate hemorrhage from wound sites and around sites of placement of intravascular catheters. In some cases, thromboembolic phenomena may follow.

TREATMENT

The goal is correction of the underlying disorder responsible for initiating the widespread clotting process. Platelet concentrates and fresh-frozen plasma may be administered as determined by measurement of the platelet count and of the prothrombin time and partial thromboplastin time, respectively. Heparin has been recommended as therapy, but its use is controversial.

ANESTHETIC CONSIDERATIONS

Avoid intramuscular injections. Avoid regional anesthesia. Monitor coagulation factors and the disseminated intravascular coagulation screen and plan to administer the necessary blood products.

GASTROINTESTINAL SYSTEM

A. Diaphragmatic Hernia

◆ ◆ ◆

DEFINITION

Incomplete embryologic closure of the diaphragm with herniation of abdominal contents into the thorax. Normal lung maturation is impaired because abdominal contents compress developing lung buds. Lungs develop with varying degrees of pulmonary hypoplasia.

INCIDENCE AND PREVALENCE

Diaphragmatic hernia occurs in 1 of 4000 live births. The mortality rate is approximately 50%.

ETIOLOGY

Diaphragmatic hernia is caused by incomplete embryologic closure of the diaphragm.

LABORATORY RESULTS

Antenatal diagnosis shows that polyhydramnios is present 30% of the time. Ultrasonography is used to detect these hernias.

CLINICAL MANIFESTATIONS

Clinical manifestations depend on the degree of the hernia and interference with ventilation. They include scaphoid abdomen, reduced to absent breath sounds on the affected side, a barrel-shaped chest, arterial hypoxia, abdominal contents in the thorax (as shown on radiographs), increased pulmonary vascular resistance, and congenital heart disease.

TREATMENT

Treatment consists of prompt decompression of the stomach and oxygen via tracheal intubation.

ANESTHETIC CONSIDERATIONS

Anesthesia should be administered via awake intubation of the trachea with invasive monitoring of blood pressure. Consider delaying surgery for

24 to 48 hours for stabilization, raising the head of the bed, and rapid sequence induction.

B. Hiatal Hernia/Gastric Reflux

◆ ◆ ◆

DEFINITION

Gastric Reflux

Reduced lower esophageal tone, which is believed to increase the risk of aspiration. Reflux symptoms are probably better to identify patients at risk. Reflux can occur without the presence of hiatal hernia. The lower sphincter is a physiologic sphincter with no specialized musculature. Tone is 15 to 35 mm Hg.

Hiatal Hernia

Herniation of the stomach and other abdominal viscera through an enlarged esophageal hiatus in the diaphragm.

INCIDENCE AND PREVALENCE

Types I to IV hiatal hernias are present in 10% of the population, usually without symptoms. Only 5% of the population have reflux symptoms along with a hiatal hernia.

ETIOLOGY

In most cases the cause is unknown—that is, whether the condition is congenital, traumatic, or iatrogenic.

LABORATORY TESTS

Radiography and barium swallow are used.

CLINICAL MANIFESTATIONS

Symptoms include heartburn; regurgitation; esophageal stricture; bleeding with a large hernia; aspiration sensation of food sticking, fullness, or bloating after eating; and sharp pain.

TREATMENT

No treatment is needed in the absence of symptoms. Larger hernias are treated to control reflux. Enlarging hernias require surgical intervention. Large hernias may require a thoracoabdominal approach.

ANESTHETIC CONSIDERATIONS

Symptomatic patients require pretreatment with a nonparticulate antacid and a histamine$_2$ blocker; elevate the head of the bed until the airway is secure, and use rapid sequence induction to prevent aspiration. Depending on the size of the hernia, one-lung anesthesia may be used to improve access to the surgical site during repair. Consult the surgeon if a double-lumen tube is required with the thoracoabdominal approach.

PROGNOSIS

Prognosis is excellent for a type I hiatal hernia (asymptomatic without reflux). Type II paraesophageal hernias are likely to enlarge. Prognosis is poor if a giant intrathoracic stomach is present.

C. Gallstone/Gallbladder Disease

◆ ◆ ◆

GALLSTONES

DEFINITION

Gallstones are cholesterol-containing stones that form in the gallbladder or bile ducts. They usually form when the bile contains more cholesterol than can be held in solution.

The gallbladder (1) concentrates bile and (2) delivers bile to the duodenum. Its capacity is 40 to 50 mL. Removing the gallbladder has little effect on the body's ability to digest fat.

INCIDENCE AND PREVALENCE

The prevalence of gallstones is high in the United States. In women they form at 20 to 30 years of age; in men, at 30 to 60 years of age.

ETIOLOGY

The two most common types of stones are: (1) cholesterol; (2) bile pigment, calcium bilirubinate, or calcium and copper. Cholesterol stones are more likely in women.

LABORATORY RESULTS

Ultrasonography and cholangiography are used to identify stones and obstruction.

CLINICAL MANIFESTATIONS

Gallstones begin with excessive cholesterol secreted in the bile. Cholesterol eventually precipitates into stones. Stones block the cystic duct, resulting in obstruction or inflammation cholelithiasis with or without jaundice.

GALLBLADDER DISEASE–CHOLANGITIS

DEFINITION

Inflammation of the biliary duct—Charcot's triad: (1) epigastric, upper abdominal pain, (2) jaundice, (3) fever and chills.

ETIOLOGY

Cholangitis is caused by obstruction or bacterial growth in the biliary tract.

LABORATORY RESULTS

The white blood cell count is 10,000 per mm^3, and bilirubin is 2 mg/dL. Hepatic alkaline phosphatase and blood urea nitrogen are elevated. Prerenal azotemia is due to dehydration. Ultrasonography, computed axial tomography, and radiography are used for diagnosis.

TREATMENT

1. Cholecystectomy, common duct exploration with open or closed surgical approach
2. Mechanical removal with forceps or baskets
3. Disintegration (dissolve stones with chemicals)
4. Fiberoptic scope

ANESTHETIC CONSIDERATIONS

The patient may require preoperative pain relief if emergent surgical intervention is required. Evaluate fluids and electrolytes if the patient is vomiting and correct imbalances.

PROGNOSIS

Prognosis is good. The surgical mortality rate is 1.7%, related to complications of infection and pancreatitis.

D. Pancreatitis

◆ ◆ ◆

DEFINITION

Pancreatitis is differentiated into edematous and necrotizing types. Plasma amylase concentrations are increased in a patient experiencing intense midepigastric pain. Chronic pancreatitis is present in alcoholics and in patients with diabetes mellitus or fatty liver infiltration.

INCIDENCE AND PREVALENCE

The incidence of pancreatitis varies in different countries, depending on the incidence of causative factors such as alchoholism, gallstones, and drug use. In the United States, acute pancreatitis is more commonly associated with alchohol abuse than gallstones. It occurs in about 0.5% of the general population.

ETIOLOGY

Biliary tract disease and alcoholism are the most common causes; other causes are obstructive pancreatic ducts, infection, primary hyperparathyroidism, uremia, renal transplantation, hyperlipemia, pregnancy, chemical substance abuse (drugs), hypothermia, idiopathic processes, and trauma.

LABORATORY RESULTS

Computed axial tomography and ultrasonography are used; complete blood count reveals leukocytosis (10,000 to 20,000 per mm^3). Serum amylase is normal. Serum lipase, urinary amylase, and urinary lipase are elevated. Analyze pleural and peritoneal fluid. Blood sugar is elevated. Calcium less than 7.5 mg/dL is associated with necrosis. Liver function enzymes are elevated. Assess coagulation studies, electrocardiogram, chest radiographs, and methemalbumin.

CLINICAL MANIFESTATIONS

Clinical manifestations are based on etiologic factors. They include an enlarged pancreas, pain, nausea, vomiting, diarrhea, bleeding, agitation, and fever.

Stages

1. *Initiating process:* bile reflux, duodenal reflux, lymphatic spread of inflammation
2. *Initial pancreatic injury:* edema, vascular drainage, rupture of pancreatic ducts, acinar damage
3. *Activation of digestive enzymes:* trypsin, lipase
4. *Autodigestion*
5. *Pancreatic necrosis:* associated with abscesses, septicemia, pulmonary failure, acute renal failure, and hyperglycemia

TREATMENT

Treatment is supportive: relieve pain; overcome shock; restore metabolic, fluid, and electrolyte balance; suppress pancreatic secretion (give nothing by mouth, gastrointestinal suction, antacids, histamine₂ blockers, calcitonin, somatostatin). Prevent secondary infection, institute optimal respiratory care, preserve renal function, and neutralize renin release.

ANESTHETIC CONSIDERATIONS

Review laboratory results. Evaluate for shock, hemorrhage, and pain relief—meperidine (Demerol) is the drug of choice. Restore fluid and electrolyte balance—give nothing by mouth, nasogastric tube, histamine$_2$ blockers, type and cross-match blood. Use plasma expanders and an invasive monitor.

PROGNOSIS

The mortality rate is 50% with hemorrhagic pancreatitis, 3% to 10% with edematous pancreatitis. One of 90 cases progresses from acute to chronic pancreatitis.

E. Carcinoid Syndrome

◆ ◆ ◆

DEFINITION

A syndrome produced by metastatic carcinoid tumors that secrete excessive amounts of vasoactive substances such as histamine, bradykinin, serotonin, and various prostaglandins.

INCIDENCE AND PREVALENCE

Carcinoid syndrome develops in about 5% of patients with a carcinoid tumor.

ETIOLOGY

Carcinoid syndrome results when carcinoid tumors in the gastrointestinal tract metastasize to the liver. The liver deactivates the hormones secreted.

LABORATORY RESULTS

Levels of vasoactive substances are increased.

CLINICAL MANIFESTATIONS

Clinical manifestations include cutaneous flushing, hypertension, tachycardia, abdominal pain, diarrhea, bronchospasm, asthma, and rarely cardiomyopathy. The exact presentation depends on the hormone secreted. Tricuspid regurgitate and pulmonic stenosis are possible. Other manifestations are premature atrial beats, cyanosis, venous telangiectasia, hepatomegaly, hyperglycemia, decreased plasma albumin concentration, and dehydration.

TREATMENT

Treatment consists of fluid resuscitation, histamine$_1$ and histamine$_2$ antagonists, steroids, and ketanserin (a serotonin antagonist). Bronchodilation is used. Histamine release is treated with bronchodilation and epinephrine.

ANESTHETIC CONSIDERATIONS

Volatile anesthetics cause bronchodilation. Avoid administering drugs associated with histamine release. Use direct-acting vasopressors. Use vasodilators as needed. Drugs that block vasoactive substances (octreotide, somatostatin) are used to treat kallikrein-releasing tumors. Avoid hypertension, which may stimulate vasoactive substance release. Avoid deep anesthesia. Avoid peripheral sympathetic nervous system block. Avoid activation of the sympathetic nervous system because catecholamines are known to activate kallikrein. Avoid ketamine. Evaluate muscle wasting related to the effect on ventilatory function.

PROGNOSIS

The prognosis is related to tumor treatment.

OTHER CONDITIONS
A. Obesity

◆   ◆   ◆

DEFINITION

Weight over 20% of ideal body weight. Brocca's index for obesity is as follows:

Women: Height (cm) − 105 = kg   *Men:* Height (cm) − 100 = kg.

INCIDENCE AND PREVALENCE

Obesity affects 25% of the population.

ETIOLOGY

Obesity is rarely a thyroid dysfunction; it is often due to a family trait, environmental factors, or psychological factors. It involves gradual accumulations of excess body weight due to a positive energy balance because of excessive caloric intake or decreased energy expenditure.

LABORATORY RESULTS

Findings include hypercholesterolemia, hypertriglyceridemia, and altered pulmonary function test results; baseline arterial blood gases, chest radiographs, electroencephalograms, and echocardiograms are used for diagnosis.

CLINICAL MANIFESTATIONS

Manifestations include increased cardiac output, blood volume, oxygen consumption, minute ventilation, work of breathing, and carbon dioxide production. Systemic hypertension, pulmonary hypertension, cardiac ventricular hypertrophy, decreased chest wall compliance, decreased lung volumes, arterial hypoxemia, diabetes mellitus, congestive heart failure, sleep apnea, fatty liver infiltration, and osteoarthritis are other manifestations.

TREATMENT

Medical treatment entails decreased calorie intake combined with exercise. A very-low-calorie, liquid-protein diet requires medical supervision. Surgical treatment entails gastroplasty, jejunoileal bypass, gastric stapling, and jaw wiring.

ANESTHETIC CONSIDERATIONS

Carefully review patient history. Evaluate for airway obstruction—sleep disturbance, snoring, cardiovascular disease (dyspnea, orthopnea, angina, hypertension, respiratory cyanosis). Gastrointestinal considerations are heartburn, reflux, and increased gastric volume.

Induction

Preoxygenate and denitrogenate for 3 to 5 minutes. Use rapid desaturation with apnea. Consider rapid sequence induction and gastrointestinal prophylaxis. Consider awake intubation.

Maintenance

Volatile anesthetic metabolism may be increased with fatty liver infiltration.

Emergency

If the patient is awake check for intact reflexes. Elevate the head of the bed. Postoperatively, oxygen may be needed by mask for transport to the postanesthesia care unit (PACU). Fasting patients may have electrolyte, fluid, and protein imbalances. Determine if the patient is using diuretics, laxatives, amphetamines, appetite suppressants, or thyroid hormone. Anesthetic medications may cause adverse drug interactions.

B. Glaucoma/Open Globe

◆　◆　◆

DEFINITION AND ETIOLOGY

Intraoccular pressure (IOP) is increased, resulting in impaired capillary flow to the optic nerve with loss of sight if left untreated.

Types of Glaucoma

1. *Open angle:* elevated IOP along with anatomically open anterior chamber angle. Sclerosed trabecular tissue impairs aqueous filtration and drainage. *Treatment:* medically produce miosis and trabecular stretching—eye drops, epinephrine, timolol.
2. *Closed angle:* peripheral iris moves in direct contact with the posterior corneal surface, mechanically obstructing aqueous flow. Caused by narrow angle between iris and posterior cornea. Swelling of crystalline lens.
3. *Congenital glaucoma* is associated with some eye diseases—retinopathy

of prematurity, aniridia, mesodermal dysgenesis syndrome. *Treatment:* surgical goniotomy or trabeculotomy to route aqueous flow into Schlemm's canal. Cyclocryotherapy decreases aqueous formation by destroying ciliary body by freezing tissue with a probe.

Open Globe

This condition usually follows traumatic injury.

DIAGNOSTIC AND LABORATORY FINDINGS

Normal IOP is 10 to 25 mm Hg, abnormal IOP is 25 mm Hg or higher. Pressure becomes atmospheric when globe is opened. Any sudden rise in IOP at this time may lead to prolapse of iris and lens, extrusion of vitreous humor, and loss of vision. Evaluate coagulation studies before instituting retrobulbar block.

CLINICAL MANIFESTATIONS

The clinical manifestations of acute glaucoma are dilated irregular pupil and pain in and around the eye.

TREATMENT

IOP is increased by (1) external pressure on the eye, including venous congestion associated with coughing or vomiting, as well as the prone position; (2) scleral rigidity—increased rigidity seen in aged persons; and (3) changes in intraoccular structure or fluids. *Pilocarpine hydrochloride* decreases resistance to improve drainage of aqueous humor. *Aczetazolamide* reduces the rate of formation of aqueous humor.

ANESTHETIC CONSIDERATIONS

Continue drug therapy to maintain miosis. Anticholinergic drugs are acceptable in preoperative medication. Avoid increases of IOP, hypercarbia, and central venous pressure. Succinylcholine causes transient increases in IOP. Rapid sequence induction generally is acceptable for patients with open globe and a full stomach. Awake intubations are not desirable because they are related to increases in IOP. Techniques associated with decreases in IOP include volatile anesthetics, intravenous anesthetics, hypocarbia, hypothermia, mannitol, glycerin, nondepolarizing muscle relaxants, and timolol. General or retrobulbar blocks are acceptable for eye surgery. General blocks are used for open globe repair.

Consider drug interactions: Echothiophate prolongs the effect of succinylcholine. Timolol may result in bradycardia. Etomidate may induce myoclonus.

Goals of Ophthalmic Surgery

The goals of ophthalmic surgery are akinesia, profound analgesia, minimal bleeding, avoidance of the occulocardiac reflex, control of IOP, awareness of drug interactions, and smooth induction and emergence without vomiting or coughing.

PROGNOSIS

The prognosis depends on control of IOP and maintenance of capillary perfusion.

C. Hypothermia

• • •

DEFINITION

Body temperature below 37°C. Hypothermia is a frequent complication of trauma.

INCIDENCE AND PREVALENCE

Patients become poikilothermic when anesthetized; 60% to 80% of patients are hypothermic when they arrive in PACU. Infants, elderly persons, and burn and trauma patients are most susceptible.

ETIOLOGY

Hypothermia is caused by trauma, burns, general anesthesia, massive resuscitation, and advanced age; it also occurs in young children, especially neonates. General anesthesia involves three phases of cooling:

Phase I   Linear decrease of 1 to 1.5°C with decrease in muscle tone, decreased metabolism, and vasodilation with volatile anesthetics, administration of blood, and exposure to wet preparations

Phase II   0.5°C decrease in the first 3 to 4 hours of anesthesia, decreasing to a core temperature of 34.5°C

Phase III Vasoconstriction prevents further decline in temperature

CLINICAL MANIFESTATIONS

Temperature is less than 37°C. Arrhythmias and respiratory depression occur as temperatures decline. Enzymatic and coagulation factor dysfunction of the humoral clotting system occurs. Bradycardia, myocardial depression, ventricular fibrillation, and shivering stops at 33°C. Coma occurs at 30°C. Relative thrombocytopenia is present.

TREATMENT

Increase room temperature 21 to 25°C and administer warm intravenous fluid with warmers. Use thermal blankets and forced hot-air heating blankets.

Use a heated, humidified breathing circuit. Use core rewarming in severe cases, gastric lavage, peritoneal lavage, and bladder lavage. Keep patients covered. Use radiant heat lamps.

ANESTHETIC CONSIDERATIONS

Anesthetized patients behave like poikilothermic patients. Coagulopathies may develop. Induced hypothermia is used for neurosurgery and cardiac surgery to decrease metabolism and oxygen consumption. Heat is lost through radiation, convection, conduction, and evaporation.

Cardiovascular

Decreased cardiac output (increased if patient is shivering) and increased systemic vascular resistance occur; central redistribution of blood may cause congestive heart failure and bradycardia.

Metabolic

Metabolic rate decreases (or increases if patient is shivering). Tissue perfusion decreases. Metabolic acidosis occurs. Glucose utilization decreases.

Pulmonary

Pulmonary vascular resistance increases, hypoxic pulmonary vasoconstriction decreases, the anatomic dead space increases, and ventilation increases.

Hematologic

Blood viscosity increases, and the oxygen dissociation curve shifts to the left.

Neurologic

Cerebrovascular resistance to cerebral blood flow increases, the electroencephalogram slows to coma status, and the minimum alveolar concentration decreases.

Drug Disposition

Hepatic blood flow decreases, hepatic metabolism decreases, renal blood flow decreases, excretion decreases, and solubility of anesthetic prolonged muscle relaxant effect increases.

Shivering

Oxygen consumption increases by up to 500%, CO_2 production increases.

D. Hyperthermia

* * *

DEFINITION

An increase in body temperature above 36°C. Temperature changes with circadian rhythms, exercise, menstruation, and the environment.

INCIDENCE AND PREVALENCE

Perioperative malignant hyperthermia is rare, occurring in 1 of 250,000 patients.

ETIOLOGY

Hyperthermia is caused by sepsis, thyrotoxicosis, pheochromocytoma, anticholinergic blockade of sweating, heat stroke, and occasionally, malignant hyperthermia syndrome.

CLINICAL MANIFESTATIONS

Temperature is elevated above 41°C because of infection or dysfunctional thermoregulation:

1. Increased heat production due to thyrotoxicosis, pheochromocytoma, exercise, neuroleptic malignant syndrome, malignant hyperthermia
2. Decreased heat dissipation due to dehydration, heat stroke, autonomic dysfunction, excessive coverings, atropine overdose
3. Hypothalamic influence—stroke, tumor, trauma, infection, antipsychotic medications

TREATMENT

Treatment consists of total body cooling and treatment or removal of source.

ANESTHETIC CONSIDERATIONS
Metabolic

Metabolism changes with increased temperature. A 1°C increase raises the basal metabolic rate by 10% to 12%. Oxygen consumption increases, CO_2 production increases, fluid and electrolyte requirements increase, and the cardiovascular workload increases.

Endocrine

Antidiuretic hormone, aldosterone, growth hormone, corticosteroids, and thyroid hormones are increased.

Central Nervous System

The level of consciousness is altered, and cellular edema occurs.

Hematologic

Platelets, prothrombin, fibrinogen, and factors V, VI, and VII are decreased; spontaneous fibrinolysis and consumption coagulopathies occur.

E. Systemic Lupus Erythematosus

♦ ♦ ♦

DEFINITION

Systemic lupus erythematosus (SLE) is a chronic inflammatory disorder of connective tissues, affecting multiple organ systems with periods of remissions and exacerbations.

INCIDENCE AND PREVALENCE

The disease occurs 8 to 15 times more often in women than in men, affecting approximately 75 cases per 1 million people every year. It occurs most often in Asians and blacks. Exacerbations are more common in spring and summer and during stresses such as infection, pregnancy, or surgery.

ETIOLOGY

The etiology of SLE is unknown. One theory is of an antibody-antigen autoimmune response. Another theory deals with predisposing factors promoting susceptibility to SLE. These include stressors such as infection, exposure to ultraviolet light, immunizations, and pregnancy. A third theory suggests that SLE may be triggered by drugs such as procainamide, hydralazine, penicillin, anticonvulsants, oral contraceptives, and sulfa drugs.

LABORATORY RESULTS

Anemia may be seen on the complete blood count with differential, the decreased white blood cell count, and the decreased platelet count. Specific tests for SLE include antinuclear antibodies, anti-DNA, and lupus erythematosus cell tests; urine analysis may show red and white blood cells. Chest radiographs may reveal pulmonary involvement, and electrocardiography may show conduction abnormalities.

CLINICAL MANIFESTATIONS

Clinical manifestations of SLE include arthritis of the upper and lower extremities as well as avascular necrosis of the femur. Systemically, SLE affects many major organ systems (heart, lungs, kidneys, liver, the neuromuscular system, and the skin.) Pericarditis, myocarditis, tachycardia, arrhythmias, and congestive heart failure may develop. Left ventricular dysfunction and endocarditis have also been associated with SLE. About 50% of SLE patients develop such cardiopulmonary abnormalities. Pneumonia, pleural effusions, cough, dyspnea, and hypoxemia are common. Glomerulonephritis and oliguric renal failure may result. Some patients develop lupoid hepatitis, which may be fatal. They may also incur intestinal ischemia. The neuromuscular system may develop myopathies, and psychological changes including schizophrenia and deterioration of the intellect. Finally, the skin may exhibit the typical lesion associated with SLE. This "butterfly rash" appears over the nose and is erythematous. Alopecia may also be seen clinically.

TREATMENT

The usual treatment of SLE is anti-inflammatory therapy with aspirin. Corticosteroids are often used to suppress adverse renal and cardiovascular system changes. For patients who do not respond well to steroids, immunosuppressive agents may be used. Antimalarial drugs have been found to be effective in treating arthritis and skin lesions in small doses.

ANESTHETIC CONSIDERATIONS

Specific anesthesia management is based on drugs being used to treat the disorder in a particular patient, as well as their specific organ involvement. Routinely, however, care must be taken in positioning and in avoiding hyperextension of the neck. These patients may be difficult to intubate because of their inflammatory changes, and they frequently have restrictive lung disease and therefore may be difficult to ventilate. Rapid rates with smaller tidal volumes may be helpful. Overall, a thorough preoperative evaluation should be performed in order to establish organ system involvement to better plan anesthetic care.

ANESTHETIC CONSIDERATIONS

Cutaneous lesions on the nose and mouth may make mask fitting difficult. Cricoarytenoid arthritis rarely occurs. Patients with advanced disease may be debilitated—check chest radiograph, complete blood count, and electrolytes. Anemia and thrombocytopenia purpura can be identified. The partial thromboplastin time may be falsely elevated because antibodies of SLE react with phospholipids used to determine partial thromboplastin time. Avoid renally excreted drugs if renal dysfunction is advanced. Use a steroid bolus if the patient is currently on steroids or has used them within 6 months.

PROGNOSIS

Early detection and treatment improves prognosis. Prognosis, however, remains poor for those who develop cardiovascular, pulmonary, renal, or neurologic complications.

F. Immunosuppression

◆ ◆ ◆

DEFINITION

Patients receiving drugs to suppress the immune response may suffer from a disease state that destroys the immune system. T4 or T helper cells are inhibited. Interleukin-2 production is inhibited. Blood transfusions cause nonspecific immunosuppression.

ETIOLOGY

Immunosuppression is caused by cancer, acquired immunodeficiency syndrome (AIDS), organ transplantation, and steroid use.

CLINICAL MANIFESTATIONS

Renal dysfunction (elevated creatinine) and liver dysfunction (elevated bilirubin) occur. The normal total lymphocyte count (TLC) is 1500 to 1800 (TLC [in cubic millimeters] = white blood cells × lymphocytes).

ANESTHETIC CONSIDERATIONS

Use good hand washing and protective isolation. Cyclosporin may potentiate barbiturates, narcotics, and vecuronium. Transplantation patients may require more time to recover from general anesthesia.

G. Malnutrition

◆ ◆ ◆

DEFINITION

Nutritional failure is associated with protein depletion in the presence of adequate calories or with combined protein-calorie deficiency. Protein-caloric depletion is a frequent finding in surgical patients and the critically ill.

INCIDENCE AND PREVALENCE

Critically ill patients experience negative caloric intake because of the hypermetabolic state produced by their illness. Trauma, fever, sepsis, and wound healing result in a drastically increased metabolism.

ETIOLOGY

Basic energy requirements are an intake of 1500 to 2000 calories/dL. An increase in body temperature of 1°C increases daily caloric requirements by 15%. Multiple fractures increase energy needs by 25%. Major burns are the greatest manifestation, increasing energy requirements by 100%. Large tumors with their growth and metabolism may cause as much of an increase.

LABORATORY RESULTS

The lack of a specific test for protein-caloric malnutrition often makes diagnosis difficult. The best single index of malnutrition is evidence of weight loss from the patient's normal level of weight. Plasma albumin levels below 3 g/dL and transferrin levels below 200 mg/dL have also been used to diagnose malnutrition. Nitrogen balance, which requires careful collection of all drainage and excretions over 24 hours, may be used to evaluate nutritional status. Nitrogen balance provides an estimate of net protein degradation or synthesis.

CLINICAL MANIFESTATIONS

Protein depletion affects the protein content of all organs. The liver and gastrointestinal tract are rapidly depleted, whereas the brain is affected less than other organs. If protein depletion is severe enough, the gastrointestinal system will be unable to tolerate or digest food because protein is needed to produce digestive enzymes. Skeletal muscle is most affected and may lose as much as 70% of its protein. Patients with malnutrition are at increased risk of infections and complications in the postoperative period.

TREATMENT

The initial step in planning a nutritional regimen is to identify the need for intervention, then to determine the route of delivery, and finally to adjust the amounts of macronutrients and micronutrients the patient requires.

ANESTHETIC CONSIDERATIONS

Enteral and parenteral are the two routes of choice. At times the two routes are combined. Enteral supplements can be sipped or administered through a nasogastric feeding tube or gastrostomy tube. If the gastrointestinal tract is nonfunctional, intravenous (parenteral) nutrition is instituted. Isotonic solutions can be delivered through peripheral veins, but if the solution is hypertonic because of a greater caloric need, a central line should be used.

Patients receiving exogenous nutritional support are prone to deficits or overabundance in certain electrolyte levels. Careful preoperative evaluation of laboratory values as well as of any function tests performed is imperative. Parenteral nutrition has the most numerous potential complications. Hypoglycemia and hyperglycemia are common. Increased carbon dioxide resulting from metabolism of large amounts of glucose may hinder early extubation postoperatively. Patients with compromised cardiac function are at risk for congestive heart failure related to fluid overload. Electrolyte abnormalities include hypokalemia, hypomagnesemia, hypocalcemia, and hypophosphatemia. If parenteral nutrition is continued intraoperatively, infusions of other fluids should be minimized. Malnutrition is a clinical finding that must be partially corrected preoperatively. Therapy must be maintained postoperatively for a substantial time based on each patient's needs.

H. Geriatrics

♦ ♦ ♦

DEFINITION

Persons aged 65 years or older.

ETIOLOGY

Peak function is reached in the late 20s. As a person ages, physiologic function declines gradually.

CLINICAL MANIFESTATIONS

Clinical manifestations include increased prevalence of age-related, concomitant disease (hypertension, renal disease, atherosclerosis, myocardial infarction, chronic obstructive pulmonary disease, cardiomegaly, diabetes, liver disease, congestive heart disease, angina, and cardiovascular accidents). Basic organ function declines.

Cardiovascular Change

There are decreases in coronary blood flow, maximum heart rate, and arterial distensibility. There are increases in peripheral vascular resistance, impediments to left-ventricular output, and systolic blood pressure. Cardiac index, resting heart rate, and ejection fraction undergo little or no change.

ANESTHETIC CONSIDERATIONS

Resting arterial oxygen pressure decreases, necessitating an increased intraoperative fractional inspiration of oxygen. Declines in the response to hypoxia and hypercapnia result in additional respiratory depression, even with small amounts of narcotics or inhalation anesthetics. Dose requirements of anesthetic agents increase because of reduced receptor sites, decreased affinity of receptors for hormones and drugs, and decreased synthesis of central nervous system neurotransmitters. Slow circulation decreases. Hypothermia is more likely. Hyperkalemia is more likely because of decreased aldosterone levels.

In terms of general pharmacology, half-lives and the volume of distribution increase; drug clearance and protein binding decrease.

Inhalation Agents

The maximum allowable concentration decreases in relation to decreased cardiac output with a faster rate of uptake. Vasodilating effects are exaggerated, and nodal dysrhythmias become more prevalent.

Muscle Relaxants

Muscle relaxants are eliminated more slowly. Their onset of action is slower.

Regional

The requirements of local anesthetics decrease in relation to decreased neuronal concentrations.

Epidural

Intervertebral spaces narrow; drugs may disperse; the incidence of spinal headaches decreases.

Spinal

Hypotension from sympathetic block increases in relation to decreased cardiac reserve and decreased intravascular volume.

Positioning

Pad bony extremities well. Arthritis may cause airway problems—assess neck mobility.

I. Scleroderma

◆　◆　◆

DEFINITION

Scleroderma entails widespread, symmetric lesions and induration of the skin, followed by atrophy and pigmentation changes. Systemic disease of muscles, bones, heart, and lungs and intestinal and pulmonary changes occur. Viral capacity is reduced, lung volumes decrease, compliance decreases, dead space decreases, the respiratory rate increases, and diffusion capacity is impaired. Pulmonary hypertension occurs.

ANESTHETIC CONSIDERATIONS

Tightening of the skin around the neck may limit the opening of the jaw. Alternate airway control with nasal intubation or fiberoptic techniques. Use pulmonary function tests and baseline arterial blood gases. Postoperative assistance may be needed. Be alert for vasospastic phenomena following induction of anesthesia—treat with a plasma expander. Regional anesthetic is acceptable. Maintain core temperature. Gastrointestinal pretreatment may be necessary because of poor gastric emptying.

COMMON DISEASES

PART 2

COMMON PROCEDURES

GASTROINTESTINAL SYSTEM
A. Cholecystectomy

◆ ◆ ◆

A. Introduction

Surgery of the upper abdomen used in the treatment of gall stones and other diseases of the gall bladder. The mortality rate for elective cholecystectomy is less than 0.5%. In patients over the age of 70, the mortality rate rises to 2% to 3%, mostly because of pre-existing cardiopulmonary disease.

B. Preoperative assessment

1. History and physical examination
   a. Standard
   b. Gastrointestinal assessment: *Pain localized in the right subcostal region. The patient may experience referred pain in the back at the shoulder level. Anorexia, nausea, and vomiting are common. Infection and fever are rare.*
2. Diagnostic tests
   a. *Complete blood count and differentials*
   b. *Diagnosis of gall stones is simple and most reliably performed with ultrasonography*
   c. *Other laboratory testing includes determination of electrolytes, glucose, prothrombin time, and partial thromboplastin time*
3. Preoperative medication and intravenous therapy
   a. *Use an antimicrobial to prevent bacteremia*
   b. *Narcotics must be used with caution to minimize potential spasm in the biliary tract and sphincter of Oddi*
   c. *Use a single, large-bore intravenous tube with fluid replacement (i.e., balanced salt solution) as indicated*

C. Room preparation

1. Monitoring equipment
   a. Standard
   b. Peripheral nerve stimulation
2. Pharmacologic agents
   a. Standard
   b. *Use narcotic agents cautiously because of changes in biliary pressure*
3. Position: supine

D. Anesthetic technique: General endotracheal anesthesia with muscle relaxation

E. Perioperative management

1. Induction
   a. *Rapid sequence induction with oral endotracheal intubation (patient is considered to have a full stomach)*
   b. *Patient may have a nasogastric tube*

2. Maintenance
  a. No specific requirements
  b. Muscle relaxation per abdominal surgery
3. Emergence: awake extubation after airway reflexes are adequate

F. Postoperative implications
1. Retraction in the right upper quadrant during surgery can lead to atelectasis in the right lower lobe; postoperative pain and splinting may lead to impaired ventilation
2. Right intercostal nerve blocks improve postoperative pain management

B. Laparoscopic Cholecystectomy

♦ ♦ ♦

A. Introduction
Surgery used in the treatment of gall stones and diseases of the gall bladder. This procedure is performed under the guidance of a laparoscope.

B. Preoperative assessment and patient preparation
1. History and physical examination
  a. Standard
  b. Gastrointestinal assessment: pain localized in the right subcostal region. The patient may experience referred pain in the back at the shoulder level. Anorexia, nausea, and vomiting are common. Infection and fever are rare.
2. Diagnostic tests
  a. Complete blood count and differentials
  b. Diagnosis of gall stones is simple and most reliably performed with ultrasonography
  c. Other laboratory testing includes determination of electrolytes, glucose, prothrombin time, and partial thromboplastin time
3. Preoperative medication and intravenous therapy
  a. Use an antimicrobial to prevent bacteremia
  b. Narcotics must be used with caution to minimize potential spasm in the biliary tract and sphincter of Oddi
  c. Use a single, large-bore intravenous tube with fluid replacement (i.e., balanced salt solution) as indicated

C. Room preparation
1. Monitoring equipment
  a. Standard
  b. Peripheral nerve stimulation
2. Pharmacologic agents
  a. Standard
  b. Use narcotic agents cautiously

COMMON PROCEDURES

3. Position
   a. *Supine*
   b. *Exposure of the operative site can be optimized with the Trendelenburg and reverse Trendelenburg positions and by tilting the table to the side*

D. Anesthetic technique: General endotracheal anesthesia with muscle relaxation

E. Perioperative management
   1. *Induction:* rapid sequence induction with oral endotracheal intubation (patient is considered to have a full stomach)
   2. Maintenance
      a. *Muscle relaxation with appropriate reversal*
      b. *The peritoneal cavity must be insufflated for surgical exposure. Insufflation with CO_2 causes a rise in the CO_2 partial pressure unless ventilation is controlled.*
      c. *Abdominal distention may lead to hypercarbia with inadequate ventilation. Special attention should be paid to possible adjustments in ventilator settings with insufflation.*
      d. *Basal measurements should be sufficient to control CO_2 partial pressure*
      e. *Insufflation leads to increased intra-abdominal pressure. An intra-abdominal pressure of 20 to 25 cm H_2O produces increases in cardiac output and central venous pressure secondary to changes in the volume of the venous return of blood. An IAP greater than 30 to 40 cm H_2O may lead to decreased central venous pressure and reduced cardiac output secondary to reduced right-ventricular preload.*
      f. *All maintenance anesthetic drugs may be used. Some surgeons request that nitrous oxide not be used to reduce the risk of bowel expansion, which could hinder surgical exposure.*
   3. *Emergence:* awake extubation after airway reflexes are adequate

F. Postoperative implications
   1. *Pain management:* this approach offers the benefit of reduced postoperative pain secondary to smaller abdominal incisions
   2. Patients usually require 24-hour hospitalization

C. Liver Resection

♦ ♦ ♦

A. Introduction
Patients presenting for hepatic surgery may have primary or metastatic tumors from gastrointestinal and other sources. Liver function may be entirely normal in these patients. Hepatocellular carcinoma is common in males over 50 years old and is associated with chronic, active hepatitis B and cirrhosis. Although most major resections can be performed by a transabdominal approach, some surgeons prefer a thoracoabdominal approach. The liver is transected by blunt

dissection utilizing the Cavitron Ultrasonic Suction Aspirator (CUSA) and Argon Beam Laser Coagulator (ABC).

As the principles and techniques of hepatic surgery have evolved, the overall mortality and morbidity rates have improved considerably. Because the normal liver can regenerate, it is possible to resect the right or left lobe along with segments of the contralateral lobe.

In patients afflicted with cirrhoses, the regeneration process is limited; thus, uninvolved liver should be preserved.

B. Preoperative assessment: the following preoperative considerations are for patients *without cirrhosis*.

1. History and physical examination

    The patient should be assessed for coexisting medical diseases. One should check for current drug therapy, previous and present jaundice, a history of blood transfusions, gastrointestinal bleeding, and previous operations and their anesthetic management. One should perform routine physical examination of organs and systems and carefully review the patient's appearance, as well as of the degree of ascites and encephalopathy.

2. Patient preparation

    a. Laboratory tests: *complete blood count, prothrombin time, partial thromboplastin time, platelet count, liver function test, albumin, creatinine, blood urea nitrogen, blood sugar, bilirubin, and electrolytes. Perform other tests as indicated per history and physical examination.*

    b. Diagnostic tests: *chest radiographs, ultrasonography, and computed tomography and magnetic resonance imaging as indicated per history and physical examination*

    c. Medications: *standard premedication that accounts for the reduced ability of the liver to metabolize drugs. Other preoperative medications include ranitidine, metoclopramide, and sodium citrate.*

C. Room preparation

1. Monitoring equipment

    a. *Standard monitoring equipment*

    b. *Arterial line and central venous pressure as clinically indicated*

    c. *Foley catheter*

2. Additional equipment

    a. *CUSA*

    b. *ABC*

    c. *Cell saver*

    d. *Consider a rapid transfusion device*

    e. *Regular operating table*

3. Drugs

    a. *Standard emergency drugs*

    b. *Standard tabletop*

    c. Intravenous fluids: *14- or 16-gauge intravenous lines (2) with normal saline or lactated ringer's solution at 10 to 20 mL/kg per hour. Warm fluids.*

    d. *Two units of packed red blood cells should be available. Blood loss can be significant, and massive transfusions may be required.*

Appropriate blood products also include 2 units of fresh frozen plasma and 10 units of platelets.

D. Perioperative management and anesthetic technique
1. Induction
   a. *General endotracheal anesthesia and appropriate postoperative analgesia*
   b. *Restore intravascular volume prior to anesthetic induction. If patient is hemodynamically unstable, consider etomidate (0.2 to 0.4 mg/kg) or ketamine (1 to 3 mg/kg).*
2. Maintenance
   a. *Standard maintenance: N_2O can be used if bowel distention is not problematic for surgical exposure and closure.*
   b. Combined epidural and general anesthesia: *Be prepared to treat hypotension with fluid and vasopressors. General anesthesia is administered to supplement regional anesthesia and for amnesia. Systemic sedatives should be minimized during this type of anesthetic because they increase the likelihood of postoperative respiratory depression. If epidural opiates are used for postoperative analgesia, a loading dose should be administered at least 1 hour before the conclusion of surgery. During surgery, maintain ventilation to avoid extremes of hypercarbia and hypocarbia.*
   c. Position: *supine, checked and padded pressure points. Avoid stretching brachial abduction to 90°.*
3. Emergence
   For major hepatic resections, the patient will be best cared for in an intensive care unit. Consider keeping the patient mechanically ventilated until the patient is hemodynamically stable and ventilatory status is optimized. If surgical resection was minimal, the patient can be extubated awake and after reflexes have returned.

E. Postoperative implications
1. Decreased liver function—patients with normal preoperative liver function may have significant postoperative impairment of liver function secondary to loss of liver mass or surgical trauma
2. Pulmonary insufficiency (atelectasis, effusion, and pneumonia): more than 90% of patients will develop some form of respiratory complication
3. Hemorrhage
4. Disseminated intravascular coagulation
5. Electrolyte imbalance
6. Hypoglycemia
7. Hypothermia

D. Pancreatectomy

◆　◆　◆

A. Introduction
Distal pancreatectomy is performed for tumors in the distal half of the pancreas, whereas subtotal pancreatectomy involves resection of the

pancreas from the mesenteric vessels distally, leaving the head and uncinate process intact. In about 95% of patients with pancreatic cancer, the cancer is ductal adenocarcinoma, with most occurring in the head of the pancreas.

Pancreatic cancer may appear as a localized mass or as a diffuse enlargement of the gland on computed tomography of the abdomen. Biopsy of the lesion is necessary to confirm the diagnosis. Complete surgical resection is the only effective treatment of ductal pancreatic cancer.

B. Preoperative assessment

Patients presenting for pancreatic surgery can be divided into three groups. (1) Those with acute pancreatitis in whom medical treatment has failed in the past. This group may be extremely ill, presenting for surgery during an exacerbation of pancreatitis or when the diagnosis is in doubt. (2) Patients with carcinoma of the pancreas, including hormone-secreting tumors such as insulinoma and gastrinoma (Zollinger-Ellison syndrome). (3) Patients suffering from the sequelae of chronic pancreatitis.

1. History and physical examination
    a. Cardiovascular: *patients with acute pancreatitis may be hypotensive and may require aggressive volume resuscitation with crystalloid and even blood prior to surgery. Patients with acute pancreatitis may show electrocardiographic change simulating myocardial ischemia. Severe electrolyte disturbances may be associated with acute pancreatitis and some hormone-secreting tumors of the pancreas.*
    b. Respiratory: *respiratory compromise such as pleural effusions, atelectasis, and adult respiratory distress syndrome progressing to respiratory failure may occur in up to 50% of patients with acute pancreatitis*
    c. Gastrointestinal: *jaundice and abdominal pain are common presenting symptoms in this group of patients. The presence of ileus or intestinal obstruction should mandate full-stomach precautions and rapid sequence induction. Electrolyte disturbances are common with acute pancreatitis and may include hypochloremic metabolic alkalosis, decreased calcium and magnesium, and increased glucose. These abnormalities should be corrected preoperatively.*
    d. Endocrine: *many patients with acute pancreatitis may have diabetes secondary to loss of pancreatic tissue. Hormone-secreting tumors of the pancreas are occasionally associated with multiple endocrine neoplasia syndromes. Insulinoma is the most common hormone-secreting tumor of the pancreas and can result in hypoglycemia.*
    e. Renal: *patients should be evaluated for renal insufficiency*
    f. Hematologic: *hematocrit may be falsely elevated because of hemoconcentration or hemorrhage. Coagulopathy may be present.*
2. Patient preparation
    a. Laboratory tests: *complete blood count, prothrombin time, partial thromboplastin time, platelet count, electrolytes, blood urea nitrogen, creatinine, blood sugar, calcium, magnesium, amylase, and urinalysis. Other tests as indicated per history and physical examination.*

       b. Diagnostic tests: *chest radiographs, pulmonary function tests, electrocardiography, and computed tomography of the abdomen. Other tests as indicated per history and physical examination.*

       c. Medication: *standard premedication that accounts for full-stomach precautions. Other preoperative medications include ranitidine, metoclopramide, and sodium citrate.*

C. Room preparation

1. Standard monitoring equipment

   a. Arterial line

   b. Central venous pressure or pulmonary artery catheter as clinically indicated

   c. Foley catheter

   d. Nasogastric tube

2. Additional equipment

   a. Patient warming device

   b. Cell saver

   c. Regular operating table

3. Drugs

   a. Standard emergency drugs

   b. Standard tabletop

   c. Intravenous fluids: 14- to 16-gauge intravenous lines (2) with normal saline or lactated Ringer's solution at 10 to 20 mL/kg per hour. Warm fluids.

   d. Blood loss can be significant, and blood should be immediately available.

D. Perioperative management and anesthetic technique

General endotracheal anesthesia is used; an epidural is used for postoperative analgesia.

1. Induction

   a. Standard

   b. Restore intravascular volume prior to anesthetic induction. If the patient is hemodynamically unstable, consider etomidate (0.2 to 0.4 mg/kg) or ketamine (1 to 3 mg/kg). The patient with bowel obstruction or ileus is at risk for pulmonary aspiration, and rapid sequence induction with cricoid pressure is indicated.

2. Maintenance

   a. Standard maintenance: *Avoid N_2O to minimize bowel distension.*

   b. Combined epidural and general anesthesia: *Be prepared to treat hypotension with fluid vasopressors. General anesthesia is administered to supplement regional anesthesia and for amnesia. Sedatives should be minimized during this type anesthetic as they increase the likelihood of postoperative respiratory depression. If epidural opiates are used for postoperative analgesia, a loading dose should be administered at least 1 hour before the conclusion of surgery.*

   c. Position: *supine, checked and padded pressure points. Avoid stretching the brachial plexus—limit abduction to 90°.*

3. Emergence

   The decision to extubate at the end of surgery depends on the patient's underlying cardiopulmonary status and extent of the surgical procedure. Patients should be hemodynamically stable,

warm, alert, cooperative, and fully reversed from any muscle relaxants prior to extubation.

E. Postoperative implications

Significant third-space and evaporative losses contribute to hypovolemia. Major hemorrhage can occur during dissection of the pancreas from the mesenteric and portal vessels. Total pancreatectomy is associated with brittle diabetes that can be difficult to control. Subtotal resections lead to varying degrees of hyperglycemia. The patient should recover in an intensive care unit or hospital ward that is accustomed to treating the side effects of epidural opiates.

Tests for postoperative management include electrolytes, calcium, glucose, complete blood count, platelets, and other tests as indicated.

Electrolyte disturbances are common with acute pancreatitis and may include hypochloremic metabolic alkalosis, decreased calcium and magnesium, and increased glucose. These abnormalities should be corrected preoperatively.

E. Whipple's Resection

◆ ◆ ◆

A. Introduction

A Whipple resection consists of a pancreatoduodenectomy followed by an anastomosis of the distal pancreatic stump into the jejunum, a choledochojejunostomy, and a gastrojejunostomy. On entering the peritoneal cavity, one determines the resectability of the pancreatic lesion. Contraindications to resection include involvement of mesenteric vessels, infiltration by tumor into the root of the mesentery, extension into the porta hepatis with involvement of hepatic artery, and liver metastasis. If the tumor is deemed resectable, the head of the pancreas is further mobilized. The common duct is transected above the cystic duct entry, and the gall bladder is removed. Once the superior mesenteric vein is freed from the pancreas, the latter is transected with care taken not to injure the splenic vein. The jejunum is transected beyond the ligament of Treitz, and the specimen is removed by severing the vascular connections with the mesenteric vessels. Reconstitution is achieved by anastomosing the distal pancreatic stump, bile duct, and stomach into the jejunum. Drains are placed adjacent to the pancreatic anastomosis. Some surgeons stent the anastomosis until it has healed.

B. Preoperative assessment

Patients presenting for pancreatic surgery can be divided into three groups: (1) Those with acute pancreatitis in whom medical treatment has failed in the past. This group may be extremely ill, presenting for surgery during an exacerbation of pancreatitis or when the diagnosis is in doubt. (2) Patients with carcinoma of the pancreas, including hormone-secreting tumors such as insulinoma and gastrinoma (Zollinger-Ellison syndrome). (3) Patients suffering from the sequelae of chronic pancreatitis.

1. History and physical examination
   a. Cardiovascular: *patients with acute pancreatitis may be hypotensive and may require aggressive volume resuscitation with crystalloid and even blood prior to surgery. Patients with acute pancreatitis may show electrocardiographic change simulating myocardial ischemia. Severe electrolyte disturbances may be associated with acute pancreatitis and some hormone-secreting tumors of the pancreas.*
   b. Respiratory: *respiratory compromise such as pleural effusions, atelectasis, and adult respiratory distress syndrome progressing to respiratory failure may occur in up to 50% of patients with acute pancreatitis*
   c. Gastrointestinal: *jaundice and abdominal pain are common presenting symptoms in this group of patients. The presence of ileus or intestinal obstruction should mandate full-stomach precautions and rapid sequence induction. Electrolyte disturbances are common with acute pancreatitis and may include hypochloremic metabolic alkalosis, decreased calcium and magnesium, and increased glucose. These abnormalities should be corrected preoperatively.*
   d. Endocrine: *many patients with acute pancreatitis may have diabetes secondary to loss of pancreatic tissue. Hormone-secreting tumors of the pancreas are occasionally associated with multiple endocrine neoplasia syndromes. Insulinoma is the most common hormone-secreting tumor of the pancreas and can result in hypoglycemia.*
   e. Renal: *patients should be evaluated for renal insufficiency*
   f. Hematologic: *hematocrit may be falsely elevated because of hemoconcentration or hemorrhage. Coagulopathy may be present.*

2. Patient preparation
   a. Laboratory tests: *complete blood count, prothrombin time, partial thromboplastin time, platelet count, electrolytes, blood urea nitrogen, creatinine, blood sugar, calcium, magnesium, amylase, and urinalysis. Other tests as indicated per history and physical examination.*
   b. Diagnostic tests: *chest radiographs, pulmonary function test, electrocardiography, and computed tomography of the abdomen. Other tests as indicated per history and physical examination.*
   c. Medication: *standard premedication that accounts for full-stomach precautions. Other preoperative medications include ranitidine, metoclopramide, and sodium citrate.*

C. Room preparation
   1. Monitoring equipment
      a. *Standard*
      b. *Arterial line*
      c. *Central venous pressure or pulmonary arterial catheter as clinically indicated*
      d. *Foley catheter*
      e. *Nasogastric tube*

2. Additional equipment
   a. *Patient warming device*
   b. *Cell saver*
   c. *Regular operating table*
3. Drugs
   a. *Standard emergency drugs*
   b. *Standard tabletop*
   c. *Intravenous fluids: 14- to 16-gauge intravenous lines (2) with normal saline or lactated Ringer's solution at 10 to 20 mL/kg per hour. Warm fluids.*
   d. *Blood loss can be significant; blood should be immediately available*

D. Anesthetic technique: general endotracheal anesthesia with an epidural for postoperative analgesia

E. Perioperative management
   1. Induction
      a. *Standard*
      b. *Restore intravascular volume prior to anesthetic induction. If the patient is hemodynamically unstable, consider etomidate (0.2 to 0.4 mg/kg) or ketamine (1 to 3 mg/kg). The patient with bowel obstruction or ileus is at risk for pulmonary aspiration, and rapid sequence induction with cricoid pressure is indicated.*
   2. Maintenance
      a. *Standard. Avoid nitrous oxide to minimize bowel distension.*
      b. *Combined epidural and general anesthesia. Be prepared to treat hypotension with fluid and vasopressors. General anesthesia is administered to supplement regional anesthesia and for amnesia. Systemic sedatives should be minimized during this type of anesthetic because they increase the likelihood of postoperative respiratory depression. If epidural opiates are used for postoperative analgesia, a loading dose should be administered at least 1 hour before the conclusion of surgery.*
      c. *Position: supine, checked and padded pressure points. Avoid stretching the brachial plexus—limit abduction to 90°.*
   3. *Emergence:* the decision to extubate at the end of surgery depends on the patient's underlying cardiopulmonary status and the extent of the surgical procedure. Patients should be hemodynamically stable, warm, alert, cooperative, and fully reversed from any muscle relaxants prior to extubation.

F. Postoperative implications
Significant third-space and evaporative losses contribute to hypovolemia. Major hemorrhage can occur during dissection of the pancreas from the mesenteric and portal vessels. Total pancreatectomy is associated with brittle diabetes that can be difficult to control. Subtotal resections lead to varying degrees of hyperglycemia. The patient should recover in an intensive care unit or a hospital ward that is accustomed to treating the side effects of epidural opiates.

Tests for postoperative management include electrolytes, calcium, glucose, complete blood count, platelets, and other tests as indicated.

COMMON PROCEDURES

F. Splenectomy

◆ ◆ ◆

A. Introduction

Typically, patients presenting for splenectomy have Hodgkin's disease or some other lymphomatous disorder. Apart from the primary disease, these patients are reasonably healthy and have not undergone irradiation or chemotherapy prior to the surgery. Patients presenting for splenectomy may be divided into two less-healthy groups: trauma patients and a more complex group that includes patients with myeloproliferative disorders and other varieties of hypersplenism. Following trauma, instead of splenectomy, a splenorrhaphy or splenic salvage is done (preservation of all or part of the spleen). This may be accomplished by the use of local hemostatic techniques (electrocoagulation, argon beam coagulator, Surgicel or Gelfoam soaked in thrombin, microfibrillar collagen, and the use of fine sutures or mattress sutures utilizing Teflon felt pledgets).

B. Preoperative assessment

1. History and physical examination
   a. Cardiovascular: *patients with systemic disease requiring splenectomy may be chronically ill and have decreased cardiovascular reserve. Patients who have received doxorubicin (Adriamycin) may have a dose-dependent cardiotoxicity that can be worsened by x-ray therapy. Manifestations include decreased QRS amplitude, congestive heart failure, pleural effusions, and dysrhythmia.*
   b. Respiratory: *patients who have splenomegaly may have a degree of left lower lobe atelectasis, which should be evaluated by physical examination. Some may have been treated with bleomycin, a chemotherapeutic drug that causes pulmonary fibrosis. Methotrexate and cytarabine may also cause pulmonary fibrosis. Toxic drug effects are potentiated by smoking, x-ray therapy, and a high fractional inspiration of oxygen.*
   c. Neurological: *patients may have neurologic deficits from receiving chemotherapeutic agents (vinblastine and cisplatin can cause peripheral neuropathies). Any evidence of neurologic dysfunction should be documented in the preoperative evaluation.*
   d. Hematologic: *patients are likely to present with splenomegaly secondary to hematologic disease. Cytopenias are common.*
   e. Hepatic: *some chemotherapeutic agents (methotrexate) may be hepatotoxic. Evaluation of liver function tests should be considered in patients deemed at risk.*
   f. Renal: *some chemotherapeutic drugs (methotrexate, cisplatin) are nephrotoxic. Patients exposed to such agents can present with renal insufficiency.*
2. Patient preparation
   a. Laboratory tests: *complete blood count, prothrombin time, partial thromboplastin time, bleeding time, platelet count, electrolytes, blood urea nitrogen, creatinine, urinalysis, and other tests as indicated per history and physical examination.*

b. Medication: *standard premedication. Administer a stress dose of steroids (100 mg hydrocortisone every 8 hours on the day of surgery) if the patient has received them as part of a chemotherapeutic regimen.*

C. Room preparation

1. Monitoring equipment
   a. *Standard*
   b. *Others as indicated by patient's status*
2. Additional equipment
   a. *Patient warming device*
   b. *Regular operating table*
3. Drugs
   a. *Standard emergency drugs*
   b. *Standard tabletop*
   c. *Intravenous fluids: 16- to 18-gauge intravenous lines (2) with normal saline or lactated Ringer's solution at 10 to 15 mL/kg per hour. Warm fluids.*

D. Anesthetic technique: general endotracheal anesthesia with or without an epidural for postoperative analgesia. If postoperative epidural analgesia is planned, it helps to place a catheter prior to induction to establish correct placement in the epidural space.

E. Perioperative management

1. Induction
   a. *Standard*
   b. *Restore intravascular volume prior to anesthetic induction. If the patient is hemodynamically unstable, consider etomidate or ketamine.*
2. Maintenance
   a. *Standard*
   b. Combined epidural and general anesthesia: *Local anesthetic (1.5% to 2% lidocaine with 1:200,000 epinephrine, 12 to 15 mL/h) can be injected incrementally into the epidural catheter to provide both anesthesia and optimal surgical exposure (contracted bowel and profound muscle relaxation). Be prepared to treat hypotension with fluid and vasopressors (ephedrine 5 to 10 mg). General anesthesia is administered to supplement regional anesthesia and for amnesia. Systemic sedatives (droperidol, opiates, benzodiazepines) should be minimized because they increase the likelihood of postoperative respiratory depression. If epidural opiates are used for postoperative analgesia, a loading dose should be administered at 1 to 2 hours before the conclusion of surgery.*
   c. Position: *supine, checked and padded pressure points. Avoid stretching the brachial plexus—limit abduction to 90°.*
3. *Emergence:* the decision to extubate at the end of surgery depends on the patient's underlying cardiopulmonary status and the extent of the surgical procedure. Patients should be hemodynamically stable, warm, alert, cooperative, and fully reversed from any muscle relaxants prior to extubation.

COMMON PROCEDURES

F. Postoperative implications
1. Bleeding
2. Atelectasis, usually in the left lower lobe
3. Pain management
   a. *Epidural analgesia (posterior cerebral artery)*
   b. *The patient should recover in an intensive care unit or a hospital ward that is accustomed to treating the side effects of epidural opiates (respiratory depression, breakthrough pain, nausea, and pruritus)*

G. Gastrectomy

◆　◆　◆

A. Introduction
Surgery performed for bleeding ulcers or adrenal ulcers. This procedure generally includes a gastroduodenostomy (Billroth I) or gastrojejunostomy (Billroth II). Gastric outlet obstruction from scarring or tumor is common.

B. Preoperative assessment and patient preparation
1. History and physical examination: *gastrointestinal assessment:* assess fluid and hydration status. The patient may be vomiting or bleeding or may have anorexia.
2. Diagnostic tests
   a. *Abdominal radiography*
   b. *Laboratory tests include complete blood count, electrolytes, blood urea nitrogen, glucose, Mg^{2+}, Ca^{2+}, PO^{4-}, prothrombin time, and partial thromboplastin time*
3. Preoperative medication and intravenous therapy
   a. *Expect moderate fluid shift with moderate to large fluid losses. Two large-bore intravenous access tubes are indicated.*
   b. *Patient may be on histamine$_2$ blocker therapy. Cytochrome P-450 inhibition is possible, especially with cimetidine.*
   c. *Antibiotic therapy*
   d. *Consider anemia from a bleeding ulcer preoperatively*
   e. *Blood transfusions*

C. Room preparation
1. Monitoring equipment
   a. *Standard*
   b. *Full warming modalities*
2. *Pharmacologic agents:* standard
3. *Position:* supine, arms extended

D. Anesthetic technique
1. Epidural (T2 to T4 level), high-abdominal exploration will produce a dull pain referred to a C5 destination (generally over the shoulders). "Light" general anesthetic with an epidural is most likely indicated.
2. Routine general anesthesia

E. Perioperative management
1. Induction
   a. *Most patients are considered to have full stomachs; therefore, rapid sequence induction is indicated*
   b. *Consider use of a nasal gastric tube prior to or immediately following induction*
2. Maintenance
   a. *Muscle relaxation is required*
   b. *Closely monitor hydration status and blood loss*
   c. *One may avoid nitrous oxide to minimize gastric or colonic distention*
3. *Emergence:* awake extubation after rapid sequence induction or placement of nasogastric tube
F. Postoperative implications
1. Pain may lead to hyperventilation, reduced cough, and splinting
2. Pain control with epidural or patient-controlled analgesia

H. Gastrostomy

♦ ♦ ♦

A. Introduction

A gastrostomy involves the placement of a semipermanent tube through the abdominal wall directly into the stomach. These tubes are used for gastric decompression or for feeding.

At the time of a laparotomy, the traditional *Stamm gastrostomy* is most common. It may also be performed through a separate, small laparotomy incision in the upper midline or transverse directly over the stomach. The gastrostomy tube is introduced into the stomach and tied securely with pursestring sutures.

The *Janeway gastrostomy* is a technical modification, also placed at the time of a laparotomy. This procedure creates a tube that arises from the main body of the stomach, which allows for permanent access to the stomach with removal of the tube between feedings. This approach is used in patients with expected long-term dependence on gastrostomy access.

Often a *percutaneous endoscopic gastrostomy* is performed. The stomach is intubated endoscopically and the gastric and abdominal walls punctured under endoscopic guidance. The gastrostomy tube is passed from the mouth and through the stomach and abdominal wall from the inside out.

Temporary gastrostomies are often used after major abdominal surgery as an alternative to nasogastric suction. Feeding gastrostomy tubes are indicated in patients unable to feed by mouth but able to absorb enteral nutrition, such as patients with advanced malignancy and intestinal obstruction, inadequate oral intake, and neurologic impairment.

B. Preoperative assessment

Patients undergoing gastrostomy often have neurologic impairment, which compromises their ability to handle oral secretions and increases their risk for aspiration.

1. History and physical examination
    a. Cardiac—*patients are likely to be hypovolemic secondary to chronically poor oral intake and malnutrition*
    b. Respiratory—*patients may have difficulty swallowing and inadequate laryngeal reflexes, which places them at high risk for aspiration of gastric contents and associated pneumonitis. Hypoxemia and decreased pulmonary reserve can present with pulmonary infections.*
    c. Neurologic—*often the patient is neurologically impaired, sick, and debilitated*
    d. Renal—*long-term indwelling urinary catheters increase the risk of infection*
2. Patient preparation
    a. Laboratory tests—*electrolytes, complete blood count; prothrombin time and partial thromboplastin time if regional is planned*
    b. Diagnostic tests—*electrocardiography; posteroanterior and lateral radiography; consider orthostatic blood pressure*
    c. Medications—*standard premedication; consider glycopyrrolate (Robinul) with percutaneous endoscopic gastrostomy*

C. Room preparation

1. *Monitoring equipment:* standard monitoring equipment
2. *Additional equipment:* endoscope, percutaneous gastrostomy kit for percutaneous endoscopic gastrostomy
3. *Drugs:* standard emergency drugs
4. Standard tabletop
5. Intravenous fluids: One 18-gauge intravenous line with normal saline or lactated Ringer's solution at 5 to 8 mL/kg per hour.

D. Anesthetic technique: maximum allowable concentration with local anesthesia to area of incision for gastrostomy; otherwise, general or regional according to the site and size of the incision, the patient's physical status, and the preferences of both the patient and the surgeon

E. Perioperative management

1. Induction
    a. *If general anesthesia is planned, use rapid sequence induction with cricoid pressure*
    b. *Awake intubation may be necessary for the patient at risk for pulmonary aspiration*
    c. *Restore volume status in a hypovolemic patient before induction*
2. Maintenance
    a. General anesthesia: *standard; muscle relaxants may be necessary to facilitate closure with laparotomy incision*
    b. Maximum allowable concentration: *titrate sedatives to effect*
    c. Position: *supine, checked and padded pressure points*
3. *Emergence:* tracheal extubation after the return of protective laryngeal reflexes

F. Postoperative implications

Mild to moderate postoperative pain intensity may be controlled with parenteral narcotics or intercostal blocks.

Postoperative complications include but are not limited to aspiration pneumonia, wound infection, and failure to function.

I. Small Bowel Resection

◆ ◆ ◆

A. Introduction

Surgery performed for abdominal trauma, abdominal structure adhesions, Meckel's diverticulum, Crohn's disease, or infection.

B. Preoperative assessment and patient preparation

1. History and physical examination: *gastrointestinal assessment:* assess fluid and hydration status. The patient may be vomiting or bleeding or may have third-spacing, diarrhea, or dehydration.
2. Diagnostic tests
   a. *Abdominal radiography*
   b. *Laboratory tests include complete blood count, electrolytes, blood urea nitrogen, glucose, Mg^{2+}, Ca^{2+}, PO^{4-}, prothrombin time, and partial thromboplastin time*
3. Preoperative medication and intravenous therapy
   a. *Patients may be on steroid therapy or immunosuppressant drugs*
   b. *Expect fluid shifts requiring moderate to large fluid resuscitation. Two large-bore intravenous access tubes are indicated.*
   c. *Preoperative hydration is essential*

C. Room preparation

1. Monitoring equipment
   a. *Standard*
   b. *Full warming modalities*
2. *Pharmacologic agents:* standard
3. *Position:* supine, arms extended

D. Anesthetic technique

1. Epidural (T2 to T4 level) with "light" general anesthetic and orogastric tube
2. General anesthesia with endotracheal tube

E. Perioperative management

1. Induction
   a. *Most patients are considered to have full stomachs; therefore, rapid sequence induction is indicated*
   b. *Consider use of a nasal gastric tube prior to or immediately following induction*
2. Maintenance
   a. *Muscle relaxation is required*
   b. *Closely monitor hydration status and blood loss*
   c. *Avoid nitrous oxide, which may cause bowel distention*

COMMON PROCEDURES

3. *Emergence:* awake extubation after rapid sequence induction or placement of nasogastric tube

F. Postoperative implications
   1. Pain may lead to hypoventilation, reduced cough, splinting, and atelectasis
   2. Pain control with epidural or patient-controlled analgesia

J. Appendectomy

♦ ♦ ♦

A. Introduction

In acute appendicitis, the long narrow tube of the appendix is obstructed, hypoxia develops, the mucosa ulcerates, and bacteria invade the wall. It is the most common surgical emergency during pregnancy.

B. Preoperative assessment and patient preparation
   1. History and physical examination
      a. Gastrointestinal: *patients point to localized pain at "McBurney's point," which is midway between the iliac crest and umbilicus; note rebound tenderness, muscle rigidity, and abdominal guarding*
      b. Pregnant female: *"Alder's sign" is used to differentiate between uterine and appendical pain. The pain is localized with the patient supine. The patient then lies on her left side. If the area of pain shifts to the left, it is presumed to be uterine.*
   2. Diagnostic tests
      a. *White blood cell count is elevated, with a shift to the left—10,000 to 16,000 mm³; 75% neutrophils*
      b. *Urinalysis shows a small number of erythrocytes and leukocytes*
      c. *Abdominal films demonstrate fecalith (formed, hard mass of feces in right-lower quadrant or localized ileus)*
      d. *Other laboratory tests include electrolytes, glucose, hemoglobin and hematocrit*
   3. Preoperative medication and intravenous therapy
      a. *Antibiotic for enteric gram-negative bacilli, anaerobic bacteria*
      b. *Single 18-gauge intravenous tube is used because patient is dehydrated from fever, anorexia, and vomiting*

C. Room preparation
   1. Monitoring equipment
      a. *Standard*
      b. *Fetal heart-tone monitoring with pregnancy*
   2. Pharmacologic agents
      a. *Standard*
      b. *For fetal safety, it is essential to avoid teratogenic anesthetic during the first trimester*

3. Position
  a. Supine
  b. Left uterine displacement with pregnancy
D. Anesthetic technique
  1. *Regional blockade:* analgesia to levels T6 to T8
  2. *General anesthesia:* endotracheal intubation is required
E. Perioperative management
  1. Induction
    a. Use general anesthesia with a rapid sequence induction because many patients have a nasogastric tube or are considered to be on a full stomach (emergency)
    b. In the pregnant patient, special care should be taken to prevent aspiration pneumonitis
  2. Maintenance
    a. No specific indications
    b. Muscle relaxation is necessary
  3. *Emergence:* awake extubation secondary to rapid sequence induction
F. Postoperative implications—none

Bibliography

Bennett JC, Plum F. *Cecil Textbook of Medicine.* 20th ed. Philadelphia, PA: W.B. Saunders Co.; 1996.

Schnider SM, Levinson G. *Anesthesia for Obstetrics.* Baltimore, MD: Williams & Wilkins; 1987.

Thompson J, et al. *Mosby's Manual of Clinical Nursing.* 2nd ed. St. Louis, MO: C.V. Mosby Co.; 1989.

COMMON PROCEDURES

K. Colectomy

◆ ◆ ◆

A. Introduction
  Surgery performed for adenocarcinomas, diverticulosis, penetrating trauma, ulcerative colitis, angiodysplasia, and infarctions.
B. Preoperative assessment and patient preparation
  1. History and physical examination: *gastrointestinal assessment:* assess hydration status, nutritional level, and electrolyte state
  2. Diagnostic tests
    a. Abdominal radiography
    b. Laboratory tests include complete blood count, electrolytes, blood urea nitrogen, creatinine, glucose, prothrombin time, and partial thromboplastin time
  3. Preoperative medication and intravenous therapy
    a. Patients may be on steroid therapy or immunosuppressant drugs
    b. Bowel preparation is usually indicated with electrolyte preparations

  c. *Expect fluid shifts requiring moderate to large fluid resuscitation. Two large-bore intravenous access tubes are indicated.*

C. Room preparation
  1. Monitoring equipment
    a. *Standard*
    b. *Full warming modalities*
  2. Pharmacologic agents: standard
  3. *Position:* supine, arms extended

D. Anesthetic technique
  1. Epidural (T2 to T4 level) with "light" general anesthetic
  2. General anesthesia with oral endotracheal tube (most common)

E. Perioperative management
  1. *Induction:* must consider possibility of full stomach with all emergency colectomies and some elective ones. Rapid sequence induction may be indicated.
  2. Maintenance
    a. *Muscle relaxation is required*
    b. *Closely monitor fluid and hydration status and blood loss*
    c. *Avoid nitrous oxide, which may cause bowel distention*
  3. *Emergence:* awake extubation after rapid sequence induction or placement of nasogastric tube

F. Postoperative implications
  1. Pain and splinting may lead to hypoventilation and decreased postoperative ventilation
  2. Pain control with epidural or patient-controlled analgesia

L. Herniorrhaphy

✦   ✦   ✦

A. Introduction
Inguinal hernias are defects in the transverse abdominal layer, where a direct hernia comes through the posterior wall of the inguinal canal and an indirect hernia comes through the internal inguinal ring.

Femoral hernia is when the hernia sac is exposed as it exits the preperitoneal space through the femoral canal. If the hernia cannot be reduced, the possibility of strangulation must be kept in mind. The peritoneal sac in most cases should be opened proximal to the femoral canal in order to gain control of the intestine before it reduces itself into the peritoneal cavity. If the bowel is ischemic, it may require resection. The repair consists of suturing the iliopubic tract to Cooper's ligament, taking care not to compromise the femoral vein.

Incisional hernias can occur after any abdominal incision, but they are most common following midline incisions. Factors leading to herniation are: wound infection, trauma, inadequate suturing, and weak tissues. Following skin incision, the skin edges and subcutaneous fat are retracted and the dissection carried down to the hernia defect. The redundant hernia sac is excised and the fascia freed up on both sides of the wound. Primary closure is preferred. In addition to primary repair, the latter may be reinforced by an only-mesh prosthesis, or the prosthesis may be used to fill the hernia sac.

B. Preoperative assessment

Predisposing factors for hernia often include increased abdominal pressure secondary to chronic cough, bladder outlet obstruction, constipation, pregnancy, vomiting, and acute or chronic muscular effort. These factors should be controlled preoperatively to avoid postoperative recurrence. The patient population may range from premature infants to the elderly with the possibility of multiple medical problems.

1. History and physical examination
   a. Musculoskeletal: *pain is likely the in area of the hernia; evaluate bony landmarks if regional anesthesia is planned*
   b. Hematologic: *if regional anesthesia is planned, check the patient's coagulation status*
   c. Gastrointestinal: *hernias may become incarcerated, obstructed, or strangulated, requiring emergency surgery; fluid and electrolyte imbalance should be assumed*
2. Patient preparation
   a. Laboratory tests: *complete blood count, electrolytes, and other tests as indicated per the history and physical examination*
   b. Diagnostic tests: *as indicated per the history and physical examination*
   c. *If necessary, use standard premedication*

C. Room preparation

1. Monitoring equipment: standard
2. Additional equipment: regular operating table
3. Drugs
   a. *Standard emergency drugs*
   b. *Standard tabletop*
   c. *Intravenous fluids: One 18-gauge intravenous line with normal saline or lactated Ringer's solution at 5 to 8 mL/kg per hour.*

D. Anesthetic technique: general, regional, or local anesthesia with sedation (maximum allowable concentration) are all appropriate. The choice depends on such factors as site of incision, the patient's physical status, and the preference of both the patient and the surgeon. General anesthesia may be preferred for incisions made above T8. Profound muscle relaxation may be needed for exploration and repair.

E. Perioperative management

1. *Standard induction:* mask general anesthesia may be suitable for the patient with a simple chronic hernia. If there is obstruction, incarceration, or strangulation, a rapid sequence induction with endotracheal intubation is indicated. General endotracheal anesthesia also may be indicated in the patient with wound dehiscence.

COMMON PROCEDURES

2. Maintenance
   a. *Standard; muscle relaxants may be necessary to facilitate surgical repair*
   b. *Position: supine, check and pad pressure points. Avoid stretching the brachial plexus. Limit abduction to 90°.*
3. *Emergence:* consider extubating the trachea while the patient is still anesthetized to prevent coughing and straining. Patients who are at risk for pulmonary aspiration and who require awake extubation after rapid sequence induction are not candidates for deep extubation.

F. Postoperative implications
   1. Wound dehiscence with coughing or straining
   2. *Urinary retention*—patients with urinary retention may require intermittent catheterization until urinary function resumes
   3. *Pain management*—surgical field block or regional anesthesia should provide sufficient analgesia postoperatively

M. Gallbladder Lithotripsy

• • •

A. Introduction
   1. Extracorporeal shock-wave lithotripsy requires endoscopic retrograde cholangiopancreatography, sphincterotomy, and placement of a nasobiliary tube. The tube opacifies the biliary tree and helps to identify common bile duct stones.
   2. Ultrasonic shock waves are delivered to the gall bladder or common bile duct to break the stones. Gallbladder contractility is of utmost importance in removal of stone fragments and debris from the biliary system.
   3. Decreased gallbladder motility and stasis are primary causes of stone formation and may hinder expulsion of stone fragments following lithotripsy.
   4. Three basic stone types are cholesterol, pigment, and mixed.

B. Preoperative history
Predisposing factors include increased age, female sex, obesity, and pregnancy.
   1. History and physical examination
      a. Cardiac: *symptoms mimic angina and myocardial infarction*
      b. Respiratory: *symptoms mimic right lower lobe pneumonia and pleurisy*
      c. Neurologic: *symptoms mimic intercostal neuritis*
      d. Renal: *symptoms mimic pyelonephritis and renal calculus*
      e. Gastrointestinal: *symptoms mimic esophagitis, pancreatitis, intestinal obstruction, perforated ulcer, peptic ulcer, and hiatal hernia*

2. Patient preparation
   a. *Laboratory tests*
      (1) Complete blood count—leukocyte count is elevated
      (2) Electrolytes—assesses effect of nausea and vomiting
   b. *Diagnostic tests*
      (1) Biliary ultrasonography
      (2) Abdominal radiographs (only 15% of stones are visible)
   c. Medications: *analgesics and sedation are not necessary, although they may help the patient to lie still for the procedure.*

C. Room preparation

1. Procedure is completed in the radiography department (usually without anesthetic support)
2. Standard monitors
3. *Additional equipment:* propofol infusion pump and airway adjuncts, nasal cannula, oxygen cylinder
4. Drugs
   a. *Fentanyl—two bolus doses of 50 to 200 μg of fentanyl*
   b. *Propofol—0.5 mg/kg loading dose followed by 50 μg/kg per min infusion*
   c. *Intravenous: 0.9% normal saline or lactated Ringer's at 2 mL/kg per hour*
   d. *Tabletop standard general anesthesia set-up*

D. Perioperative management and anesthetic technique

1. No anesthesia
2. Monitored anesthesia care with sedation
3. *Maintenance:* propofol drip as necessary

E. Postoperative implications

1. Transport to recovery room if patient has been sedated
2. Transport to room if no anesthesia was given

N. Esophagoscopy/Gastroscopy

◆   ◆   ◆

A. Introduction

Flexible, diagnostic esophagogastroduodenoscopy, a common procedure in pediatrics, is usually performed under heavy sedation in an endoscopy suite or special procedure area. Rigid esophagoscopy is usually performed for therapeutic indications such as removal of a foreign body, dilation of an esophageal stricture, or injection of varices. The procedure is similar for each diagnosis and generally is performed with endotracheal intubation. Foreign-body removal is normally a short procedure, whereas dilation and variceal injection can be prolonged and may require multiple insertions or removals of the endoscope. Compression of the trachea distal to the endotracheal tube by the rigid esophagoscope is not uncommon.

B. Preoperative assessment

Esophagoscopy for foreign-body removal is usually performed in healthy infants and children, although esophageal lodging of a foreign body can occur in any age group. All these patients should be treated with full-stomach precautions. Esophageal dilation usually is performed in two distinct patient populations: (1) those with prior tracheoesophageal fistula repair and (2) those with prior ingestion of a caustic substance.

1. History and physical examination
   a. Cardiovascular: *there may be persistent congenital cardiac anomalies in the patient with a tracheoesophageal fistula*
   b. Respiratory: *patients with prior caustic ingestion may have a history of pulmonary aspiration, with resultant chemical pneumonitis, fibrosis, or both. Prolonged intubation after tracheoesophageal fistula repair may lead to subglottic stenosis. Check any recent anesthesia records for endotracheal intubation.*
2. Patient preparation
   a. Laboratory tests: *no routine laboratory analyses are required if the patient has no underlying chronic illness*
   b. Diagnostic tests: *as indicated per history and physical examination*
   c. Medications: *for foreign-body removal, intravenous access may be necessary before induction. No premedication is used if the patient is less than 1 year old.*

C. Room preparation

1. Monitoring equipment: standard
2. Additional equipment
   a. *Regular operating table*
   b. *Esophagoscope with forceps and dilators*
3. Drugs
   a. *Standard emergency drugs*
   b. *Standard tabletop*
   c. *Intravenous fluids: One 20- to 22-gauge intravenous line with normal saline or lactated Ringer's solution at 4 to 6 mL/kg per hour.*

D. Anesthetic technique

Use general endotracheal anesthesia. For the pediatric patient, one may use a pediatric circle or a non-rebreather circuit. Room temperature can be maintained at 65 to 70°F as long as the patient is covered.

E. Perioperative management

1. *Induction:* a rapid sequence induction is usually appropriate for this patient population, unless the patient is presenting for dilation alone and has no evidence to suggest reflux
2. Maintenance
   a. *Maintain anesthesia with a volatile agent, N_2O, and O_2. Opiates are unnecessary because postprocedural pain is negligible. Maintain neuromuscular blockade. Movement must be avoided, particularly with rigid esophagoscopy.*
   b. *Position: supine, check and pad pressure points. Avoid stretching the brachial plexus—limit abduction to 90°.*

3. *Emergence:* extubate when patient is fully awake. Do not attempt reversal of neuromuscular blockade until first twitch of train of four has returned.

F. Postoperative implications
1. Pneumothorax—esophageal perforation is more common with rigid esophagoscopy and will lead to pneumothorax.
2. Aspiration
3. Accidental extubation
4. Stridor secondary to subglottic edema
5. Postoperative pain is negligible; if the patient reports marked substernal discomfort, suspect esophageal perforation

O. Colonoscopy

◆ ◆ ◆

A. Introduction
Procedure used to examine the colon and rectum to diagnose inflammatory bowel disease, including ulcerative colitis and granulomatous colitis. Polyps can be removed through the colonoscope. The colonoscope is also helpful in diagnosing or locating the source of gastrointestinal bleeding; a biopsy of lesions suspected to be malignant may be performed.

B. Preoperative assessment and patient preparation
1. History and physical examination: *Gastrointestinal:* assess patient's hydration status, nutritional level, and electrolyte state
2. Diagnostic tests
   a. *Radiographs of the abdomen*
   b. *Laboratory tests include electrolytes, glucose, hemoglobin and hematocrit, prothrombin time, and partial thromboplastin time*
3. Preoperative medication and intravenous therapy
   a. *Patients may be on steroid therapy or immunosuppressants*
   b. *Bowel preparation is required for visualization of the mucosa. Use colon electrolyte lavage preparations (Colyte, GoLYTELY).*
   c. *One 18-gauge intravenous tube; minimal fluid replacement*
   d. *Patient is lightly sedated with the use of medazepams because the procedure lasts less than 30 minutes and is an outpatient procedure*

C. Room preparation
1. *Monitoring equipment:* standard
2. Pharmacologic agents
   a. *Standard*
   b. *Glucagon*
3. *Position:* left lateral decubitus; occasionally, position changes are required to aid advancement of the scope at the descending sigmoid colon junction and splenic fixture

D. Anesthetic techniques
   1. Sedation
   2. Intravenous sedation: midazolam (Versed), fentanyl or propofol in sedative doses
E. Perioperative management
   1. *Induction:* oxygenate the patient with the use of nasal cannulae or a face mask
   2. *Maintenance:* no specific indications
   3. *Emergence:* no specific indications
F. Postoperative implications
   Complications of the procedure include perforation of the bowel, abdominal pain and distention, rectal bleeding, fever, and mucopurulent drainage.

P. Esophageal Resection

◆   ◆   ◆

A. Introduction
   Esophagectomy is commonly performed for malignant disease of the middle and lower thirds of the esophagus. It may also be indicated for Barrett's esophagus (peptic ulcer of lower esophagus) and for peptic strictures that do not respond to dilatation. Lesions in the lower third are usually approached via a left thoracoabdominal incision, whereas middle-third lesions are best approached via the abdomen and right side of the chest. Resections of the esophagogastric junction for malignant disease are best performed through a left thoracoabdominal approach in which a portion of the proximal stomach is removed along with a coeliac node dissection.
   Blind esophagectomy is done via the abdomen and neck by blunt dissection. This is useful primarily for benign esophageal lesions or malignant lesions of the pharynx and larynx in which the pharynx and/or upper esophagus require resection.
   Total esophagectomy may be done via an abdominal and right thoracotomy approach with colonic interposition and anastomosis in the neck. Either the right or the left side of the colon can be mobilized for interposition. Both depend on the middle colic artery and the marginal artery of the colon for their vascular supply. When the proximal portion of the right colon is utilized, the interposed segment of bowel is isoperistaltic, but when the left colon is brought up, the segment is antiperistaltic. Although the colonic interposition is said to function primarily as a conduit for food, the isoperistaltic colonic segment functions better. In either case, the colonic segment is connected to the body of the stomach following suturing of the esophageal colonic anastomosis.

B. Preoperative assessment
  1. History and physical examination
     a. Cardiovascular: *the patient may be hypovolemic and malnourished from dysphagia or anorexia. Chemotherapeutic drugs (daunorubicin, adriamycin) may cause cardiomyopathies. Chronic alcohol abuse may also produce a toxic cardiomyopathy. Congestive heart failure, if present, may be refractory to treatment, although preoperative optimization of cardiac status is essential.*
     b. Respiratory: *a history of gastric reflux suggests the possibility of recurrent aspiration pneumonia, decreased pulmonary reserve, and increased risk of regurgitation and aspiration during anesthetic induction. If a thoracic approach is planned, the patient should be evaluated to ensure that one-lung ventilation can be tolerated.*

     Determine if the patient has been exposed to bleomycin, which may cause pulmonary toxicity; toxicity may be made worse by high concentrations of oxygen. Many patients with esophageal cancer have a long history of smoking with consequent respiratory impairment.

     Pulmonary function tests and arterial blood gases can be helpful in predicting the likelihood of perioperative pulmonary complications and whether the patient may require postoperative mechanical ventilation. Patients with baseline hypoxemia/hypercarbia on room-air arterial blood gases have a higher likelihood of postoperative complications and a greater need for postoperative ventilatory support. Severe restrictive or obstructive lung disease will also increase the chance of pulmonary morbidity in the perioperative period.
     c. Hematologic: *encourage preoperative autologous blood donation.*
  2. Patient preparation
     a. Laboratory tests: *type and cross-match packed red blood cells, electrolytes, glucose, blood urea nitrogen, creatinine, bilirubin, transaminase, alkaline phosphatase, albumin, complete blood count, and platelet count. Prothrombin time, partial thromboplastin time, urinalysis, arterial blood gases, and other tests as indicated per history and physical examination.*
     b. Diagnostic tests: *chest radiographs, electrocardiography, pulmonary function tests, and other tests as indicated per history and physical examination. If congestive heart failure or cardiomyopathy is suspected, consider cardiac or medical consultations.*
     c. Medications: *midazolam and morphine. Consider histamine₂ antagonists, metoclopramide, and sodium citrate.*

C. Room preparation
  1. Monitoring equipment
     a. *Standard monitoring equipment*
     b. *Arterial line*
     c. *Central venous pressure or pulmonary arterial catheter as clinically indicated*
     d. *Foley catheter*
  2. Additional equipment
     a. *Patient warming device*
     b. *Regular operating table*
     c. *Axillary roll if lateral decubitus position is used*

COMMON PROCEDURES

3. Drugs
   a. *Standard emergency drugs*
   b. *Standard tabletop*
   c. *Intravenous fluids: 14- to 16-gauge (2) normal saline or lactated Ringer's solution at 8 to 12 mL/kg per hour, fluid warmer*
   d. *Blood loss can be significant, and blood should be immediately available*

D. Anesthetic technique

General endotracheal anesthesia (with or without epidural anesthetic for postoperative analgesia). If postoperative epidural analgesia is planned, placement and testing of the catheter prior to anesthetic induction is helpful. If the thoracic or abdominothoracic approach is used, placement of a double-lumen tube is indicated, because one-lung anesthesia provides excellent surgical exposure.

E. Perioperative management

1. Induction

   Patients with esophageal disease are often at risk for pulmonary aspiration; therefore, the trachea should be intubated with the patient awake or after rapid sequence induction with cricoid pressure. Awake intubation can be done by either blind nasal or fiberoptic bronchoscopy. If the patient is clinically hypovolemic, restore intravascular volume prior to induction and titrate induction dose of sedative/hypnotic agents.

2. Maintenance

   a. *Standard maintenance without N_2O. Alternatively, a combined technique may be used. A local anesthetic (1.5% to 2% lidocaine with 1:200,000 epinephrine 12 to 15 mL every 60 min) can be injected into an epidural catheter to provide both anesthesia and optimal surgical exposure (contracted bowel and profound muscle relaxation). Be prepared to treat hypotension with fluid and vasopressors. General anesthesia is administered to supplement regional anesthesia and for amnesia. Systemic sedatives (droperidol, opiates, benzodiazepines) should be minimized during administration of epidural opiates because they increase the likelihood of postoperative respiratory depression. If epidural opiates are used for postoperative analgesia, a loading dose should be administered at least 1 hour before the conclusion of surgery.*

   b. *Position: supine, check and pad pressure points. Avoid stretching the brachial plexus—limit abduction to 90°. If the lateral decubitus position is used, an axillary roll and arm holder are needed. Check pressure points, including ears, eyes, and genitals. Check radial pulses to ensure correct placement of axillary roll (a misplaced axillary roll will compromise distal pulses). Problems that can arise include: brachial plexus injuries, and damage to soft tissues, ears, eyes, and genitals from malpositioning.*

3. Emergence

   The decision to extubate at the end of surgery depends on patient's underlying cardiopulmonary status and the extent of the surgical procedure. The patient should be hemodynamically stable, warm, alert, cooperative, and fully reversed from any muscle relaxants prior to extubation. With patients who require postoperative ventilation, the double-lumen tube should be changed to a single-lumen endotracheal tube prior to transport to postanesthesia intensive care unit. Weaning from mechanical ventilation should begin when the patient is awake and cooperative, is able to protect the airway, and has adequate pulmonary function.

F. Postoperative implications
1. For atelectasis or aspiration, recover the patient in Fowler's position
2. Hemorrhage—check coagulation times; replace factors as necessary
3. Pneumothorax/hemothorax—decreased partial oxygen pressure, increased partial carbon dioxide pressure, wheezing, coughing; confirm with chest radiograph, institute chest tube drainage as necessary. In an emergency (tension pneumothorax), use needle aspiration, supportive treatment; oxygen, vasopressors, endotracheal intubation, positive-pressure ventilation.
4. Hypoxemia/hypoventilation—ensure adequate analgesia and supplemental oxygen
5. Esophageal anastomotic leak—begin surgical repair for esophageal anastomotic leak
6. Pain management—patient-controlled analgesia or epidural analgesia; patient should recover in the intensive care unit or a hospital ward that is accustomed to treating the side effects of epidural opiates (respiratory depression, breakthrough pain, nausea, and pruritus)

Q. Exploratory Laparotomy

◆ ◆ ◆

A. Introduction
Exploratory laparotomy is indicated primarily in patients suffering from penetrating or severe abdominal blunt trauma. A thorough and systematic intra-abdominal examination must be carried out to prevent missing significant injuries. Any active bleeding should be controlled prior to a systematic examination. Other indications for laparotomy include certain patients with fever of undetermined origin or those in whom a specific diagnosis cannot be made.

An urgent laparotomy may be indicated in hypotensive patients who respond poorly to volume resuscitation. Patients may arrive in the operating room without benefit of adjunctive diagnostic tests. For stab wounds of the anterior and lateral abdomen, a local exploration of the wound in the emergency department followed by peritoneal lavage is usually performed to determine the need for formal intraoperative exploration. For gunshot wounds suspected of penetrating the peritoneum, formal intraoperative exploration is usually indicated. The objectives of any laparotomy for trauma are to examine the intraperitoneal space and to control bleeding rapidly. The midline incision is standard in trauma surgery because of its constant features, rapidity of achieving entry, and ease of closure.

B. Preoperative assessment

1. History and physical examination

   a. Cardiovascular: *blood pressure and heart rate should be followed, and trends and responses to fluid resuscitation should be noted. Tachycardia can maintain an adequate blood pressure with reduced pulse pressure, despite a 25% to 30% loss of blood volume. Attempt to quantitate overt blood loss (scalp laceration, open fracture sites). Blunt chest trauma (steering-wheel contact) may result in myocardial contusion with various dysrhythmias, most often premature ventricular or atrial complexes.*

   b. Respiratory: *associated injuries such as hemothorax and/or pneumothorax may be present, requiring thoracostomy tube placement. A widened mediastinum, apical pleural capping, or fracture of the first or second rib often occur with serious vascular injuries. Multiple rib fractures suggest possible pulmonary contusions, which may not be evident on initial chest radiographs but can progressively impair oxygenation and ventilation with time and fluid resuscitation.*

   c. Neurologic: *seek physical evidence of open or closed head injuries such as palpable depressions of the skull or scalp lacerations, abrasions, or contusions. Pupil size and reactivity should be noted. Intubation in the emergency room is necessary for patients who are unable to protect their airway, require hyperventilation, or are combative and unable to cooperate with medical staff for examination and treatment. In general, any patient with a Glasgow Coma Scale score of <7 to 9 requires intubation. This patient typically has no spontaneous eye opening, inappropriate or incomprehensible speech, and only reflexive motor responses. Motor and sensory deficits may reflect spinal cord injury and may be associated with neurogenic (spinal) shock, particularly with upper thoracic or cervical cord injuries.*

   d. Musculoskeletal: *known or suspected cervical spine injuries require intubation precautions. In urgent cases, intubation without neck extension is achieved with an assistant providing axial traction on the head. If time permits, awake, blind, or fiberoptically assisted intubation may be attempted. Basilar skull fractures contraindicate passage of nasal endotracheal or nasogastric tubes. Pelvic and femur fractures may be sources of significant (>1000 mL) occult blood loss.*

   e. Hematologic: *depending on estimations of prior, ongoing, and anticipated surgical blood losses, preoperative blood type and cross-match may be desired.*

2. Patient preparation

   a. Laboratory tests: *complete blood count, electrolytes, type and cross-match, and other tests as indicated from history and physical examination or suspected injuries*

   b. Diagnostic tests: *chest radiography, cervical spine radiography, and other tests as indicated from history and physical examination or suspected injuries*

c. Medication: *premedication is rarely useful because of the urgency of the procedures and the need to have an alert, responsive patient for serial evaluations of mental status or abdominal pain. Sedative premedication should be avoided in patients who are hemodynamically unstable and those with probable head injuries. Virtually all patients are considered to have a full stomach, and any compromise of the ability to protect the airway is inappropriate. Although sodium citrate may be administered to patients at risk for aspiration, histamine blockers and metoclopramide may not reach effective levels in the short interval before induction.*

C. Room preparation
1. Monitoring equipment
   a. *Standard monitoring equipment*
   b. *Arterial line as clinically indicated*
   c. *Central venous pressure or pulmonary arterial catheter as clinically indicated*
   d. *Foley catheter*
   e. *Nasogastric tube if indicated*
2. Additional equipment
   a. *Patient warming device*
   b. *Regular operating table*
   c. *Cell saver and rapid transfusion device if clinically indicated*
3. Drugs
   a. *Standard emergency drugs*
   b. *Standard tabletop*
   c. *Intravenous fluids: 16- to 18-gauge intravenous lines (2) with normal saline or lactated Ringer's solution at 8 to 10 mL/kg per hour. Warm fluids.*
   d. *Blood loss can be significant, and blood should be immediately available*

D. Anesthetic technique
General endotracheal anesthesia with full-stomach precautions.

E. Perioperative management
1. Induction
   Before induction, a variety of laryngoscope blades (Miller 1 and 2, Macintosh 3 and 4) and endotracheal tubes with styles (7.0 and 8.0 mm) should be ready. Most often, preoxygenation is followed by a rapid sequence intravenous induction with a cricoid pressure (Sellick's maneuver) using sodium thiopental (3 to 5 mg/kg) and succinylcholine (1.0 to 1.5 mg/kg). If hypotension is present or a concern, alternative induction agents (ketamine 0.5 to 2 mg/kg or etomidate 0.1 to 0.3 mg/kg) may be used. Axial head and neck traction is necessary if cervical spine injury is present or suspected.

   Patients who are profoundly hypotensive may enter the operating room already intubated. Induction consists of verifying endotracheal tube placement by auscultation and end-tidal carbon dioxide monitoring. Ventilation with 100% oxygen and muscle relaxation with pancuronium or vecuronium (0.1 mg/kg) is appropriate. Ongoing fluid resuscitation should be continued during this time.

2. Maintenance
   a. *Oxygen/air, muscle relaxants, narcotics, and volatile agents are titrated as tolerated. Avoid N_2O in the presence of pneumothorax, pneumocephalus, bowel distention, or prolonged procedures. Shorter-acting agents (volatile agents, fentanyl, vecuronium), carefully titrated, may be preferred with head injuries to facilitate early postoperative assessment of neurologic status. Heated humidifiers should be used, particularly in prolonged cases. Heating blankets and elevated room temperatures may also be necessary if hypothermia becomes problematic.*
   b. Position: *supine, check and pad pressure points. Avoid stretching the brachial plexus—limit abduction to 90°.*

3. Emergence
   Prior to extubation, the patient should be awake, able to protect the airway, and hemodynamically stable and spontaneously ventilating with ease through the endotracheal tube. Patients who should not be extubated at the end of the case include elderly persons with rib fractures, hemodynamically unstable patients, those who have received massive amounts of fluid, and those with coagulopathy.

F. Postoperative implications
1. Active warming of blood products, warming blankets, and warm room temperatures should be continued in the postanesthesia care unit if hypothermia persists.
2. Atelectasis, ventilation-perfusion mismatch
3. Pulmonary compliance is often increased with large volumes of fluid replacement. Pulmonary contusions may aggravate this problem and severely compromise oxygenation and ventilation, requiring high inspired oxygen concentration, high positive inspiratory pressure, and positive end-expiratory pressure.
4. Coagulopathy—coagulation products may be necessary according to platelet counts, prothrombin time and partial thromboplastin time, and ongoing red blood cell transfusion requirements
5. Pain management—patients with rib fractures benefit from epidural narcotic infusions

R. Anal Fistulotomy/ Fistulectomy

◆　◆　◆

A. Introduction
The great majority of perianal fistulae arise as a result of infection within the anal glands located at the dentate line (cryptoglandular fistula). Fistulae may also arise as the result of trauma, Crohn's disease,

inflammatory processes within the peritoneal cavity, neoplasms, or radiation therapy. The ultimate treatment of fistula-in-ano is determined by the etiology and the anatomic course of the fistula. The principle behind treatment of cryptoglandular fistulae is to excise the offending gland and lay open or excise all infected tissue. Fistulae that track above the majority of the sphincter mechanism must be treated by procedures that either do not cut the overlying sphincter, cut the sphincter and repair it, or cut the sphincter gradually. A fistula may be treated at the time of drainage of a perianal abscess or as a separate elective operation. The route of a fistula tract is best determined by exploration at the time of operation. Although local anesthesia is acceptable for simple fistulae with known routes, many fistula operations require regional or general anesthesia because the ultimate route and depth of the fistula will not be known. Special consideration is given to fistulae that arise in the setting of Crohn's disease. Poor wound healing, the likelihood of recurrent or multiple fistulae, and the premium on sphincter function in patients with chronic diarrhea dictate that only the most superficial fistulae can be laid open. The primary goal is palliation, specifically to drain abscesses and prevent their recurrence. This is often accomplished by placing a Silastic seton (a ligature placed around the sphincter muscles) around the fistula tract and leaving it in place indefinitely. In the absence of active Crohn's disease in the rectum, attempts at fistula cure may be undertaken.

B. Preoperative assessment
 1. History and physical examination
   a. Respiratory: *a careful evaluation of respiratory status is important. If the patient has decreased respiratory reserve, the lithotomy position may be better tolerated than the prone or jack-knife positions.*
   b. Musculoskeletal: *pain is likely at the surgical site and should be considered when positioning patient for anesthetic induction (if the patient has pain while sitting, perform regional anesthesia in the lateral decubitus position)*
   c. Hematologic: *if regional anesthesia is planned and the patient is taking acetylsalicylic acids, nonsteroidal anti-inflammatory drugs, or dipyridamole, check the platelet count and bleeding time*
 2. Patient preparation
   a. Laboratory tests: *as indicated per history and physical examination*
   b. Diagnostic tests: *as indicated per history and physical examination*
   c. Medication: *standard premedication*

C. Room preparation
 1. *Monitoring equipment:* standard
 2. *Additional equipment:* regular operating table
 3. Drugs
   a. *Standard emergency drugs*
   b. *Standard tabletop*
   c. *Intravenous fluids, 18-gauge, normal saline/lactated Ringer's at 5 to 8 mL/kg per hour*

D. Anesthetic technique
   General anesthesia; spinal or epidural techniques may be used.

E. Perioperative management
1. *Induction:* standard induction. Procedures done in the jack-knife position may require endotracheal intubation for airway control if a regional technique is not performed.
2. Maintenance
   a. *Standard maintenance*
   b. Position: *chest support or bolster to optimize ventilation in the jack-knife position; take care in positioning the patient's extremities and genitals after turning the patient into jack-knife position. Avoid pressure on the eyes and ears after turning the patient. Avoid stretching the brachial plexus—limit abduction to 90°.*
3. *Emergence:* no special consideration. Patient is extubated awake and after return of airway reflexes.

F. Postoperative implications
1. Lithotomy position can lead to damage to the peroneal nerve, which can lead to foot drop
2. Urinary retention
3. Poor wound healing
4. Atelectasis

S. Hemorrhoidectomy

◆ ◆ ◆

A. Introduction
Hemorrhoids are masses of vascular tissue found in the anal canal. Internal hemorrhoids are found above the pectinate line, arise from the superior hemorrhoidal venosus plexus, and are covered with mucosa. External hemorrhoids are found below the pectinate line, arise from the inferior hemorrhoidal venosus plexus, and are covered by anoderm and perianal skin.

B. Preoperative assessment and patient preparation
1. History and physical examination: *rectal:* bright red blood on toilet paper or surface of the stool; iron-deficiency anemia; prolapsed mass of tissue that protrudes from the anus; and thrombosis—blood clot within the hemorrhoidal vein, causing pain
2. *Diagnostic tests:* complete blood count
3. Preoperative medication and intravenous therapy
   a. *Consider a narcotic with premedication if the patient experiences pain*
   b. *18-gauge intravenous tube with minimal fluid replacement*

C. Room preparation
1. *Monitoring equipment:* standard
2. *Pharmacologic agents:* ephedrine
3. *Position:* prone or lithotomy

D. **Anesthetic techniques**
   1. Regional blockade and general anesthesia
   2. *Regional blockade:* analgesic to S2–S5 required
      a. *Hypobaric spinals—lithotomy position*
      b. *Hypobaric spinals—flexed prone or knee-chest position*
   3. *General anesthesia:* mask in lithotomy position (endotracheal intubation is necessary for the prone position)
E. **Perioperative management**
   1. Induction
      a. Prone: *general anesthesia induction performed on the stretcher*
      b. *Position the patient onto operating table with adequate support and padding of extremities, head, and neck*
      c. Spinal: *review principles of sympathetic blocks*
   2. Maintenance: *general anesthesia:* deep planes of anesthesia or muscle relaxants are required to relax the anal sphincter
   3. *Emergence:* if the prone position is used and general anesthesia is implemented, patients are usually repositioned onto the stretcher prior to emergence
F. **Postoperative implications: bearing down to void will be painful—keep fluids to a minimum**

Bibliography

Firestone LL, Lebowitz PW, Cook CE. *Clinical Anesthesia Procedures of the Massachusetts General Hospital.* Boston, MA: Little, Brown & Co.; 1982.

Thompson J, et al. *Mosby's Manual of Clinical Nursing.* 2nd ed. St. Louis, MO: C.V. Mosby Co.; 1989.

T. Adrenalectomy

◆ ◆ ◆

A. **Introduction**
   1. A procedure in which the glands are removed by sharp or blunt dissection. The left adrenal is exposed by manipulating the spleen and pancreas. The right adrenal is exposed by retracting the liver cephalad. Adrenal veins are exposed and ligated prior to removal.
   2. *Pathophysiology:* the procedure is performed for medullary or cortical tumors, Cushing's syndrome due to adrenal calcium or hyperplasia, pituitary hypersecretion, pheochromocytoma, primary hyperaldosteronism, and adenocarcinoma
B. **Preoperative assessment**
   1. History and physical examination
      a. Cardiac: *Cushing's syndrome: hypervolemia, hypertension, hypokalemia, polycythemia*
      b. Respiratory: *Cushing's syndrome may cause truncal obesity and*

buffalo hump. Assess for shortness of breath. May function as a restrictive disease.

    c. Neurologic: *Cushing's syndrome: headache, mood changes, psychosis, muscular wasting, possibly increased response to muscle relaxants*

    d. Renal: *Cushing's syndrome: Na retention and K^+ excretion, glucose intolerance from excess steroids*

    e. Gastrointestinal: *Cushing's syndrome: truncal obesity, muscle wasting. The patient may need rapid sequence induction and aspiration prophylaxis.*

    f. Endocrine: *Cushing's syndrome: hypokalemia, hyperglycemia, diabetes, excess steroid production, impaired Ca^{2+} absorption*

  2. Patient preparation

    a. Laboratory tests—*electrolytes, complete blood count, glucose*

    b. Diagnostic tests: *Cushing's syndrome will cause elevated plasma and urinary cortisol levels, plasma adrenocorticotropic hormone, and 17-hydroxycorticosteroids. Hyperadrenocorticism is diagnosed when endogenous cortisol is not suppressed after exogenous dexamethasone is given. Computed tomography or magnetic resonance imaging may be useful.*

    c. Medications—*Cushing's syndrome: Spironolactone inhibits excess aldosterone effects, mobilizes fluid, and increases K^+ level. Hydrocortisone dose: 100 mg every 8 hours.*

C. Room preparation

  1. *Monitoring equipment:* electrocardiogram, oxygen saturation, arterial line; consider monitoring central venous pressure and inserting a Foley catheter

  2. *Additional equipment:* Positioning devices: patient may be supine or in nephrectomy or prone jack-knife position. Careful padding is needed for Cushing's syndrome patients because of their easy bruisability, thin skin, and osteopenia.

  3. Drugs

    a. Continuous infusions. Intravenous fluids—large fluid loss is possible. Use isotonic crystalloid at 10 mL/kg per hour.

    b. Blood—*estimated blood loss is 200 to 300 mL, but can be significant. Type and crossmatch are needed.*

    c. Tabletop—standard. Have atropine available for unopposed parasympathetic response, lidocaine for ventricular arrhythmias (hypokalemia), syringes of vasoactive available (ephedrine).

D. Perioperative management and anesthetic technique

  1. *Induction:* thiopental (Pentothal) 3 to 5 mg/kg or etomidate 0.2 to 0.4 mg/kg depending on left-ventricular function. Use a nondepolarizer if rapid sequence induction is not used. Consider decreased muscle mass.

  2. *Maintenance:* volatile gas, opiates, muscle relaxant. Epidural anesthesia can improve surgical exposure by contracting the bowel.

  3. *Emergence:* The patient may be hemodynamically labile and may have large third-space fluid accumulation. Consider postoperative ventilation.

E. Postoperative complications

Complications include hypoadrenocorticism after tumor resection, hypoglycemia, pneumothorax, and hypertension. Continue steroid therapy after the procedure.

U. Pheochromocytoma

◆ ◆ ◆

A. Introduction

1. Surgical procedure is 90% curative; 10% to 25% of patients have bilateral tumors. Adrenalectomy is possible, depending on tumor location.
2. *Pathophysiology:* pheochromocytomas are highly vascular tumors associated with adrenal medulla chromaffin tissue that secrete mostly norepinephrine but also epinephrine. Tumors usually are in the abdomen (95%) but may be found anywhere that chromaffin tissue arises. They are malignant in 10% of patients. An inherited autosomal dominant trait is involved 5% of the time. These tumors can be associated with multiple endocrine neoplasia syndrome. They are most common in young to mid-adult life. Catecholamine release does not depend on neurogenic control.

B. Preoperative assessment

1. History and physical examination
   a. Cardiac: *paroxysmal severe hypertension, dysrhythmia, myocardial infarction, orthostatic hypotension, hypovolemia, catecholamine-induced cardiomyopathy, decreased sensitivity to catecholamines*
   b. Respiratory: *none*
   c. Neurologic: *cerebrovascular accident from hypertension, headache, tremors, sweating, hypertension retinopathy, mydriasis*
   d. Renal: *impairment from hypertension*
   e. Gastrointestinal: *none*
   f. Endocrine: *hyperglycemia*
2. Patient preparation
   a. Laboratory tests: *complete blood count—elevated hematocrit is common; electrolytes*
   b. Diagnostic tests: *electrocardiogram—left-ventricular hypertrophy and nonspecific T-wave changes are common; echocardiogram for left-ventricular function; chest radiography—assess cardiomegaly; magnetic resonance imaging or computed tomography to localize tumors; urinary vanilylmandelic acid, norepinephrine, and epinephrine levels usually are elevated in 24-hour collection*
   c. Medications: *alpha-adrenergic blockade is recommended 10 to 14 days prior to surgery. Use phenoxybenzamine 80 to 200 mg/day or prazosin 6 to 20 mg/day. Beta-blockers are added only after alpha-blockade to help manage tachydysrhythmias that are caused from*

alpha-blockade. If beta-blockers are begun prior to alpha-blockade, unopposed alpha response is possible.

C. Room preparation

1. *Monitoring equipment:* electrocardiogram, arterial line, oxygen saturation, pulmonary arterial catheter (optional), Foley catheter
2. *Additional equipment:* positioning devices—may be supine, nephrectomy, or prone jack-knife position, depending on whether incision is midline abdominal, bilateral subcostal, curved posterior, or dorsal flank oblique
3. Drugs
   a. *Continuous infusions—nitroprusside, phentolamine, and esmolol for severe hypertension and tachycardia during tumor manipulation. Hypotension after ligation of tumor's venous supply can be treated with phenylephrine, dopamine, and fluids.*
   b. Intravenous fluids: *prehydrate prior to surgery, because patient is usually intravascularly depleted. Large third-space loss and blood loss is possible; use isotonic fluids at 10 mL/kg per hour.*
   c. Blood: *type and cross-match 2 units of packed red blood cells*
   d. Tabletop: *have vasoactive drugs available for prompt treatment (lidocaine, nitroglycerine, nitroprusside, esmolol, phenylephrine). Syringe boluses may be used.*

D. Perioperative management and anesthetic technique

1. *Induction:* slow and controlled to avoid sympathetic nervous system response to laryngoscopy. One may pretreat with esmolol. Avoid histamine-releasing drugs, ketamine, or vagolytics.
2. *Maintenance:* avoid halothane for increased ventricular irritability. Use isoflurane or enflurane with intravenous opiates. Desflurane may increase the heart rate. Epidural combination can also be used; however, avoid using epinephrine in test dose.
3. *Emergence:* pay careful attention to labile hemodynamics

E. Postoperative complications

Catecholamine levels normalize in several days. Pneumothorax, hypoglycemia, cardiac dysfunction, hypoadrenocorticism are possible.

GENITOURINARY SYSTEM

A. Transurethral Resection of the Prostate

❖ ❖ ❖

A. Introduction

Application of a high-frequency current to a wire loop with fragments of obstructive tissue removed under direct endoscopic vision. Hemostasis is effected by sealing vessels with the coagulating current. Continuous irrigation with fluids is required to improve visibility through the cystoscope, distend the prostatic urethra, and maintain the operative field free of blood and dissected tissue. Glycine 1.5% or cytol 3.2% may be used.

B. Preoperative assessment and patient preparation

1. History and physical examination: elderly patient population—assess for coexisting medical diseases
2. Diagnostic tests
   a. *Blood urea nitrogen, creatinine, electrolytes*
   b. *Postpone procedure if serum sodium is 128 mEq/L or less*
3. Preoperative medication and intravenous therapy
   a. *Use an 18-gauge intravenous tube with minimal fluid replacement*
   b. *Antibiotics*

C. Room preparation

1. *Monitoring equipment:* standard
2. *Pharmacologic agents:* standard
3. *Position:* lithotomy

D. Anesthetic technique

1. Regional blockade or general anesthesia; for regional blockade, analgesia to T10 is required. An awake patient can provide early warning of complications (hypervolemia, hypernatremia).
2. *Technique of choice:* spinal anesthesia

E. Perioperative management

1. *Induction:* no specific indications
2. Maintenance
   a. Blood loss: *difficult to assess because the irrigating fluid dilutes the blood. The average loss is about 4 mL/min of resection time.*

    b. Intravascular absorption of irrigating fluid: *open venous sinuses of the prostate bed causes absorption of irrigating fluid. The primary determinants of fluid absorption are:*
        (1) Height of irrigation container
        (2) Number and size of venous sinuses opened
        (3) Duration of resection
    c. Limit resection time to less than 1 hour (10 to 30 mL of fluid is absorbed per minute of resection time) and monitor resection time closely
    d. Absorption of large volumes of irrigating fluids results in increased intravascular volume and dilutional hyponatremia with early symptoms of hypertension and reflex tachycardia. Symptoms in an awake patient include restlessness, nausea and vomiting, mental confusion, and visual disturbances.
  3. Treatment
    a. Terminate surgical procedure
    b. Send blood for serum Na^+; if Na^+ level is 120 mEq/L or less, administer furosemide and limit fluids
    c. If hyponatremia is severe with neurologic symptoms, administer hypertonic saline (3% to 5%) at a rate no faster than 100 mL/h
        (1) *Bladder perforation*—suspect perforation of prostatic capsule if irrigation fluid fails to return. Initial symptoms include hypertension and tachycardia followed by hypotension. An awake patient will experience suprapubic fullness and pain in the upper abdomen or referred from the diaphragm to the precordial region or shoulders
        (2) Prepare for a possible open surgical procedure
        (3) *Glycine toxicity*—a metabolite of glycine is ammonia. Glycine absorption can produce central nervous system symptoms such as mild depression, confusion, and transient blindness to coma
  4. *Emergence:* no specific indications
F. Postoperative considerations
Hyponatremia may not be suspected until postoperatively.

B. Extracorporeal Shock Wave Lithotripsy (ESWL)

◆ ◆ ◆

A. Introduction
Noninvasive technique that pulverizes renal stones with shock waves. Disintegrated stones are passed in the urine. Patients are placed in a hydraulically operated chair-lift device and submerged from the clavicles down into a tub of water. The impact of the shock waves at

the flank entry site is painful, requiring anesthesia. Procedure length is 30 to 90 minutes.

B. Preoperative assessment and patient preparation

1. Routine preoperative assessment with laboratory tests based on any abnormalities found in the history and physical examination. Consider cardiac status—many hemodynamic changes are associated with this procedure.
2. Relative contraindications include aortic aneurysm, spinal tumors, orthopedic implants in the lumbar region, pregnancy, morbid obesity, presence of a cardiac pacemaker, uncontrolled arrhythmias, and coagulation disorders incl. BLOOD THINNERS.
3. Urinary track obstruction distal to stone prevents passage of stone fragments and is an absolute contraindication
4. Ureteral stent placement prior to ESWL may be used to move the stone upward in the ureter, where it is amenable to therapy
5. Prophylactic antibiotics may be given

C. Room preparation

1. Lithotripsy suite may be located away from the main operating room. All anesthetizing equipment must be available.
2. Plan emergency and resuscitative measures in advance (emersed anesthetized patient)
3. Gas and monitor tubings must be long enough to extend between the patient in the tank and the anesthesia machine
4. Position the electrocardiogram electrode on the trunk and cover with transparent dressings—this results in less artifact. The R wave of the electrocardiogram is used to trigger shock waves.
5. To minimize treatment times, atropine may be used to increase the heart rate (continue with cardiac patients)
6. Use waterproof dressings to cover intravenous tubes and epidural catheters
7. Start an 18-gauge intravenous tube of dimenhydrinate (Hydrate) preoperatively to ensure passage of stones
8. Esophageal or precordial stethoscopes are impractical because of shock discharge noise
9. Have vasopressors available to treat hemodynamic changes
10. Monitor the temperature of the patient and bath—the bath should be kept at 37°C

D. Anesthetic techniques

Use local anesthetic with sedation; general or regional anesthesia usually is required.

E. Perioperative management

1. Regional anesthesia
   a. *Analgesia to T4 is required*
   b. *An awake patient can cooperate in positioning and requires less attachment of anesthetic equipment*
2. *Epidural anesthesia:* produces a slower onset of sympathetic block with less hypotension; can be used along with pre-ESWL cystoscopy and stent placement
3. *Spinal anesthesia:* results in more profound circulatory changes during positioning

4. General anesthesia
   a. *Preferred when close cardiopulmonary control is needed*
   b. *Intubation is mandatory*
   c. *Stones may move during ventilation of lungs—use low tidal volume and increase the respiratory rate*
5. Position
   a. *Patient is supported in a padded metal frame in a "lawn-chair position" and lowered into the water*
   b. *Allow shock waves to hit the kidneys and disintegrate stones but not to reach the lungs*
6. Considerations
   a. *Prevent patient movement—patient may be paralyzed if general anesthesia is used; sedate with regional anesthesia*
   b. *Hemodynamic responses to the procedure vary. Sitting position and warm water cause vasodilation, venous pooling, and decreased cardiac output. Immersion counteracts this—hydrostatic pressure on vessels increases venous return.*
   c. *Slowly remove the patient from the tub or profound hypotension may occur*
   d. *Pressure on the chest from immersion decreases vital capacity and functional reserve capacity and causes ventilation-perfusion mismatch*
   e. *Cardiac arrhythmias may occur during immersion or emergence because of rapid changes in hemodynamics and during the procedure from the discharge of shock waves independent of the cardiac cycle*
7. *Emergence:* use maintenance anesthesia or sedation until the patient is removed from the tub

F. Postoperative implications—none

C. Cystectomy

◆   ◆   ◆

A. Introduction

The bladder is usually removed for cancer but may also be removed for severe hemorrhagic or radiation cystitis. In a radical cystectomy for invasive cancer, the female's uterus, the fallopian tubes, the ovaries, and a portion of the vaginal wall are removed. In males, the ampulla of the vas deferens, prostate, and seminal vesicles are removed. There is also lymph node dissection, and a urinary diversion is created (via intestine).

B. Preoperative assessment

1. *Cardiac/respiratory/neurologic/endocrine:* routine. Keep in mind that these patients may be elderly.
2. *Renal:* gross hematuria may be a presenting symptom. Check renal function tests as well as evidence of a urinary tract infection.

3. *Gastrointestinal:* patients are at risk for fluid and electrolyte imbalance because of bowel preparation

C. **Patient preparation**
1. *Laboratory tests:* complete blood count, electrolytes, blood urea nitrogen, creatine, glucose, prothrombin time, partial thromboplastin time, type and screen for 2 to 4 units, urinalysis
2. *Diagnostic tests:* electrocardiography and chest radiography for most of this patient population
3. *Medication:* sedation as needed

D. **Room preparation**
1. Standard
2. *Monitors:* standard, arterial line, and central venous pressure. Urine output cannot be measured during this procedure. Have two large-bore, reliable intravenous lines.
3. *Additional equipment:* epidural insertion and infusion supplies, if using, and warming devices for the patient and fluids
4. *Positioning:* supine
5. *Drugs and fluids:* 6 to 10 mL/kg per hour of crystalloid for maintenance. Have 2 to 4 units of blood readily available.

E. **Perioperative management**   ⟶TOTₕ
Combined general/epidural or general anesthesia. Standard introduction. The patient may be anemic because of hematuria and hypovolemic because of bowel preparations. Attempt to correct these conditions before induction. Maintenance is routine, with special attention paid to fluid calculations and keeping the patient warm. Plan to extubate immediately postoperatively unless the patient is unstable during the procedure or prior respiratory complications prevent early extubation.

F. **Postoperative considerations**   JAFFE PAIN OP 10
Epidural or patient-controlled analgesia should be planned for preoperative use. Watch patients for signs of hypovolemia, anemia, or pulmonary edema due to fluid shifts intraoperatively.

D. Nephrectomy

♦ ♦ ♦

A. **Introduction**
Indications for nephrectomy include calculus, hemorrhage, hydronephrosis, hypertension, neoplasms, renal donation, trauma, and vascular disease. Partial nephrectomy is performed to preserve as much renal function as possible. Surgery of the kidney is usually accomplished through a flank incision.

B. Preoperative assessment and patient preparation
 1. History and physical examination (based on renal disease
    potentials)
    a. Respiratory: *pulmonary edema, pleural effusions*
    b. Cardiac: *pericarditis, congestive heart failure, hypertension, capillary
       fragility, dysrhythmias (abnormal electrolytes)*
    c. Neurologic: *peripheral neuropathy, lethargy*
    d. Renal: *decreased renal blood flow and glomerular filtration rate*
    e. Gastrointestinal: *nausea, vomiting; ileus, peptic, and colonic
       ulceration*
    f. Endocrine: *glucose intolerance, pancreatitis; parahormone,
       aldosterone antidiuretic hormone and growth hormonal alterations*
    g. Musculoskeletal: *generalized muscle weakness, metastatic
       calcification, gout*
    h. Integument: *pruritus, hyperpigmentation*
    i. Hematologic: *anemia, diminished erythrocyte survival, platelet
       dysfunction, shift in P_{50} of oxyhemoglobin dissociation curve*
       (right → acidosis)
 2. Diagnostic tests
    a. Intravenous pyelography with nephrotomography: *identify
       renal mass*
    b. Ultrasonography: *differentiates simple cysts from solid tumor*
    c. Arteriography: *determine suitable kidney for renal transplantation*
    d. Computed tomography
    e. Laboratory tests
       (1) Prothrombin time, partial thromboplastin time, complete
          blood count, electrolytes, glucose
       (2) Glomerular filtration rate
          (a) Blood urea nitrogen
          (b) Plasma creatinine
          (c) Creatinine clearance
       (3) Renal tubular function
          (a) Urine concentration ability
          (b) Sodium secretion
          (c) Proteinuria
          (d) Hematuria urine sediment
          (e) Urine volume
 3. Preoperative medications and intravenous therapy
    a. Discuss date of last hemodialysis
    b. Epidural catheter: *perform test dose in preoperative area*
    c. Antibiotics
    *d. Small incremental doses of benzodiazepines to ease operating room
       preparation*
    *e. Minimum of two peripheral intravenous tubes (18- and 16-gauge)
       with moderate fluid replacement*
C. Room preparation
 1. Monitoring equipment
    *a. A line and central venous pressure monitoring may be necessary to
       trend volume status, especially if the patient is elderly with coexisting
       medical disease*

   b. *Noninvasive blood pressure cuff (if used) not in a line with arteriovenous fistula*
2. Pharmacologic agents
   a. *Dopamine—low dose (2 to 5 μg/kg) to increase urinary output*
   b. *Furosemide (Lasix) and/or mannitol for stimulation of urinary output*
   c. *Indigo carmine or methylene blue administration (intravenously to assess urinary flow)*
   d. *Hetastarch (Hespan)/albumin*
   e. *With renal failure patients, administer hypotonic solutions: 5% dextrose in water or 5% dextrose and 0.45% saline*
      (1) Avoid normal saline—may increase sodium levels
      (2) Avoid plasmolyte or lactated Ringer's solution—may increase K^+ levels
      (3) Restrict fluids, and consider using microdrip tubing
   f. *Heparin and protamine—with donor kidneys*
3. Position
   a. *Lateral decubitus position with the kidney bar raised and the table fluid*
   b. *With low calcium levels, skin and nerve damage occur easily*
   c. *Inadequate support of the head may lead to Horner's syndrome postoperatively*
   d. *Evaluate radial pulse after placement of axillary roll*
   e. *Respiration is impaired secondary to ventilation-perfusion mismatching, decreased functional reserve capacity, decreased vital capacity, and decreased thoracic compliance*
   f. *Reassess breath sounds post-movement; an endotracheal tube may migrate into the mainstem bronchus during positioning*

D. Anesthetic techniques
1. Regional blockade, general anesthesia, or a combination of both
2. *Technique of choice:* general anesthesia with endotracheal intubation because the flank position results in significant hemodynamic compromise and general discomfort
3. *Regional blockade:* epidural catheter placement preoperatively; analgesia to T6–T8
4. *General anesthesia:* endotracheal intubation
5. *Regional blockade with general anesthesia:* smaller doses of each are needed

E. Perioperative management
1. Induction
   a. *Opioids can be used because only a small amount of the drug is excreted unchanged by the kidneys*
   b. *Succinylcholine is contraindicated if K^+ is elevated*
   c. *Atracurium does not require a functional kidney because it is degraded by ester hydrolysis and Hoffman elimination*
   d. *Vecuronium (Norcuron) has a kidney metabolism rate of 10% to 20%*
   e. *Regardless of blood volume status, renal patients may respond to induction of anesthesia as if they are hypovolemic*
   f. *Induction of anesthesia and intubation of the trachea can be safely accomplished with intravenous drugs plus a nondepolarized muscle relaxant*

2. Maintenance
   a. Maintain normal end-tidal carbon dioxide levels
   b. If working on a donor nephrectomy, expect the 11th rib to be removed—pneumothorax is a complication; therefore, nitrous oxide is best avoided
   c. Maintain urinary output—use medications if necessary
   d. Volatile anesthetic is used to control intraoperative hypertension
3. Emergence
   a. If hypertension occurs on emergence, administer a vasodilator
   b. Renal patients are considered to have a full stomach, so some practitioners require an "awake" patient prior to extubation
   c. Initiate regional blockade through the epidural catheter for postoperative analgesia prior to the end of the case

F. Postoperative implications
1. Continue to assess volume status
2. Obtain chest film—rule out pneumothorax or pulmonary edema, which may occur after administration of large volumes of fluid in the flank position
3. For renal failure patients, normeriperidine, the major metabolite of meripidine, may accumulate and result in prolonged depression of ventilation and seizures

E. Cystoscopy

◆   ◆   ◆

A. Introduction
The use of instrumentation to examine the urinary tract. A cystoscope may be used for diagnostic or therapeutic procedures, such as the work-up of hematuria, structure, and tumor; removal and manipulation of stones; placement of stents; and follow-up of therapy. Retrograde pyelography and other dye studies may be used. This procedure is usually performed on outpatient basis.

B. Preoperative assessment and patient preparation
1. History and physical examination: standard
2. Diagnostic tests: standard
3. Preoperative medication and intravenous therapy
   a. Prophylactic antibiotics
   b. 18-gauge intravenous tube with minimal fluid replacement

C. Room preparation
1. Monitoring equipment: standard
2. Pharmacologic agents: indigo carmine, methylene blue
3. Position: lithotomy

D. Anesthetic techniques
1. Intramuscular opioid premedication, topical anesthetic jelly, intravenous sedation, regional blockade, and general anesthesia

2. Technique of choice—regional blockade or general anesthesia
   a. *Intravenous sedation: versed, fentanyl, or propofol in sedation doses*
   b. Regional blockade: *analgesia to T9 required*
   c. General anesthesia: *administered by mask or oral endotracheal tube*

E. Preoperative management
1. *Induction:* no specific indications
2. Maintenance
   a. *Diagnostic dyes may be administered. Use indigo carmine dye (alpha-sympathomimetic effects) cautiously with hypertension or cardiac ischemia. Methylene blue dye may cause hypertension. Oxygen saturation readings may be altered by dye administration.*
   b. *Persistent erection may occur in younger males, preventing manipulation of the cystoscope—use deeper anesthesia*
   c. *Water or irrigation solution may be used to distend the bladder (see Chapter A in this section)*
   d. *Quadriplegics or paraplegics may undergo repeated cystoscopies—autonomic hyper-reflexia is possible if the injury is above level T5*
3. *Emergence:* no specific indications

F. Postoperative considerations—none

F. Radical Prostatectomy

◆ ◆ ◆

A. Introduction

Open prostatectomy refers to removal of the prostate with or without the prostatic capsule. Several surgical approaches may be used, including suprapubic, transvesical, retropubic, perineal, and transcoccygeal. In the suprapubic or transvesical procedures the prostate is removed through the cavity of the bladder. Retropubic prostatectomy is performed through a low abdominal incision without opening the bladder. The transcoccygeal approach allows maximal surgical access to the posterior lobes of the prostate. Perineal prostatectomy is most often performed for cancer of the prostate when it is confined to the capsule.

B. Preoperative assessment and patient preparation
1. *History and physical examination:* symptoms of metastatic disease include bone pain, weight loss, spinal cord compression, and acute renal failure secondary to bilateral hydronephrosis
2. Diagnostic tests
   a. *Plasma concentration of prostate-specific antigen is increased in prostate cancer*

COMMON PROCEDURES

      b. *Blood urea nitrogen, creatinine, electrolytes, complete blood count, prothrombin time, partial thromboplastin time, type and cross-match*

      c. *Ultrasonography*

   3. Preoperative medication and intravenous therapy

      a. *Bowel preparation will render the patient in a dehydrated state*

      b. *Minimum of two peripheral intravenous lines (18- and 16-gauge) with moderate fluid replacement*

      c. *Epidural catheter—perform test dose in preoperative area*

      d. *Antibiotics*

      e. *Small incremental doses of benzodiazepines may be given to ease patient preparation*

C. Room preparation

   1. Monitoring equipment

      a. *A line and central venous pressure monitoring may be necessary to tend volume status, especially if the patient is elderly with coexisting medical diseases*

      • b. *Warning modalities*

   2. Pharmacologic agents

      a. *Dopamine—may need low dose (2 to 5 $\mu g/kg$) to increase urinary output*

      b. *Hetastarch (Hespan) and albumin*

   3. *Position:* supine—surgeon may request use of kidney rest and for the patient's body to be partially fluxed. Expect to need to rotate the patient from side to side for optimal surgical viewing.

D. Anesthetic techniques

   1. *Regional blockade,* general anesthesia, or a combination of both

   2. *Technique of choice:* general anesthesia with endotracheal intubation

   3. *Regional blockade:* epidural catheter placement in preoperative area; analgesia to T6–T8

   4. *General anesthesia:* endotracheal intubation

   5. *Regional blockade with general anesthesia:* smaller doses of each with combination technique

E. Perioperative management

   1. *Induction:* The patient may be dehydrated and show an exaggerated response to medications

   2. Maintenance

      a. *Initiate warming modality*

      b. *The Foley catheter is discontinued during the case, and volume status (blood loss) is difficult to quantify*

      c. *Muscle relaxation is necessary*

   3. Emergence

      a. *Initiate regional blockade through the epidural catheter for postoperative analgesia prior to the end of the case*

      b. *Base extubation on the patient's general health, amount of blood loss, and overall status after the procedure*

      c. *An awake or deep extubation may be appropriate*

F. Postoperative implications

   1. Obtain hemoglobin and hematocrit

   2. Continue to trend volume status

G. Dilation and Curettage

• • •

A. Introduction

Dilation and curettage is the expansion of the cervix and scraping of the uterine endometrium. It is performed for diagnostic or therapeutic purposes, such as the removal of retained products of conception.

B. Preoperative assessment and patient preparation

1. *History and physical examination:* for an incomplete abortion, women may complain of:
   a. *Bleeding—vaginal hemorrhage*
   b. *Pain—pelvic and low back*
   c. *Infection—foul odor of vaginal drainage, fever, and hematuria*
2. Diagnostic tests
   a. *Laboratory tests include: serum human chorionic gonadotropin, hemoglobin and hematocrit, electrolytes, and type and screen*
   b. *Ultrasonography*
3. Preoperative medication and intravenous therapy
   a. *The patient can be lightly sedated with the use of benzodiazepines and short-acting narcotics because the procedure lasts less than 20 minutes*
   b. *Aspiration prophylaxis*
   c. *One 18-gauge intravenous line with minimal fluid replacement*

C. Room preparation

1. *Monitoring equipment:* standard
2. *Pharmacologic agents:* standard
3. *Position:* lithotomy

D. Anesthetic techniques

1. Local infiltration, regional blockade, and general anesthesia
2. Technique of choice—general anesthesia
   a. Regional blockade: *analgesia to T6–T8*
   b. General: *may be administered by mask (preferred) or endotracheal intubation (e.g., full stomach, poor airway, obesity)*

E. Perioperative management

1. *Induction:* consider rapid sequence induction with an obese patient or a patient with a full stomach
2. *Maintenance:* gynecologic procedures may cause nausea and vomiting. Consider administration of droperidol (Inapsine) and low-dose N_2O.
3. *Emergence:* if rapid sequence induction is used, awake extubation is indicated

F. Postoperative implications—none

Bibliography

Schnider SM, Levinson G. *Anesthesia for Obstetrics.* Baltimore, MD: Williams & Wilkins; 1987.

Thompson J, et al. *Mosby's Manuel of Clinical Nursing.* 2nd ed. St. Louis, MO: C.V. Mosby Co.; 1989.

COMMON PROCEDURES

H. Vulvectomy

* * *

A. Introduction

Cancer of the vulva usually strikes women in their 60s or 70s. Radical vulvectomies are done for invasive cancers. The incision and excised portion can reach to the groin, necessitating skin grafts.

B. Preoperative assessment

1. *Cardiac/Respiratory/Neurologic/Endocrine/Renal:* routine, keeping in mind that these women most likely are elderly.
2. *Gastrointestinal:* fluid and electrolyte imbalance are a risk because of bowel preparation.

C. Patient preparation

1. *Laboratory tests:* complete blood count, electrolytes, blood urea nitrogen, creatinine, glucose, prothrombin time, partial thromboplastin time, urinalysis, type and cross-match for 2 to 4 units
2. *Diagnostic tests:* electrocardiography and chest radiography for most of this patient population
3. *Medication:* sedation as needed

D. Room preparation

1. *Monitors:* standard, Foley, arterial line. Use central venous pressure or pulmonary arterial catheter if history warrants.
2. *Additional equipment:* epidural insertion and infusion supplies, if using; warming devices for patients and fluids
3. *Position:* lithotomy
4. *Drugs and fluids:* 6 mL/kg per hour of crystalloid for maintenance. Have 2 to 4 units of blood readily available.

E. Anesthesia and perioperative management

General/epidural or general: If history warrants, regional anesthesia is option. Patients may be anemic because of hematuria, hypovolemic because of bowel preparations, or both. Attempt to correct these conditions before instituting regional anesthesia or induction. Maintenance is routine with special attention paid to fluid calculations and keeping the patient warm. Plan to extubate immediately postoperatively.

F. Postoperative considerations

Epidural or patient-controlled analgesia should be planned for preoperative use. Watch patients for signs of hypovolemia, anemia, or pulmonary edema due to fluid shifts intraoperatively.

I. Penile Procedures

* * *

A. Introduction

Penile procedures are usually done for three different indications. First, for congenital defect—hypospadias, which is usually a pediatric procedure. Second, for penectomy/penile resection as a result of penile cancer. Third, for implants to compensate for impotence. Organic impotence is often secondary to diabetes, hypertension and its treatment, or spinal cord trauma.

B. Preoperative assessment

1. *Cardiac:* pay special attention to the presence of hypertension and compliance with antihypertensive medications (many have impotence as a side effect)

2. *Neurologic:* if the patient is impotent as a result of spinal cord trauma, assess for level of injury and history of autonomic hyper-reflexia

3. *Renal/Genitourinary:* if hypospadias is present, assess for history of frequent urinary tract infections. If penile cancer is present, assess for history of lymph-node involvement or known metastasis.

4. *Endocrine:* assess for history of diabetes, level of compliance, and usual blood glucose values

C. Patient preparation

Twelve-lead electrocardiography is indicated for patients with hypertension, electrolytes for those on diuretics. Glucose level must be monitored on the day of surgery for all diabetic patients. Preoperatively, most patients will benefit from an anxiolytic, such as midazolam. Pediatric patients (usually over the age of 1 year) may receive midazolam orally 30 minutes prior to surgery.

D. Room preparation

1. *Monitoring:* standard

2. *Position:* supine

3. *Drugs and tabletop:* atropine and succinylcholine should be drawn up on the tabletop for pediatric cases

E. Anesthesia and perioperative management

For pediatric patients, use an inhaled induction for general anesthetic. Intubation is desired because hypospadias repair generally takes longer than 2 hours. For penectomy or prosthetic insertion, regional or general anesthetic may be used, depending on the preferences of the patient and anesthetist and on the medical condition. Muscle relaxation is not required, and blood loss is minimal. Some practitioners will perform a caudal block for pediatric patients just prior to awakening for postoperative pain control.

F. Postoperative implications

Urinary retention is common and may be intensified with use of a regional anesthetic.

J. Scrotal Procedures

♦ ♦ ♦

A. Introduction

Scrotal procedures are considered minor operative procedures and can be done on an outpatient basis unless there are pre-existing medical conditions. In adults, most elective scrotal procedures can be done under local anesthesia with sedation. The most common procedures include surgery for infertility, hydrocele, undescended testicle, or orchiectomy for cancer.

The most common emergency scrotal surgery is for testicular torsion. These patients will be in acute pain and should be considered to be on a full stomach.

B. Preoperative assessment

Most patients who present for infertility concerns, hydrocele, and minor procedures are essentially healthy. Those who present for orchidectomy require careful preoperative evaluation for possible metastasis.

No specific laboratory tests or medications are required except those that are suggested from the preoperative evaluation.

C. Room preparation

1. *Monitoring:* standard
2. *Positioning:* supine. Arms usually are out at the sides. Lithotomy position may be requested.
3. *Drugs and tabletop:* sedatives and narcotics. Tabletop should be set up for emergency general anesthetic.

D. Anesthesia and perioperative management

The patient may receive local anesthesia with sedation, regional anesthesia, or general anesthesia depending on condition and anesthetist preference. There are no specific considerations because muscle relaxation is not required and blood loss is minimal.

E. Postoperative considerations

Pain management may be commenced intraoperatively by use of narcotics, ketorolac, or both. Some patients, especially if being treated for malignancy, may experience nausea and vomiting.

NEUROSKELETAL SYSTEM

A. Lumbar Laminectomy

◆ ◆ ◆

A. Introduction

Lumbar laminectomy is most commonly performed for symptomatic nerve root or cord compression. Compression may occur from protrusion of an intervertebral disk or osteophyte bone into the spinal canal. An intervertebral disk usually herniates at the L4–L5 or L5–S1 intervertebral spaces.

B. Preoperative assessment and patient preparation

1. History and physical examination: *neurologic:* assess and document neurologic deficits of lower extremities
2. *Diagnostic tests:* type and screen blood, T + S, complete blood count
3. Preoperative medication and intravenous therapy
    a. *Consider a narcotic with premedication if the patient experiences pain*
    b. *Use a 16- or 18-gauge intravenous tube with minimal fluid replacement*

C. Room preparation

1. *Monitoring equipment:* standard
2. *Pharmacologic agents:* vasopressors, steroids, antibiotic
3. Position
    a. *Prone, lateral, knee-chest*
    b. *Have doughnut, axillary roll, and indicated padding available*
    c. *Specially designed frames may be used to aid in positioning*

D. Anesthetic techniques

1. Local infiltration, regional blockade, and general anesthesia
2. Technique of choice—general anesthesia
    a. Regional blockade: *analgesia to T7–T8 is required; regional anesthesia cannot be used if nerve function will be tested*
    b. Epidural: *must be in single dose with the catheter removed*
    c. Spinal: *hypotension may be accentuated with position change*

E. Perioperative management

1. Induction
    a. *If the prone or knee-chest position is used, anesthesia is inducted on the stretcher*
    b. *Position changes may be done in stages to avoid hemodynamic compromise. A vasopressor may be needed to treat hypotension.*

       c. Tape the endotracheal tube to the side of the mouth that will be positioned up

  2. Maintenance

      a. Question the surgeon regarding the use of muscle relaxants. Nerve function may be tested. An intermediate nondepolarizing muscle relaxant may be used for induction

      b. Blood loss is rarely sufficient to necessitate deliberate hypotension. The wound may be infiltrated with an epinephrine solution to decrease intraoperative blood loss.

      c. The wound may be infiltrated with a local anesthetic to decrease postoperative pain

  3. *Emergence:* extrication is performed when the patient is supine. The patient may need to be awake at the end of the procedure to allow the surgeon to assess for neurologic deficits.

F. Postoperative considerations

The patient can usually be transported in any position because stability of the back is rarely compromised.

B. Anterior Cervical Diskectomy/Fusion

❖ ❖ ❖

A. Introduction

Anterior cervical fusion is most commonly performed for symptomatic nerve root or cord compression. Compression may occur from protrusion of an intervertebral disk or osteophytic bone into the spinal canal. An intervertebral disk usually herniates at the fifth or sixth cervical levels. A bone graft may be taken from the iliac chest.

B. Preoperative assessment and patient preparation

  1. Airway assessment should include thorough assessment of the range of motion of the neck. Neurologic deficits should be documented. Neurologic deficits with limited neck movement may require intubation with the head in a neutral position. Limited neck mobility may require special intubation techniques.

  2. Patients may have considerable pain preoperatively and require a narcotic with premedication. If a difficult airway is anticipated premedication should be used sparingly.

JAFFE PASN
3-4/10

C. Room preparation

  1. Standard tabletop setup

  2. Supine position, arms tucked at side; a small roll may be placed under the shoulders. A doughnut may be placed under the head.

  3. Use a single 18-gauge intravenous with minimal fluid replacement

[handwritten margin notes:] IF TENSION PNEUMO FROM MAJOR ENTRAINMENT OR OROPHARYNGEAL LAC 18ga NEEDLE IN 2nd ICS · IF AIRWAV OBSTRUCTION 2° TO BLOOD IN WOUND REOPEN & EVACUATE, DON'T REINTUBATE 5/8 : PPV EXHALING IS SLOW 5/5 : PPV EXHALING IS FAST.

D. Perioperative managment and anesthetic techniques
1. General anesthesia with endotracheal intubation
2. Tape tube to the side opposite of where the surgeon stands—keep tape out of the sterile field
3. Wound retraction may impinge on the airway or carotidal artery. Palpate the temporal artery to monitor for carotidal artery occlusion.
4. Ask the surgeon if muscle relaxation may be used because nerve function may need to be assessed *[handwritten:]* NMR DOSE ×1 AT BEGINNING IS HELPFUL
5. Administer lidocaine prior to extubation. Prevent coughing or bucking on the tube. The neck must remain in a neutral position. A neck brace may be applied. Extubate prior to application of the neck brace—jaw lift may be required. The patient should be awake before leaving the operating suite because the surgeon may want to assess neurologic function.
6. If a nerve stimulator is used on the face, limit twitch application to when the surgeon is not operating—the face may move with twitches

[handwritten:] - SHOULDER ROLL, TONGS + TRACTION 5 -10, OR STRAP ON CHIN AND OCCIPUT

C. Posterior Spinal Instrumentation and Fusion

♦   ♦   ♦

A. Introduction

Posterior spinal instrumentation refers to implanted metal rods affixed to the spine to correct and internally splint the deformed spine. Originally designed for scoliosis, posterior spinal instrumentation is commonly performed simultaneously with spinal fusion for a variety of diagnoses, including fracture, tumor, degenerative changes, and developmental spinal deformity. The original Harrington rod is the simplest and still considered by many to be the standard.

Harrington rodding or similar extensive surgical procedures to correct spinal column deformities put the spinal cord at risk for ischemia secondary to mechanical compression of its blood supply. This complication has been mitigated with methods to assess spinal cord function intraoperatively. These include "wake-up" intraoperative testing of neurologic function and sensory evoked potential monitoring. Wake-up testing requires an informed cooperative patient and a practice trial of patient responses after awake positioning, and it may necessitate complete or partial reversal of muscle relaxants and other anesthetic drugs. Problems with awake testing, beyond ensuring a cooperative patient, include recall, coughing that may disrupt the surgical correction, and inadvertent tracheal extubation.

B. Preoperative assessment

Patients presenting for spinal reconstruction usually have either idiopathic or acquired scoliosis. Scoliosis is a complex deformity involving both lateral curvature and rotation of the spine, as well as an associated deformity of the rib cage. Types of scoliosis include idiopathic, congenital, neuromuscular, myopathic, trauma, tumor-related, and mesenchymal disorders. Most cases are idiopathic and the male-to-female ratio is 1:4. Normally, the cervical spine and lumbar spine are lordotic, whereas the thoracic spine is kyphotic. Surgery is indicated when the curvature is severe (angulation beyond 40° in the thoracic or lumbar spine) or progressing rapidly. Nonscoliotic patients presenting for this surgery may have spinal instability as a result of trauma, metastatic carcinoma, or infection. These patients are usually healthy apart from their underlying pathology. The patients with disseminated lung or breast cancer may need a careful work-up with regard to respiratory, nutritional, and chemotherapeutic status.

1. History and physical examination
    a. Cardiovascular: *high incidence of congestive heart disease. Pulmonary vascular resistance is increased independent of the severity of scoliosis.*
    b. Respiratory: *respiratory impairment proportional to angle of lateral curvature. There is a restrictive pattern (decreased total lung capacity and vital capacity). If vital capacity is greater than 70% predicted, respiratory reserve is adequate. If vital capacity is less than 40% predicted, postoperative ventilation usually is required.*
    c. Neurologic: *some surgeons may request that the patient be awakened intraoperatively to test anterior cord funtion. Practice wake-up testing preoperatively to reveal any baseline deficits and reassure the patient that no pain will be felt during intraoperative testing. Tuberculosis spondylitis frequently presents with focal neurologic lesions ranging from loss of bowel and bladder control to paraplegia. Careful preoperative documentation of the neurologic status is essential because surgery may worsen these symptoms.*
    d. Musculoskeletal: *when the angle of lateral curvature of the spine is greater than 25°, the degree of respiratory impairment will be significant and postoperative ventilatory support becomes more likely. Patients with muscular dystrophy may be more sensitive to myocardial depression from anesthetic agents and may require postoperative ventilation secondary to muscle weakness. Succinylcholine may cause severe rhabdomyolysis with hyperkalemia. These patients may also be at risk for malignant hyperthermia.*
    e. Hematologic: *avoid use of platelet inhibitors for 2 to 3 weeks before surgery. Encourage autologous blood donation. Consider use of intraoperative hemodilution, controlled hypotension, and cell saver devices.*
2. Patient preparation
    a. Laboratory tests: *complete blood count, prothrombin time, partial thromboplastin time, arterial blood gases, electrolytes, and other tests as indicated per history and physical examination*

   b. Diagnostic tests: *chest radiographs, pulmonary function test, spine studies, and other tests as indicated per history and physical examination*
   c. Medication: *standard premedication, if appropriate*
C. Room preparation
   1. Monitoring equipment
      a. *Standard monitoring equipment*
      b. *Arterial line*
      c. *Foley catheter*
      d. *Central venous pressure line if indicated*
   2. Additional equipment
      a. *Patient-warming device*
      b. *Cell saver*
      c. *Somatosensory evoked potential monitor, if indicated*
      d. *Regular operating table with spinal frame or bolster*
   3. Drugs
      a. *Standard emergency drugs, standard tabletop*
      b. *Intravenous fluids via 16- to 18-gauge intravenous with normal saline at 8 to 10 mL/kg per hour with fluid warmer*
      c. *Blood loss can be significant, and blood should be immediately available*
D. Anesthetic technique
   General endotracheal anesthesia. For pediatric cases, preheat room to 78°F.
E. Perioperative management
   1. *Induction:* standard
   2. Maintenance
      a. *Standard maintenance. It is important to use low concentrations and minimize changes of potent inhalational agents during measurement of somatosensory evoked potentials. Continue muscle relaxation. Droperidol is avoided because its alpha-blocking effect reduces the effectiveness of the epinephrine injected at the beginning of surgery to reduce incisional bleeding.*
      b. Position: *prone on spinal frame or bolster. Avoid abdominal compression. Check eyes and neck. Check and pad pressure points. Pressure points must be carefully padded and checked frequently, especially during controlled hypotension.*
      c. Wake-up test: *needs 40 to 60 minutes advance warning from the surgeon; decrease inhalational agents; reverse muscle relaxants and narcotics if necessary; monitor train of four; request hand squeeze; if present, elicit bilateral foot movement. Uncontrolled patient movement during a wake-up test can result in accidental extubation or dislodgement of the spinal instrumentation. Unrestrained inspiratory efforts may provoke venous air embolism. The anesthetist must be prepared to rapidly reanesthetize the patient.*
      d. *Somatosensory evoked potential indications of spinal cord ischemia should be treated by restoring normal blood pressure and by decreased cord traction. Prompt transfusion may be necessary, and blood should be available in the room.*

COMMON PROCEDURES

F. Postoperative implications
1. Pulmonary insufficiency—postoperative ventilation may be required in patients with severe respiratory impairment.
2. Neurologic sequelae—neurologic sequelae probably remain the most feared complication, and it is important to document the postoperative neurologic examination
3. Hypothermia
4. Pneumothorax
5. Dislodgement of internal fixation

D. Spinal Cord Injuries

✦ ✦ ✦

A. Introduction
Spinal cord transection is the description of damage to the spinal cord manifested as paralysis of the lower extremities (paraplegia) or all the extremities (quadriplegia). Spinal cord transection above the level of C2–C4 is incompatible with survival, because innervation to the diaphragm is likely to be destroyed.

The most common cause of spinal cord transection is the trauma associated with a motor vehicle or diving accident, resulting in fracture dislocation of cervical vertebrae. Occasionally, rheumatoid arthritis of the spine leads to spontaneous dislocation of the C1 vertebra on the C2 vertebra, producing progressive quadriparesis. These patients can suddenly become quadriplegic. The most frequent nontraumatic cause of spinal cord transection is multiple sclerosis. In addition, infections or vascular and developmental disorders may be responsible for permanent damage to the spinal cord.

B. Preoperative assessment
Spinal cord transection initially produces flaccid paralysis, with total absence of sensation below the level of injury. In addition, temperature regulation and spinal cord reflexes are lost below the level of injury. The phase after the acute transection of the spinal cord is known as spinal shock and typically lasts 1 to 3 weeks. Several weeks after acute transection of the spinal cord, the spinal cord reflexes gradually return, and patients enter a chronic stage, characterized by overactivity of the sympathetic nervous system and involuntary skeletal muscle spasms. Mental depression and pain are pressing problems after spinal cord injury.
1. History and physical examination
   a. Cardiovascular: *electrocardiographic abnormalities are common during the acute phase of spinal cord transection and include ventricular premature beats and ST–T wave changes suggestive of myocardial ischemia. Decreased systemic blood pressure and bradycardia are also*

common secondary to loss of sympathetic tone. Generally, this condition can be treated effectively with crystalloid and colloid infusion and atropine to increase the heart rate. Around 85% of patients with spinal cord transection above T6 exhibit autonomic hyper-reflexia, a disorder that appears after the resolution of spinal shock and in association with the return of the spinal cord reflexes.

b. Respiratory: spontaneous ventilation is impossible if the level of spinal cord transection results in paralysis of the diaphragm. A transection between the levels of C2 and C4 may result in apnea due to denervation of the diaphragm. The ability to cough and clear secretions from the airway is often impaired because of decreased expiratory reserve volume. Vital capacity also is significantly decreased if the transection of the spinal cord is at the cervical level. Furthermore, arterial hypoxemia is a consistent early finding during the period after cervical spinal cord injury. Tracheobronchial suctioning has been associated with bradycardia and cardiac arrest in these patients, emphasizing the importance of establishing optimal arterial oxygenation before undertaking this maneuver. Acute respiratory insufficiency and the inability to handle oropharyngeal secretions necessitates immediate tracheal intubation. Before intubation is initiated, the neck must be stabilized. The objective is to not flex or extend the head or move it laterally during the course of tracheal intubation.

c. Neurologic: patients with spinal cord trauma at the T1 level are paraplegic, whereas traumas above C5 may result in quadriplegia and loss of phrenic nerve function. Injuries between these two levels result in varying loss of motor and sensory functions in the upper extremities. A careful documentation of preoperative sensory and motor deficits is important.

d. Musculoskeletal: prolonged immobility leads to osteoporosis, skeletal muscle atrophy, and the development of decubitus ulcers. Pathologic fractures can occur when these patients are moved. Pressure points should be well protected and padded to minimize the likelihood of trauma to the skin and the development of decubitus ulcers.

e. Renal: renal failure is the leading cause of death in the patient with chronic spinal cord transection. Chronic urinary tract infections and immobilization predispose to the development of renal calculi. Amyloidosis of the kidney can be manifested as proteinuria, leading to a decrease in the concentration of albumin in the plasma.

2. Patient preparation
   a. Laboratory tests: arterial blood gases to substantiate the degree of respiratory impairment, urinalysis, complete blood count, prothrombin time, partial thromboplastin time, electrolytes, and other tests as indicated per history and physical examination
   b. Diagnostic tests: computed tomography, magnetic resonance imaging, radiography of the injured parts, and other tests as indicated per history and physical examination
   c. Medications: premedication is useful in this patient population. Midazolam and fentanyl prior to entering the operating room makes patients amnestic and tractable.

COMMON PROCEDURES

C. Room preparation

1. Monitoring equipment
   a. *Standard monitoring equipment*
   b. *Foley catheter*
   c. *Arterial line*
   d. *Central venous pressure line as clinically indicated*
2. Additional equipment
   a. *Patient warming device*
   b. *Regular operating table*
   c. *Cervical traction, tong traction, or pins; shoulder rolls as clinically indicated*
3. Drugs
   a. *Standard emergency drugs*
   b. *Standard tabletop*
   c. *Intravenous fluids via 16- or 18-gauge I.V. with normal saline at 4 to 6 mL/kg per hour with fluid warmer*
   d. *Regardless of the technique selected for anesthesia, a drug such as nitroprusside must be readily available to treat precipitous hypertension. Nitroprusside administration as a rapid injection (1 to 2 µg/kg per minute) is an effective method of treating sudden hypertension.*

D. Anesthetic technique

Use general endotracheal anesthesia. Management of anesthesia in the patient with transection of the spinal cord is largely determined by the duration of the injury. Regardless of the duration of spinal cord transection, preoperative hydration helps prevent hypotension during the induction and maintenance of anesthesia.

E. Perioperative management

1. *Induction:* If the patient's neck is unstable, with the head in tongs, a halo device, or a body jacket or if findings on the history and physical examination suggest that tracheal intubation may be difficult, it is preferable to place the endotracheal tube with fiberoptic laryngoscopy under local anesthesia before the induction of general anesthesia. Once the endotracheal tube is in place, anesthesia is induced with sodium thiopental 3 to 5 mg/kg or propofol 1.5 to 2.5 mg/kg.
2. Maintenance
   a. *Standard maintenance. It is helpful to surgeons if a single dose of neuromuscular blocking drug (vecuronium 10 mg) is administered to relax the neck muscles. Additional doses of relaxants are rarely necessary.*
   b. Position: *for the anterior approach, the patient is positioned supine with a roll under the shoulders and moderately hyperextended. Check and pad pressure points. A cervical strap is placed below the chin and behind the occiput, and attached to a weight of 5 to 10 lbs hung over the head of the bed. For the posterior approach, the patient is positioned either prone (on a Wilson frame or on bolsters) or sitting with the head in three-point fixation. The major disadvantage of the sitting position is the risk of venous air embolism.*

3. *Emergence:* if a cervical fusion has been performed and the patient is returned to a halo device or body jacket, it is desirable to leave the endotracheal tube in place until the patient is fully awake and able to manage her or his own airway. To permit tolerance of the endotracheal tube and minimize coughing during emergence, it is useful to spray lidocaine (4 mL of 4%) down the orotracheal tube. Extubation may lead to immediate airway obstruction secondary to soft tissue occlusion or superior laryngeal nerve damage. A useful way to test for airway patency is to deflate the cuff of the tracheal tube and determine that the patient is able to breathe around the tube as well as through it.

F. Postoperative implications

1. Airway obstruction/hematoma/neurologic deficit—the cause of the airway obstruction is usually from soft tissue falling back against the posterior pharyngeal wall, which cannot be corrected by forward displacement of the mandible because of the neck fusion or postoperative traction/stabilization device (halo or body jacket). An oral or nasal airway may be required.

2. Tension pneumothorax—Delayed respiratory insufficiency is usually caused by either development of a tension pneumothorax from entrainment of air via the surgical wound, an unsuspected oropharyngeal laceration during tracheal intubation, or bleeding into the neck at the surgical site with progressive compression and occlusion of the airway.

COMMON PROCEDURES

NEUROLOGIC SYSTEM

A. Cerebral Aneurysm

• • •

A. Introduction

An intracranial aneurysm is a localized dilation most frequently located at vessel bifurcations that develop secondary to a weakness of the arterial wall. No single mechanism has been identified in the pathogenesis of intracranial aneurysm. Possible causes are congenital structural defects in the media and elastica of the vessel wall, incomplete involution of embryonic vessels, and secondary factors such as arterial hypertension, atherosclerotic changes, hemodynamic disturbances, and polycystic disease.

Aneurysmal rupture is prevented by maintaining a stable or low transmural pressure (TMP) within the aneurysm. TMP is defined as the difference between the mean systemic pressure (MAP) and the intracranial pressure (ICP). The relationship between the transmural pressures and the wall stress or tension of the aneurysm is linear. Either an increase in the MAP or a fall in the ICP increases the transmural pressure, the wall stress, and risk rupture. Cerebral perfusion pressure (CPP) is also equal to MAP-ICP; therefore, when one attempts to maintain a low TMP, one should be careful not to decrease the CPP and compromise cerebral blood flow.

B. Preoperative assessment and patient preparation

1. History and physical examination—findings depend on hemorrhage location—*neurologic focus:*

    a. *Level of consciousness—brief loss of consciousness to persistent coma*

    b. *Meningeal irritation—nuchal rigidity, positive Kernig's and Brudzinski's signs, fever, irritability, restlessness*

    c. *Visual disturbance—blurred vision, double vision, or both; visual field defects*

    d. *Cranial nerve involvement—ptosis and dilation of the pupil, inability to move the eye upward or inward, papilledema, photophobia*

    e. *Autonomic function—diaphoresis, chills, heart rate and blood pressure changes, slight temperature elevation, altered respiratory rhythm*

    f. *Motor function—onset and worsening of hemiparesis, aphasia, dysphagia hemiplegia, unilateral or bilateral transient paralysis of lower extremities*

    g. *Increased ICP—restlessness and lethargy, changes in level of consciousness and vital signs (Cushing's response, increased blood pressure, wide pulse pressure, decreased pulse rate), pupillary changes* (mydriasis), impaired pupillary reflex, papilledema, vomiting, fluctuations in temperature, seizures, and respiratory changes

    h. Pain—sudden onset of a violent headache—usually begins locally at frontal or temporal region, generalizing to entire head

 2. Diagnostic tests

    a. Computed tomography shows blood in the subarachnoid space

    b. Magnetic resonance imaging shows blood in the subarachnoid space

    c. Cerebral arteriogram identifies local or general vasospasm, outlining of cerebral vasculature

    d. Skull radiographs reveal calcified walls of aneurysm and areas of bone erosion

    e. Electroencephalogram reveals shifts in midline structure

    f. Brain scan shows local diminution of flow

    g. Lumbar puncture is controversial—increased opening pressures, elevated protein count, elevated white blood cells, cerebrospinal fluid with anthochromia (hemolyzed red blood cells)

    h. Regional cerebral blood flow—mean flow values for both hemispheres and determination of cerebral vasospasm

    i. Laboratory tests—complete blood count, electrolytes, glucose, blood urea nitrogen, creatinine, urinalysis, prothrombin time, partial thromboplastin time, type and cross-match

 3. Perioperative medications and intravenous therapy

    a. Anticonvulsants—phenytoin or phenobarbital

    b. Antihypertensives—hydralazine or methyldopa

    c. Antifibrinolytic agents—aminocaproic acid (Amicar); not given with coagulopathies

    d. Corticosteroids—dexamethasone

    e. Analgesics/antipyretics—acetaminophen

    f. Pituitary hormone—vasopressin injection

    g. Narcotic analgesics—acetaminophen with codeine

    h. Stool softeners—ducosate sodium

    i. Agents to control vasospasms—calcium antagonist

    j. Antibiotic

    k. Premedication—should not obscure signs of neurologic deterioration. However, some sedation is advisable to prevent anxiety and hypertension.

    l. Two large-bore (16- to 18-gauge) intravenous tubes with variable fluid management

C. Room preparation

 1. Monitoring equipment

    a. Central venous pressure or pulmonary artery catheter monitors cardiac function, adequacy of fluid, and blood replacement and allows access to treat venous air embolism

    b. A line—right or left radial artery depending on access requirement

    c. Doppler—monitors venous air embolism

      (1) Place between second and third intercostal spaces just to right of sternum

      (2) Use a 50-mL syringe to remove air

    d. Foley catheter—assess global renal function

    e. Peripheral nerve stimulator—monitor muscle blockade

COMMON PROCEDURES

    f. Warming modalities—minimal. Hypothermia (32°C) enhances the brain's ability to tolerate ischemia and reduces the cerebral metabolic requirement

  2. Pharmacologic agents

    a. Prepare infusions of nitroglycerin, nitroprusside, phenylephrine, and dopamine

    b. Drugs—mannitol, furosemide, lidocaine intravenous push, beta-blockers: esmolol

    c. Volume—isotonic salt solution; glucose and water solutions are not recommended because they are rapidly and equally distributed throughout total body water

      (1) Administer minimal volume prior to aneurysm clipping (2 to 3 mL/kg). The goal is to maintain hemodynamic stability, accounting for preoperative fluid and electrolyte status.

      (2) When the aneurysm is secured, deficits are replaced with additional volume as needed

      (3) At the time of aneurysm dissection, blood must be available in case of rupture

  3. Position—sitting or supine with the head of the bed raised

    a. Plan on the use of head-holder pins

    b. The airway most likely will be away from immediate reach

D. Anesthetic techniques and perioperative management

Use general anesthesia with endotracheal tube placement.

  1. *Induction:* the goal is smooth, rapid, gentle intubation and induction with control of blood pressure

    a. During induction and laryngoscopy, avoid wide swings and variances in MAP and ICP due to noxious stimuli, thus increasing the risk of rupture

    b. Preoxygenate, followed by a combination of thiopental (3 to 5 mg/kg) and a nondepolarizing muscle relaxant with minimal cardiovascular effects

    c. To block the cardiovascular and increased ICP response to laryngoscopy, use additional thiopental, fentanyl, sufentanyl, or intravenous lidocaine

    d. Sympathetic stimulation may be blocked with use of beta-blockers: esmolol, which is ultra-short-acting, may be preferred

    e. Use of succinylcholine in open-globe injuries is controversial because it has been shown to raise ICP

  2. Maintenance

    a. Any spontaneous movement during surgery can be disastrous; therefore, adequate depth of anesthesia and muscle paralysis is crucial

    b. Prepare for noxious stimuli—application of head device and scalp incision

    c. Anesthesia can be maintained with O_2/air, a volatile anesthetic, and intravenous supplementation with opioids, barbiturates, or both

    d. Use caution with volatile anesthetics. Their cerebral vasodilating effects may increase CBF and thus increase ICP.

    e. Isoflurane is the least potent cerebral vasodilating of the common inhalation anesthetics

f. Total dose of fentanyl should not exceed 10 to 12 μg/kg unless postoperative ventilation is planned

g. Nitrous oxide is controversial because venous air embolism is possible

h. Venous air embolism—associated with procedure when the operative site is above the level of the heart

  (1) Signs and symptoms

    (a) Decreased Et_{CO_2} (end-tidal carbon dioxide) and Et_{N_2} (end-tidal nitrogen)

    (b) Hypertension

    (c) Mill-wheel murmur by Doppler

    (d) Dysrhythmias

    (e) Increased right atrial and pulmonary arterial pressures

  (2) Treatment

    (a) Alert the surgeon

    (b) Aspirate from central venous pressure/pulmonary arterial catheter

    (c) Use the Trendelenburg position with the left side down

    (d) Flood the field with saline or occlude an open vein or venous sinus

    (e) Consider continuous positive airway pressure or positive end-expiratory pressure

    (f) Compress the jugular vein

i. Arterial carbon dioxide pressure—maintain between 25 and 30 mm Hg; hypocarbia decreases cerebral blood flow and ICP

j. Controlled hypotensive technique is used to facilitate surgical exposure and control intracranial aneurysms

  (1) Blood-pressure parameters need to be individualized

  (2) It is suggested that MAP be decreased by 30% below a patient's usual MAP

  (3) Deepen anesthesia with volatile anesthetic

  (4) Initiate drip: nitroprusside (seldom >3 μg/kg per min) or nitroglycerin

  (5) Nitroprusside may cause systemic toxicity due to production of cyanide, which is manifested by metabolic acidosis and high venous oxygen pressure

  (6) Whichever agent is used, one should be prepared for exaggerated responses in patients made relatively hypovolemic by diuretics

  (7) Strict attention to calibration and positioning of the arterial line transducer is necessary

  (8) CPP decreases approximately 0.7 mm Hg for each centimeter the head is elevated above the heart

  (9) Some suggest placing the transducer the same level as the circle of Willis—the level of the external auditory canal

k. Slack brain—improves lesion exposure, reduces retractor ischemia, and decreases the chance of rupture

  (1) Hyperventilate the lungs

  (2) Administer thiopental

  (3) Administer osmotic diuretics: mannitol (0.25 to 2 g/kg)

  (4) Optimize venous drainage

COMMON PROCEDURES

l. *Aneurysm rupture—likely times of rupture include:*
  (1) Dura incised and decreased ICP
  (2) Excessive brain retraction and increased blood pressure
  (3) Dissection of aneurysm
  (4) Clip placed onto neck of aneurysm
  (5) Removal of clip holder from clip
  (6) Must immediately replace blood losses
  (7) Maintain MAP between 40 and 50 mm Hg—decrease the rate of bleeding
  (8) Alternatively, one or both carotids may be compressed against vertebral bodies for up to 3 minutes to decrease blood in the field
  (9) Intravenous thiopental (Pentothal) for cerebral protection
m. *Post aneurysm clipping, assess hemodynamics—recommendations: Pulmonary capillary wedge pressure PCWP 15 to 18 mm Hg, central venous pressure taken 10 to 12 times monthly, hematocrit of 30 to 35*

3. *Emergence:* the goal is to avoid coughing, straining, hypercarbia, and hypertension
  a. *Unless the patient is to be ventilated postoperatively, deep extubation is the preferred method*
  b. *Patients require monitoring in the intensive care unit for assessment of hemodynamics and neurologic status*

E. Postoperative implications
Delayed ischemia—vasospasm; in areas of dysfunctional autoregulation, cerebral perfusion passively depends on systemic arterial pressure.
1. Therapy is directed at improving cerebral perfusion by increasing systemic arterial pressure to approximately 150 mm Hg with either dopamine or phenylephrine
2. Increase central venous pressure approximately 10 to 12 mm Hg. Colloid is preferred to crystalloid because of the impermeability of the blood-brain barrier to low-molecular-weight proteins
3. Use calcium channel blockers, especially nimodipine, to prevent or treat delayed ischemia
4. Potential for rebleed—usually occurs in the first 24 hours

Bibliography

Allen MB. A Manual of Neurosurgery. Baltimore: University Park Press, 1987.

B. Posterior Fossa Procedures

A. Introduction
Posterior fossa craniotomies are performed for treating infratentorial tumors. The posterior fossa is a limited area that contains the medulla,

pons, cerebellum, major motor and sensory pathways, lower cranial nerve nuclei, and primary respiratory and cardiovascular centers.

B. Preoperative assessment and patient preparation

1. History and physical examination

   a. Neurologic: *the history and physical examination should include a thorough neurologic evaluation with documentation. Pay special attention to signs and symptoms of brain stem involvement such as focal neurologic deficits, depressed respiration, and cranial nerve palsies. Changes in level of consciousness may be secondary to increased intracranial pressure due to obstructive hydrocephalus of the fourth ventricle.*

   b. Cardiovascular: *evaluate for cardiovascular disease and hypertension*

   c. Pulmonary: *assess for a coexisting disease process*

   d. Renal: *correct fluid and electrolyte abnormalities, if present*

   e. Gastrointestinal: *infratentorial tumors may involve the glossopharyngeal and vagus nerves. This may impair the gag reflex, increasing chances of aspiration.*

   f. Endocrine: *steroid therapy may be in use*

2. *Laboratory tests*—complete blood count, electrolytes, blood urea nitrogen, creatinine, glucose, prothrombin time, partial thromboplastin time

3. *Diagnostic tests:* computed tomography and magnetic resonance imaging

4. *Preoperative medications:* anxiolytics may be given to alert and anxious patients. Patients who are lethargic or have an altered level of consciousness do not receive premedication.

5. *Intravenous therapy:* Central line, two 16- to 18-gauge intravenous tubes; consider a pulmonary arterial catheter. Estimated blood loss is 25 to 500 mL.

C. Room preparation

1. *Monitoring equipment:* standard monitors, A-line, central venous pressure, urinary catheter, with possible intracranial pressure monitoring, precordial Doppler, electroencephalography, electromyography, and sensory/somatosensory/brain stem auditory evoked potential monitoring

2. *Additional equipment:* depending on the position of the patient, have appropriate padding available (ie., prone pillow, doughnut, chest and axillary rolls); fluid warmer

3. Drugs

   a. Miscellaneous pharmacologic agents: *vasoconstrictors, vasodilators, inotropes, adrenergic antagonists, steroids, osmotic and loop diuretics, thiopental, lidocaine, fentanyl, nondepolarizing muscle relaxants, and antibiotic*

   b. Intravenous fluids: *use isotonic crystalloid solutions. Avoid glucose- or dextrose-containing solutions. Limit normal saline to less than or equal to 10 mL/kg plus replacement of urinary output. If volume is required, administer 5% albumin or hetastarch and limit to less than or equal to 20 mL/kg. Maintain hematocrit at 30 to 35. Transfuse for a hematocrit of less than 25.*

   c. Blood: *type and cross-match for 2 units packed red blood cells*

   d. Tabletop: *standard*

COMMON PROCEDURES

D. Anesthetic technique and perioperative management

1. General anesthesia

2. *Induction:* the goal is to minimize increases in blood pressure and intracranial pressure. Once an airway has been established, induce with thiopental (4 to 6 mg/kg), an opioid (fentanyl 3 to 5 μg/kg), and a nondepolarizing muscle relaxant (vecuronium 0.1 to 0.5 mg). To deepen the anesthetic, consider supplementing with fentanyl in 50-μg increments to a total of 10 to 15 μg/kg, midazolam, and lidocaine 1.5 mg/kg 90 seconds prior to intubation.

3. *Maintenance:* most commonly used maintenance anesthetics are nitrous oxide–opioid and nitrous oxide–volatile inhalational agents. The most common opioid is fentanyl and most common inhalational agent is isoflurane. High-dose narcotic technique may be also considered. Maintain arterial carbon dioxide pressure between 25 and 30 mm Hg. Cardiovascular instability secondary to surgical stimulation of the trigeminal, glossopharyngeal, or vagus nerves is common.

4. *Positioning:* patient may be placed in the sitting, lateral, prone, park-bench, or three-quarters prone position. If the sitting position is utilized, one must consider the increased incidence of venous air embolism and cardiovascular instability

5. *Emergence:* emergence should be as smooth as possible. Avoid bucking or straining on the endotracheal tube. Consider lidocaine 1.5 mg/kg 90 seconds prior to suctioning or extubation. Antihypertensive medications are administered to control systemic hypertension.

E. Postoperative implications

Complications: closely observe for the occurrence of seizures, hemorrhage, edema, increased intracranial pressure, neurologic deficits, and tension pneumocephalus. Impairment of cranial nerves or respiratory center in the brain stem may require postoperative mechanical ventilation.

C. Transsphenoidal Tumor Resections

◆   ◆   ◆

A. Introduction

A procedure to access the pituitary gland. It has an advantage over craniotomy because it results in less blood loss. It involves an incision over the maxillary gingiva or along the side of the nose.

B. Preoperative assessment and patient preparation

1. *History and physical examination:* see Chapters D (Craniotomy) and G (Pituitary Tumors) in this section.

   a. Respiratory: *airway changes can occur with acromegaly (the patient may require a smaller oral endotracheal tube). Problems occur with* mask fit. Thoroughly evaluate the airway; check for dyspnea, stridor, hoarseness.

b. Cardiac: *common findings are hypertension, coronary artery disease, congestive heart failure acromegaly*

c. Neurologic: *a nonfunctional gland usually is discovered because of increased size, resulting in neurologic changes. A hypersecreting gland is found when small.*

d. Renal: electrolyte imbalance

e. Diagnostic tests: *complete blood count. Patients with panhypopituitarism require hormone replacement prior to surgery. They should be euthyroid and should be receiving corticosteroids (assess for diabetes mellitus); patients may be on intranasal vasopressin. Diabetes insipidus occurs after corticosteroid is introduced. Check electrolytes and random blood sugar as indicated by history and physical examination.*

f. *Preoperative medications and intravenous therapy:* replace deficits and hourly surgical loss; one intravenous large-bore

C. Room preparation

1. *Monitoring equipment:* standard if sitting position is used; central venous pressure and precordial Doppler; consider a-line, Foley catheter. Visual or auditory evoked potentials may be monitored.

2. *Additional medications and continuous infusions:* adjunct medicines to treat hypertension and tachycardia; cocaine, epinephrine preparation

3. *Position:* supine, head elevated 30 degrees, table turned

D. Anesthetic technique

Use general anesthesia, oral endotracheal intubation (RAE or anode tubes).

E. Perioperative management

See Chapters D (Craniotomy for Tumors) and G (Pituitary Tumors) in this section.

1. *Induction:* see Chapter D (Craniotomy for Tumors) if increased intracranial pressure is a concern

2. *Maintenance:* no further neuromuscular blocking agent is required; normocapnia is desired

3. *Emergence:* one must decide whether the patient will be extubated. If so, deep extubation is the method of choice unless contraindicated by airway management at induction.

F. Postoperative considerations

The patient's nose is packed, and the patient thus is breathing by mouth.

D. Craniotomy

♦ ♦ ♦

A. Introduction

An opening is made into the cranium for removal of a tumor, relief of intracranial pressure, or to control bleeding. A flap is created by

COMMON PROCEDURES

leaving the bone attached to the muscle so that the tissue can be turned down. The dura is then incised in the opposite direction so its base is near the midline. After the surgery is complete, closure is performed in layers: dura, muscles, fascial, galea, and scalp. Craniotomies are classified as supratentorial or subtentorial. (See Chapter A, Cerebral Aneurysm, for in-depth explanations on the following information.)

B. Perioperative assessment and patient preparation

1. *History and physical examination:* attempt to establish the presence or absence of intracranial hypertension; *neurologic focus:* level of consciousness, meningeal irritation, visual disturbances, cranial nerve involvement, autonomic function, motor function, and pain

2. Diagnostic tests

   a. *Computed tomography, magnetic resonance imaging, cerebral arteriogram, echoencephalogram, brain scan, regional cerebral blood flow*

   b. Laboratory tests: *complete blood count, electrolytes, glucose, blood urea nitrogen, creatinine, urinalysis, prothrombin time, partial thromboplastin time, anticonvulsant levels, type and cross-match*

3. Preoperative medications and intravenous therapy

   a. *Premedication is best avoided when intracranial hypertension is suspected; hypercapnia and second-degree respiratory depression increases intracranial pressure (ICP) and may be lethal*

   b. *Patients with a normal ICP may be given a benzodiazepine*

   c. *Steroids and anticonvulsant therapy is continued up to the time of surgery*

   d. *Two large-bore intravenous tubes*

C. Room preparation

1. Monitoring equipment

   a. *Central venous pressure for patients requiring vasoactive drugs; also allows access for treating venous air embolism*

   b. *A-line ensures optimal cerebral perfusion*

   c. *Somatosensory evoked potential or electroencephalogram evaluates cerebral status and prevents optic nerve damage during resections of large pituitary tumors*

   d. *Doppler—monitor venous air embolism*

   e. *Foley catheter—guides fluid therapy and frequent use of diuretics*

   f. *Peripheral nerve stimulation—monitor on nonaffected side*

   g. *Intracranial pressure—usually via ventriculostomy or subdural blot*

2. Pharmacologic agents

   a. *Prepare infusions of nitroglycerine, phenylephrine, nitroprusside, and dopamine*

   b. Drugs: *mannitol, furosemide, lidocaine, calcium channel blocker*

   c. Volume: *glucose-free isotonic salt solutions*

      (1) Hyperglycemia is common in this patient population (steroid effect) and has been implicated in increasing ischemic brain injury

      (2) Colloid solutions restore intravascular volume deficits

      (3) Isotonic crystalloid solutions are used for maintenance fluid requirements

(4) Intraoperative fluid replacement should be calculated and kept at a minimum unless otherwise indicated

3. Position—supine
   a. Plan to use head-holder pins
   b. Head elevated 15 to 30 degrees to facilitate venous and cerebrospinal fluid drainage
   c. Head may be turned to the side to facilitate exposure; be careful not to impede jugular venous drainage, which will increase ICP
   d. Table is usually turned 90 to 180 degrees away from anesthesia. Secure endotracheal tube and breathing circuit connections.

D. **Anesthetic techniques and perioperative management**
   General anesthesia with endotracheal tube placement.
   1. *Induction:* goal is to intubate the trachea in a slow, controlled fashion without compromising cerebral blood flow or increasing ICP
      a. Induction of anesthesia and endotracheal intubation are critical periods for the patient with compromised intracranial compliance or an increased ICP. Intracranial compliance can be improved by:
         (1) Osmotic diureses
         (2) Steriods
         (3) Removal of cerebrospinal fluid via ventriculostomy
      b. Do not allow arterial hypertension, which increases cerebral blood volume, promotes cerebral edema, and increases intracranial pressure.
      c. Most common induction technique employs thiopental together with hyperventilation to lower ICP and blunt the noxious effects of laryngoscopy and intubation
      d. Muscle relaxant is given to facilitate ventilation and prevent straining and coughing, which can abruptly increase ICP
      e. An intravenous narcotic (fentanyl 5 to 10 $\mu g/kg$) just prior to thiopental attenuates the sympathetic response
      f. Intravenous lidocaine (1 to 1.5 mg/kg) following thiopental but prior to intubation blunts the noxious effects of laryngoscopy
      g. Avoid succinylcholine, which may increase ICP, especially if intubation is attempted prior to establishment of deep anesthesia and hyperventilation
   2. Maintenance
      a. Any spontaneous movement during surgery can be detrimental; therefore, adequate depth of anesthesia and muscle paralysis is crucial
      b. Prepare for noxious stimuli: application of head device and scalp incision
      c. Anesthesia can be maintained with oxygen/air, a volatile anesthetic, and intravenous supplementation with opioids, barbiturates, or both
      d. Isoflurane and desflurane are the least potent cerebral vasodilators of the volatile agents
      e. Arterial carbon dioxide pressure is maintained at 25 to 30 mm Hg; hypocarbia decreases cerebral blood flow and ICP; severe hypocarbia may result in ischemia
      f. Controlled hypotensive technique is used to facilitate surgical exposure
      g. Venous air embolism is possible at the operative site above the heart
      h. Slack brain improves lesion exposure, reduces retraction ischemia

3. Emergence
   The goal is to avoid coughing, straining, hypercarbia, and hypertension.
   a. *Most patients can be extubated at the end of the procedure as long as intracranial hypertension is no longer present*
   b. *Patients left intubated should remain sedated, paralyzed, and hyperventilated*
   c. *Patients require intensive care unit monitoring for assessment of hemodynamics and neurologic status*

E. **Postoperative implications—delayed ischemia, bleeding, and infection**

E. Stereotactic Surgery

♦   ♦   ♦

A. **Introduction**
   Stereotactic neurosurgery is a neurosurgical technique that makes detailed use of the relationship between the three-dimensional space occupied by intracranial structures or lesions and an extracranial reference system to accurately and precisely guide instruments to such targets. This type of technique is used when the lesion is small or is located deep within brain tissue or as a means of obtaining a biopsy of a lesion for diagnosis.

   All current stereotactic procedures begin with the attachment of a frame to the patient's head. The frame is anchored to the skull with either four pins or four screws. This procedure typically is done outside the operating room using local anesthetic. In the cooperative adult, frame application takes only 5 to 10 minutes. For children, general anesthesia is used.

B. **Preoperative assessment**
   1. History and physical examination: *neurologic:* neurologic symptoms vary, depending on the site and size of the lesion; they should be carefully documented. In addition to the routine test, computed tomography is performed preoperatively with the frame in place to determine stereotactic coordinates. Once the coordinates are established, the frame must not be moved on the head until the operation is complete.
   2. *Laboratory tests:* complete blood count and other tests as indicated per the history and physical examination
   3. *Diagnostic tests:* computed tomography of the head and other tests as indicated per the history and physical examination
   4. *Medication:* usually not required

C. **Room preparation**
   1. *Monitoring equipment:* standard
   2. Additional equipment
      a. *Stereotactic instruments*
      b. *Monitoring, ventilation, and oxygenation equipment during transport*

3. Drugs
   a. *Standard emergency drugs*
   b. *Standard tabletop*
   c. *Intravenous fluids: 18-gauge intravenous with standard replacement therapy*

D. Anesthetic technique

General endotracheal anesthesia or monitored anesthesia care is used. In adults, the stereotactic frame is placed the morning of operation under local anesthesia, and the patient is taken to the radiologic suite for computed tomography to determine stereotactic coordinates. The patient is then brought to the operating room with the frame still in place. If operation is to be a biopsy, it is generally done under monitored anesthesia care. If a complete resection is planned, such as in the removal of an arteriovenous malformation, general endotracheal anesthesia is used. In children, it is usually necessary to induce general anesthesia before placing the frame, thus necessitating the maintenance of general anesthesia during the computed tomography. The child is then moved to the operating room still anesthetized, and the operation is completed.

E. Perioperative management

1. Induction

   If monitored anesthesia care is planned, oxygen is administered by nasal prongs, and the patient is lightly sedated with combinations of droperidol to prevent nausea and vomiting, midazolam to provide amnesia, and meperidine or fentanyl to provide analgesia. The patient must be able to communicate with the surgeon as needed throughout the operation. If general endotracheal anesthesia is needed, fiberoptic laryngoscopy is necessary before inducing anesthesia because the frame precludes intubation by direct laryngoscopy. Once endotracheal intubation is established, anesthesia may be induced with sodium thiopental or propofol, followed by a nondepolarizing blocking drug to facilitate positioning of the patient.

2. Maintenance

   If general anesthesia is used, the ideal drug is one that decreases intracranial pressure and the cerebral metabolic rate of oxygen, maintains cerebral autoregulation, redistributes flow to the potentially ischemic areas, and provides protection of the brain from focal ischemia. If children are to be transported from the site of placement of the stereotactic frame to the radiologic suite and then the operating room, it is best to use inhalational anesthesia with isoflurane and 100% oxygen with spontaneous ventilation to ensure adequate ventilation during transport and study. Opiates and non-neuromuscular blocking drugs should not be administered until the child is in the operating suite.

3. Emergence

   No special consideration. The patient is extubated awake and after the return of airway reflexes. If the surgeon suspects that the patient may have a slow recovery or a neurologic injury, or if the anesthetist believes that recovery from the anesthesia may be delayed, it is advisable to leave the endotracheal tube in place at least overnight.

COMMON PROCEDURES

F. Postoperative implications
Focal bleeding may occur postoperatively, causing onset of a neurologic deficit.

F. Cranioplasty

♦   ♦   ♦

A. Introduction
Cranioplasty can be performed for a bony tumor resulting from traumatic injury (depressed skull fracture) or, more rarely, resulting from a congenital malformation (fused suture lines). These defects may occur anywhere on the head, so the surgery may take place in varying positions such as supine, sitting, prone, or supine with the head turned. Patients range widely in age, from newborn to elderly.

B. Preoperative assessment and patient preparation
1. *Cardiac:* if the patient is an infant, assess for congenital defects, marked murmurs, maternal pregnancy history. If the patient is elderly, assess for myocardial infarction, hypertension, coronary artery disease, angina, and exercise tolerance. Use 12-lead electrocardiography and further cardiac work-up if the history suggests and if time permits.
2. *Respiratory:* infants—assess for periods of apnea, pregnancy history, meconium complications. Elderly—assess for history of smoking, pneumonia, chronic obstructive pulmonary disease, and exercise tolerance. With traumatic injuries, assess the pattern and depth of respiration.
3. *Neurologic:* infants—assess for congenital defects, pregnancy history, delivery history, reflexes. With traumatic injuries, assess for Glasgow Coma Scale, pupils, reflexes. Also ensure that cervical spine injury has been ruled out or is stabilized. Elderly—assess history of stroke, seizure, mentation. Alway assess for the document preoperative focal neurologic deficits.
4. *Gastrointestinal:* consider patients to be on a full stomach if they present with trauma

C. Patient preparation
Complete blood count, electrolytes, blood urea nitrogen, creatinine, glucose, prothrombin time, partial thromboplastin time (D-dimer or fibrin split products if disseminated intravascular coagulation needs to be ruled out). Type and cross-match (for at least 2 units). Arterial blood gases if the patient is being ventilated.

D. Room preparation
1. *Monitoring equipment:* standard. Arterial line and central line if history suggest. Use a Foley catheter if surgery is scheduled for more than 2 hours. Some patients may have an intracranial pressure monitor in place.
2. *Additional equipment:* determine the position the surgery will be in if supine or supine with the head turned; a foam support aids in

positioning the head. Longer ventilation tubing is needed because the table will be turned. With the sitting position, a Doppler and a central line (with a 60-mL syringe attached) are needed to assess and treat venous air embolism. With the prone position, use prone foam rest shoulder rolls and multiple pads. In all cases, a nasal endotracheal tube assists in clearing the surgical field and in stabilizing the endotracheal tube.

3. *Drugs and tabletop:* thiopental and etomidate are useful in cranioplasty because of their cerebral protective properties. Propofol is known to decrease intracranial pressure. Most surgeons desire antibiotics during surgery, and they should be questioned about steroids and diuretics.

4. *Blood and fluid requirements:* glucose-containing solutions are best avoided in neurologic surgery. It is better to err on the side of underhydration. Fluid usually is replaced with normal saline or lactated Ringer's solution at 2 to 4 mL/kg per hour. Blood loss may be substantial, and blood should be immediately available to avoid hypotension or crystalloid overload.

E. Anesthetic technique

Induction is intravenous, with one of the agents known to decrease intracranial pressure. If the patient is significantly obtunded preoperatively, an inhaled induction with isoflurane, possibly supplemented with a narcotic, may be beneficial. With severe trauma, one may wish to use only oxygen and to paralyze the patient. Avoid nasal intubation if there is any chance of a basilar skull fracture. For maintenance, keep the patients mean arterial blood pressure slightly below the baseline and maintain normocarbia to slight hypocarbia. A constant infusion of thiopental, etomidate, or propofol with or without inhalation of isoflurane will help to maintain cerebral perfusion and maximize the cerebral oxygen consumption. Muscle relaxation is not necessary if the procedure is confined to the skull and the head is immobilized with tongs or some other type of fixator. Most practitioners leave the endotracheal tube in place until the neurologic status is certain to allow for regular respiration. Lidocaine is useful in minimizing cough.

F. Postoperative implications

Assess postoperative neurologic functions. Pain usually is controlled in the altered patient with parenteral agents or a passive cutaneous anaphylaxis pump in selected patients. One must be watchful to avoid hypercarbia in neurologic patients receiving opiates.

G. Pituitary Tumors

◆ ◆ ◆

A. Introduction

Transsphenoidal resection of the pituitary gland is performed either through a nasal or a labial incision and is associated with fewer

COMMON PROCEDURES

complications than a craniotomy. A tunnel to the sphenoid sinus is created, and it is entered by removing a piece of the vomer. The mucosa of the sphenoid sinus is removed, and the sella is entered by removing a portion of the sella floor. The tumor is removed with microdissectors and suctioned under fluoroscopic guidance and with the aid of the operating microscope. Fat from the abdomen or thigh may be harvested and placed in the sella to graft and seal the dura if cerebrospinal fluid is found. The floor of the sella may be reconstructed with bone salvaged from the exposure. Uncontrollable bleeding is rare but can be massive, requiring frontal craniotomy to achieve hemostasis.

B. Pathophysiology

The pituitary gland is located at the base of the skull in the sella turcica, a bony cavity within the sphenoid bone, and it is divided into the anterior (adenohypophysis) and posterior (neurohypophysis) lobes. The anterior pituitary secretes growth hormone, prolactin, gonadotropins (follicle-stimulating hormone, luteinizing hormone), adrenocorticotropic hormone, beta-lipotropin, and thyroid-stimulating hormone. The posterior pituitary stores and secretes antidiuretic hormone and oxytocin.

Nonfunctioning pituitary adenomas are the most common tumor type. Rarely, some patients have endocrine deficiencies due to hypothalamopituitary compression. Various hyperpituitary syndromes may accompany a functioning adenoma. The most frequently occurring are prolactinomas, followed by growth hormone–and adrenocorticotropic hormone–secreting adenomas.

C. Preoperative assessment

1. *Cardiac:* no special considerations unless the patient has acromegaly (growth hormone–secreting adenoma), in which case they may have hypertension, ischemic heart disease, cardiomegaly, congestive heart failure, or diabetes.

2. *Respiratory:* mask fit and visualization of the larynx may be difficult in patients with acromegaly due to hypertrophy of facial bones, nasal turbinates, tongue, tonsils, epiglottis, and larynx. Hoarseness and dyspnea may be caused by glottic stenosis from soft tissue overgrowth; these patients may require a smaller endotracheal tube and may be predisposed to postextubation edema. Awake intubation with a fiberoptic laryngoscope is recommended for patients with glottic abnormalities and difficult airways; this obviates the need for a tracheostomy in all but the most severe cases.

3. *Neurologic:* secretory tumors are usually small and rarely cause intracranial pressure (ICP). Nonfunctional tumors, however, are not usually diagnosed until they extend beyond the boundaries of the sella, causing headaches, visual field defects, ICP, or cranial nerve palsies by mass effect.

4. *Endocrine:* adrenocorticotropic hormone–secreting adenomas can produce Cushing's disease, which has multiple systemic effects, including insulin-resistant hyperglycemia, hyperaldosteronism with hypokalemia and metabolic alkalosis, and obesity. Prolactin-secreting tumors may present with lactation and amenorrhea.

Patients with growth hormone–secreting adenomas may have large hands, feet, and head.

D. Patient preparation
1. *Laboratory tests:* preoperative endocrine studies including serum and urinary levels of pituitary, thyroid, and adrenal hormones. Hematocrit and others as indicated from the history and physical examination.
2. *Diagnostic tests:* computed tomography or magnetic resonance imaging to delineate tumor size and site. Radiography of the neck to analyze airway conformation and lumen diameter in patients with dyspnea, hoarseness, or stridor.
3. *Medications:* Ampicillin (or vancomycin) 1 g IV + cefotaxime 1 g. Appropriate replacement therapy should be established in patients with endocrine deficiencies before proceeding with surgery.

E. Room preparation
1. *Monitoring equipment:* standard monitors, arterial line, central venous pressure line, urine output, Doppler to monitor for venous air embolism in semi-sitting position
2. Additional equipment: anesthetic circuits and intravascular lines must be long enough to be accessible at patient's feet. Anode or right-angle endotracheal tube may be helpful.
3. *Tabletop:* table turned 180 degrees, anesthetist will be at patient's feet
4. Drugs
   a. Continuous infusion: *vasoactive infusions to maintain mean arterial pressure and thus cerebral perfusion pressure should be readily available (phenylephrine, nitroglycerine, nitroprusside)*
   b. Intravenous fluids: *one 16- to 18-gauge tube, normal saline or lactated Ringer's solution 4 to 8 mL/kg per hour*
   c. Blood: *estimated blood loss is usually less than 250 mL, unless bleeding from the internal carotid artery or cavernous sinus occurs during the course of dissection and drilling into the sella*
   d. Tabletop: *measures to lower ICP should be readily available (dexamethasone, mannitol, sodium thiopental)*

F. Perioperative management
1. *Anesthetic technique:* general endotracheal anesthesia is required for this operation
2. *Induction:* if difficult intubation is anticipated, orotracheal intubation will need to be accomplished before the induction of general anesthesia. Awake fiberoptic is the best choice. Because tumors are generally confined to the sella turcica and ICP is usually normal, standard induction techniques are appropriate. If ICP is of concern, induction should be similar to that used for patients with other kinds of brain tumors. (See Anesthetic Considerations in Chapter D, Craniotomy, in this section.) Lidocaine may be administered by topical spray or intravenously (1.5 mg/kg) to lessen cardiovascular responses to intubation.
3. *Maintenance:* isoflurane (maximum allowable concentration is 1.15%) titrated to effect, fentanyl. Basic neuroanesthetic principles apply whether the transsphenoidal or transcranial approach is used.

With the transcranial approach, measures to control ICP are instituted because brain retraction and greater blood loss are necessary. (See Anesthethic Considerations in Chapter D, Craniotomy, in this section.) Lumbar cerebrospinal fluid drainage is commonly used in transcranial procedures, and in transsphenoidal procedures subarachnoid air injection may facilitate tumor delineation. When air is injected, N_2O should be discontinued because it may increase the volume of the air-filled closed space. Neuromuscular blocking drugs are generally not necessary, because with adequate anesthesia and the head in Mayfield-Kees skeletal fixation, movement is unlikely. Ventilation is controlled with the arterial carbon dioxide pressure in the normal range.

4. *Position:* supine, head elevated 30 degrees, shoulder role. Access to the patient's head is obstructed by the operating microscope, so the endotracheal tube must be firmly secured.

5. *Emergence:* when surgical conditions permit, reverse the residual muscle relaxant when at least one twitch is present in train of four ratio. Discontinue N_2O/volatile agents and administer 100% O_2.

6. *Extubation:* if the patient evidences normal emergence from anesthesia, the endotracheal tube can be removed after suctioning the oropharynx and ensuring that the throat packs placed by the surgeon have been removed. Nasal breathing will be obstructed by packs; therefore if there is any question about airway patency because of a large tongue, small mouth, or redundant soft tissue in the oropharynx, the endotracheal tube should be left in place until the patient is fully awake.

G. Postoperative implications

Diabetes insipidus, evidenced by polyuria and decreased urine specific gravity, may occur after transsphenoidal hypophysectomy. Treatment with intravenous fluids or vasopressin may be necessary.

Corticosteroids may be needed postoperatively for several days until testing shows an intact pituitary-adrenal axis.

H. Arteriovenous Malformation Neurosurgery

♦ ♦ ♦

A. Introduction

Arteriovenous malformations (AVMs) are congenital abnormalities that form direct communications between cerebral arteries and veins. Arterial blood flows directly into veins, causing an irregular resistance without an intervening capillary bed, leaving surrounding brain tissue ischemic (intracerebral steal). Ninety-five per cent of AVMs occur supratentorially and present as subarachnoid or intracerebral hemorrhage, focal deficits, or seizures.

B. Preoperative assessment and patient preparation

1. History and physical examination
   a. Neurologic: *a documented thorough neurologic examination is essential. Altered level of consciousness, focal deficits, seizure disorders, and headaches are occasionally seen.*
   b. Cardiovascular: *Assess for past history, usually negative. Electrocardiographic changes might reflect the degree of brain injury.*
   c. Pulmonary: *assess for history of smoking or other respiratory complications*
2. Patient preparation
   a. Laboratory tests: *complete blood count, prothrombin time, partial thromboplastin time, electrolytes, blood urea nitrogen, creatinine, bleeding time, and urinalysis*
   b. Diagnostic tests: *cerebral angiogram, computed tomography, magnetic resonance imaging, and lumbar puncture*
   c. Preoperative medications: *titrate anxiolytics to alert, anxious patients. Avoid premedicating patients with altered level of consciousness.*
   d. Intravenous therapy: *central line, two 16-gauge tubes, consider pulmonary arterial catheter. Estimated blood loss is 500 to 3000 mL.*

C. Room preparation

1. *Monitoring equipment:* standard, A-line, central venous pressure, and urinary catheter
2. *Additional equipment:* fluid warmer, cell-saver, special frame to support the head, surgical microscope
3. Drugs
   a. Miscellaneous pharmacologic agents: *osmotic and loop diuretics, sodium nitroprusside, phenylephrine, ephedrine, atropine, esmolol, labetalol, lidocaine, fentanyl, nondepolarizing muscle relaxants, antibiotic and thiopental infusion*
   b. Intravenous fluids: *non–dextrose containing crystalloids. Normal saline/lactated Ringer's solution not to exceed 10 mL/kg plus urinary output. Transfuse for a hematocrit of less than 30. If patient is hypovolemic, give 5% albumin. Avoid hetastarch.*
   c. Blood: *type and cross-match for 6 units of packed red blood cells*
   d. Tabletop: *standard*

D. Perioperative management and anesthetic technique

Use general anesthesia.

1. *Induction:* thiopental 3 to 5 mg/kg, fentanyl 5 to 10 μg/kg, vecuronium 0.1 to 0.15 mg/kg, lidocaine 1.5 to 2 mg/kg. If the patient is in a stereotactic frame, endotracheal intubation via fiberoptics, is done prior to induction.
2. *Maintenance:* isoflurane or desflurane of maximum allowable concentrations less than 1% with O_2 fentanyl. Consider a bolus of thiopental, 3 to 5 mg/kg, followed by a continuous infusion of 3 to 5 mg/kg when the risk of cerebral ischemia is increased. Esmolol boluses can be used to prevent reflex tachycardia, rebound hypertension, or both. Techniques to reduce intraoperative

bleeding, decrease cerebral blood flow, and decrease AVM wall tension include deliberate hypotension and intentional hypothermia. Deliberate hypotension may be incorporated to maintain a mean arterial pressure of 50 to 65 mm Hg. One may utilize sodium nitroprusside 0.5 to 0.8 μg/kg per minute, increasing inhalational agent to 2% to 3% of maximum allowable concentration, or nitroglycerine 0.5 to 8.0 μg/kg per minute. Intentional hypothermia of 28° to 35°C can be achieved by using ice packs, a thermal blanket, or a cool air blower, or by lowering the operating room temperature. Resection of AVMs can be facilitated by hyperventilation (arterial carbon dioxide pressure of 25 to 35 mm Hg), diuretics, and cerebrospinal fluid drainage.

3. *Positioning:* most common position is supine with the head turned lateral with a shoulder roll. Lateral or modified prone positions are also used.

4. *Emergence:* ensure full reversal from neuromuscular blockade and closely regulate blood pressure. Suppress cough, remove the endotube, or do both. The patient is placed supine with the head of the bed elevated 30 degrees, and supplemental O_2 is administered.

E. Postoperative implications

Complications include neurologic deficits, cerebral edema and increased intracranial pressure, and intracerebral hemorrhage.

I. Electroconvulsive Therapy

• • •

A. Introduction

Used in the treatment of endogenous depression in patients in whom an adequate course of antidepressant drugs has failed and those who suffer from severe melancholia or are suicidal. It involves placement of electrodes on the scalp and application of a stimulus to elicit a brief grand mal seizure: a 2- to 3-second latent phase, followed by a tonic phase lasting 10 to 12 seconds, and finally by a clonic phase of 30 to 50 seconds. The clinical outcome from electroconvulsive therapy correlates with both duration of individual seizures and cumulative seizure time.

B. Preoperative assessment and patient preparation

1. History and physical examination

   a. Cardiovascular: *assess baseline status*

      (1) Parasympathetic nervous system response to electroconvulsive therapy is immediate and may cause asystole, bradycardia, premature ventricular contractions, hypotension, and ventricular escape

(2) Sympathetic nervous system discharge follows within seconds manifested as increased heart rate, premature ventricular contractions, bigeminy, tachycardia, and severe hypertension

(3) Myocardial oxygen consumption often increases significantly

b. Endocrine: *assess status of diabetes and glucose levels—neuroendocrine response is manifested by increased levels of adrenocorticotropic hormones, cortisol, and catecholamine*

c. Musculoskeletal: *assess for long bone of vertebral fractures and severe osteoporosis—convulsions may exacerbate skeletal trauma*

2. Relative contraindications
   a. *Angina pectoris*
   b. *Congestive heart failure*
   c. *Chronic obstructive pulmonary disease*
   d. *Thrombophlebitis*
   e. *Glaucoma and retinal detachment*

3. Absolute contraindications
   a. *Recent myocardial infarction*
   b. *Recent stroke*
   c. *Intracranial mass*
   d. *Pheochromocytoma*

4. *Laboratory tests:* electrolytes, glucose

5. Preoperative medications and intravenous therapy
   a. *Antipsychotic agents may compound the sedating properties of anesthesia*
   b. *Monoamine oxidase inhibitors predispose to hemodynamic oxidase inhibitors, hemodynamic instability, hypertensive crisis*
   c. *Patients receiving lithium may show delayed awakening, memory loss, and confusion postictally*
   d. *Antacids and metoclopramide reduces the risk of aspiration of gastric contents*
   e. *Anticholinergics modify parasympathetic nervous system response—glycopyrrolate causes USS tachycardia and central nervous system confusion*
   f. *18-gauge intravenous line with minimal fluid replacement*

C. Room preparation
1. *Monitoring equipment:* electrocardiogram, blood pressure cuff, pulse oximeter, and tourniquet
2. *Pharmacologic agents:* standard
3. *Position:* supine, arms safely tucked to the side or secured on armboards

D. Anesthetic techniques
Use general anesthesia and skeletal muscle paralysis.

E. Perioperative management
1. Induction
   a. *Methohexital (0.75 to 1.0 mg/kg IV)—its redistribution is more rapid than that of thiopental, thus decreasing recovery time; etomidate (0.3 to 0.4 mg/kg IV) may be an alternative*
   b. *Ventilate lungs with oxygen by mask*

c. *Inflate a tourniquet on the arm opposite the intravenous catheter—permits seizure visualization because the arm is isolated from the muscle relaxant*

d. *Administer a muscle relaxant, usually succinylcholine (1 mg/kg IV)*

2. Maintenance

a. *Ventilation continues by mask with 100 mL oxygen*

b. *An oral airway may be inserted to prevent tongue and tooth damage*

c. *An electrical charge is applied to the head—avoid contact with the patient and stretcher*

d. *Severe hypertension is expected: a short-acting intravenous agent may be needed*

3. Emergence: mask ventilation is resumed until spontaneous recovery occurs

F. Postoperative implications—none

J. Ventriculoperitoneal Shunt

◆ ◆ ◆

A. Introduction

A ventriculoperitoneal shunt is placed to relieve increasing cerebrospinal fluid pressures. The hydrocephalus may be caused by a congenital defect, cyst, tumor, trauma, infection, or cerebral blood flow absorption abnormality. Therefore, patients undergoing this procedure range in age from the newborn to the elderly. Besides a conduit to the peritoneum, the ventricle can also be drained into the pleura or right atrium.

B. Preoperative assessment

Neurologic intracranial pressure (ICP) monitoring is routine. Assess for level of consciousness, headaches, nuchal rigidity seizures, and any presurgical neurologic defects such as stroke, spina bifida, and focal defects. Review results of computed tomography of the head. Review blood pressure and heart rate trends in relation to ICP. Cushing's triad—increased ICP-increased blood pressure and decreased heart rate.

C. Patient preparation

Complete blood count, electrolytes (especially if the patient is receiving diuretics), glucose (especially if the patient is on steroids such as dexamethasone), prothrombin time, partial thromboplastin time, type and screen. Use 12-lead electrocardiography and chest radiography if the history suggests. Review the results of head computed tomography. Communicate with the neurologist if steroid and diuretic therapy are anticipated during surgery. Usually, preoperative medication is not given to patients with increased ICP.

D. Room preparation

1. *Monitors:* standard and ICP monitor

2. *Position:* supine with the head turned. A shoulder roll may be used. A foam head rest aids positioning.
3. *Additional equipment:* table will probably be turned, requiring an adequate length of ventilation tubing. Because much of the patient will be exposed, it is helpful to have a fluid warmer and the room temperature adjusted warmer.
4. *Drugs and tabletop:* standard. Fluids are usually run at approximately 4 mL/h.

E. Anesthesia and perioperative management

Use general anesthesia with endotracheal intubation. Thiopental and etomidate are good choices for induction because of their cerebral protective properties. Muscle relaxation is desirable. Normocarbia aids the surgeon in cannulating the ventricles. It is wise to have the thiopental or etomidate immediately available during the "tunneling," which is the most stimulating part of this procedure. Extubation is performed at the end of the procedure.

F. Postoperative implications

Assess neurologic status. Pain can usually be managed with oral preparations.

—JAFFE PAIN 4-6/10
— CUSHING'S TRIAD (↑ICP) → ↓↓HR, ↑BP, RESP. ARREST

SECTION V

INTRATHORACIC AND EXTRATHORACIC

A. Mediastinoscopy

◆ ◆ ◆

CHAMBERLAIN PROCEDURE USED FOR LEFT SIDE OF MEDIASTINUM

A. Introduction

→ Performed to diagnose and stage the spread of carcinoma of the bronchus. Permits biopsy of the subcarinal, peritracheal, and superior tracheobronchial lymph nodes under direct visualization. A small transverse incision is made above the suprasternal notch. The patient's head is turned to the left, and the mediastinoscope is placed in the space between the anterior surface of the trachea and the posterior border of the suprasternal notch.

B. Preoperative assessment and patient preparation

1. History and physical examination

   a. *Respiratory*

   (1) Search for potential airway obstructions and distortions *CAN PT. LIE SUPINE?*

   (2) Assess smoking history

→ (3) Mediastinoscopy may cause recurrent laryngeal nerve injury

   b. *Cardiac*

   (3) BLEEDING (INADVERTENT GREAT VESSEL PUNCTURE)

   (1) Assess for hypertension, angina, dysrhythmias, congestive heart failure, etc.

   (2) Reflex bradycardia and arrhythmias may be caused by mechanical compression on the aorta

   c. *Neurologic*

   (1) Assess for evidence of impaired cerebral circulation: stroke, carotid bruits, transient ischemic attacks

→ (2) The mediastinoscope can exert pressure against the innominate artery and cause diminished blood flow to the right carotid and subclavian arteries

   √RGP

2. Diagnostic tests

   a. *Review Eaton-Lambert syndrome resulting from oat cell carcinoma because mediastinoscopy is used as a diagnostic test*

   b. *Posterior chest radiography*

   c. *Laboratory tests: complete blood count, electrolytes, glucose, prothrombin time, partial thromboplastin time, type and cross-match*

224

3. Preoperative medications and intravenous therapy
   a. *Sedatives and narcotics—use with caution in patients with poor respiratory reserve*
   b. *18-gauge peripheral intravenous with minimal fluid replacement* ⟵

   · RIGHT A line
   · LARGE IV IN LEFT
   · X2 LUMEN TUBE?

C. **Room preparations**
1. Monitoring equipment
   a. *Pulse oximeter on the right and a noninvasive blood pressure monitor on the left arm*
   b. *Continuous assessment to identify compression of the innominate artery: repositioning of the mediastinoscope is necessary*
   c. *Peripheral nerve stimulator*
2. Pharmacologic agents
   a. *Atropine—vagal mediated reflexes*   JAFFE PAIN 2-3
   b. *Cardioactive drugs*
3. *Position: supine—arms may need to be tucked to the side*

D. **Anesthetic techniques**
   Local anesthetic with intravenous sedation and general anesthetic.
1. *Local anesthetic with sedation: mediastinum has extensive autonomic nerve supply but few pain fibers. This technique allows continuous monitoring of the level of consciousness in a patient with cerebrovascular disease or an airway obstruction.*
2. *General anesthetic: endotracheal intubation*
3. *Technique of choice: general anesthesia*

E. **Perioperative management**
1. *Induction: consider the use of reinforced/armored tubes—avoids tracheal compression from the mediastinoscope*
2. Maintenance
   a. *After endotracheal intubation, either an inhalation or a balanced anesthetic may be used*   NO N₂O!
   b. *Although the procedure is not very stimulating, the patient must remain motionless* ⟵ JAFFE 3/10 PAIN
   c. *A muscle relaxant may be used to prevent the patient from coughing because this may produce venous engagement in the chest or trauma by the mediastinoscope*
   d. *Patients with Eaton-Lambert syndrome are sensitive to succinylcholine and nondepolarizing muscle relaxants; therefore, reduce the dosage*
   e. *Positive-pressure ventilation of the lungs minimizes the risk of venous air embolism*
3. Emergence
   a. *Extubate after full return of airway reflexes*
   b. *Consider evaluation of vocal cord movement (extubate under direct vision)*

   AIRWAY OBSTRUCTION (VAGAL RESPONSE)
   AIR EMBOLISM
   ALSO GREAT VESSEL RUPTURE

F. **Postoperative implications**
   Obtain chest radiographs—pneumothorax is a complication; it is ⟵ usually right-sided. Signs and symptoms are tracheal shift, decreased blood pressure, cyanosis, decreased oxygen saturation (SpO_2), decreased chest movement, decreased blood sugar. Treatment—100% oxygen and prepare for chest-tube insertion.

B. Open Lung Biopsy (Wedge Resection of Lung Lesion)

◆ ◆ ◆

A. Introduction

This procedure involves the removal of a mass and 1-cm margins in a manner that does not remove an entire pulmonary segment. This procedure is appropriate for a patient with limited pulmonary reserve who cannot tolerate a lobectomy.

B. Preoperative assessment

1. *Cardiovascular:* electrocardiography (watch for right-ventricular hypertrophy, conduction defects, and prior ischemia)
2. *Respiratory:* pulmonary function tests as with an open thoracotomy. Chest radiographs if computed tomography of the chest is not available. Look for airway obstruction, which could interfere with double-lumen tube (DLT) placement.
3. *Musculoskeletal:* patients diagnosed with lung cancer may have myasthenic (Eaton-Lambert) syndrome, causing an increased sensitivity to nondepolarizing muscle relaxants
4. *Hematologic:* patients are often anemic because of their primary disease. Preoperative blood transfusions may be a consideration.
5. *Premedication:* when epidural opioids are planned, avoid opioid or other sedative medications, which may potentiate the respiratory effects of the spinal opioids

C. Room preparation

1. Routine monitors and room set-up. Consider a DLT if one-lung ventilation is needed. If so, have a fiberoptic bronchoscope available for checking tube placement. An arterial line is needed occasionally.
   The patient will be positioned in the lateral decubitus or supine position. If the patient is supine, a wedge will be placed under the back of the operative side.
2. One large-bore intravenous tube will be needed.
3. *Fluid requirements:* normal saline or lactated Ringer's at 2 mL/kg per hour

D. Perioperative management and anesthesia

Routine induction and maintenance. Use a balance technique of oxygen, isoflurane, and intravenous opioids (if an epidural catheter is not used). Nitrous oxide may be used with two-lung ventilation, but discontinue with one-lung ventilation.

Extubate in the operating room, transfer the patient in the head-up position to the postanesthesia care unit or intensive care unit with oxygen via mask.

E. Postoperative management

Postoperative complications include atelectasis, pneumonia, and fluid overload.

C. Thoracotomy

A. Introduction

Thoracotomy is usually performed in an attempt to resect malignant lung tissue but may also be performed for trauma, infections, and parenchymal abnormalities such as recurrent blebs. Because thoracotomy involves incising the pleura, all patients require a chest tube postoperatively. Most patients are above the age of 40 years with a history of smoking. Many also have associated cardiovascular disease.

B. Preoperative assessment

1. *Cardiac:* exercise tolerance is an excellent assessment for cardiopulmonary reserve. Also question the patient about heart failure or arrhythmias. A 12-lead electrocardiogram is needed. Echocardiography and cardiac catheterization may also be useful in certain patients.

2. *Respiratory:* pulmonary function tests are routine for elective cases involving resections. Arterial blood gases are mandatory but cannot often predict postoperative functioning. Chest radiographs are mandatory. Most patients also have computed tomography of the chest. Question the patient about smoking history, bronchospasm, exercise tolerance, pneumonia. Auscultate the chest carefully immediately preoperatively. Confer with the surgeon about one-lung anesthesia preferences and whether there are any foreseeable problems with tube placement (e.g., tumor in the mainstem bronchus).

3. *Neurologic:* the incidence of Eaton-Lambert syndrome is increased in patients with lung cancer. Assess patients for any generalized weakness or any focal weaknesses that may be the result of stroke.

4. *Gastrointestinal, renal, endocrine:* routine

C. Patient preparation

Laboratory tests include complete blood count, electrolytes, blood urea nitrogen, creatinine, glucose, prothrombin time, partial thromboplastin time, arterial blood gases; type and cross-match for at least 2 units (depending on the type of surgery and the patient's hemoglobin.) Other tests are electrocardiography, chest radiography, pulmonary function tests, and others indicated by history. Keep preoperative medications, especially narcotics, to a minimum in patients who are carbon dioxide retainers. Digitalization is recommended during pneumonectomy to help prevent postoperative heart failure. It will also reduce tachyarrhythmias intraoperatively. Have bronchodilators, especially inhalants, readily available. Many practitioners administer them prophylactically. Administer an anti-sialagogue, such as glycopyrrolate, to ease placement and verification of the double-lumen endobronchial tube.

D. Room preparation

1. *Monitoring:* standard with a reliable arterial line. Central venous pressure or pulmonary arterial catheter for patients with pre-existing

heart disease. Keep in mind that central venous pressure readings may be inaccurate while the chest is opened, and the pulmonary arterial catheter may interfere with a pneumonectomy.

2. *Additional equipment:* Double-lumen endobronchial tubes, at least two. (Balloon rupture upon insertion is common.) Fiberoptic endoscope to check tube placement. Equipment to add continuous positive airway pressure and positive end-expiratory pressure intraoperatively. Epidural catheter insertion and infusion supplies, if used. Warming devices for the patient and fluids.

3. *Positioning:* lateral or supine with lateral tilt. Bean bag, arm "sled," and axillary rolls may be used. Check for lack of pressure on down arm, eye, ear. Ensure that arms are not hyperextended.

4. *Drugs and fluids:* it is preferable to err on the side of underhydrating because these patients are prone to pulmonary edema. Usually use no more than 4 to 5 mL/kg per hour. Have ephedrine/phenylephrine available to treat hypotension. Usual blood loss will not exceed 1000 mL.

E. Perioperative management and anesthetic techniques
Use standard induction techniques keeping in mind that the positioning and placement of a double-lumen endobronchial tube require more time than a standard tube placement. Preoxygenate these patients. Arterial blood gases are obtained after the induction for baseline so that they may be compared with later results on one-lung ventilation. During one-lung ventilation, maintain tidal volume and place patient on 100% oxygen. If hypoxemia is present (verify tube placement first), add 5 cm of continuous positive airway pressure to the "up" (surgical) lung. If hypoxemia is still present, add 5 cm of positive end-expiratory pressure to the "down" (ventilated) lung. Extubation at the end of the procedure is preferable unless the patient had a preoperative respiratory indication for remaining intubated (e.g., bronchospasm) or there were large fluid shifts. If the patient needs to remain intubated, the double-lumen tube must be replaced with a standard endotracheal tube.

F. Postoperative considerations
Epidural anesthesia, patient-controlled analgesia, or another type of pain control (e.g., nerve block) should be planned preoperatively. The patient must understand and be able to perform deep-breathing exercises. Institute intensive care unit monitoring for at least 24 hours.

D. Bronchopulmonary Lavage

♦   ♦   ♦

A. Introduction
This procedure consists of irrigation of the lung and bronchial tree. It is performed under general anesthesia with a double-lumen tube.

Bronchopulmonary lavage can be used to treat alveolar proteinosis, cystic fibrosis, bronchiectasis, radioactive dust inhalation, and asthma or bronchitis.

B. Preoperative assessment and patient preparation
Routine preoperative assessment, including a ventilation-perfusion scan. The lavage is performed on the most severely affected lung first. If both lungs are affected equally, the left lung is lavaged first because of better exchange on the larger right lung.

C. Room preparation
A fiberoptic bronchoscope is needed to check for accurate placement of the double-lumen tube. Monitors are routine, including an arterial line. A stethoscope should be placed over the nondependent lung to check for rales, which may indicate leakage of the lavaged fluid into this lung. The patient is positioned in the left or right down position.

D. Perioperative management and anesthetic technique
After intravenous induction, anesthesia is maintained with an inhalation agent. Keep the fractional inspired oxygen as high as possible. The cuff seal on the double-lumen tube should be checked and should maintain perfect separation at a pressure of 90% of the fluid cm H_2O to prevent leakage of fluid from around the cuff.

With the patient in the head-up position, 700 to 1000 mL of warmed heparinized isotonic saline is instilled from a reservoir 30 cm above the midaxillary line into the catheter to the dependent lung. When the fluid ceases to flow, the patient is placed in the head-down position and the fluid is allowed to drain out.

With each lavage, inflow and outflow volumes are measured to prevent excess absorption and leakage to the ventilated side. At least 90% of the fluid should be recovered with each lavage. Two-lung ventilation is reestablished and as compliance improves air may be added to maintain alveolar patency. Patients can be extubated in the operating room if stable.

COMMON PROCEDURES

E. Thymectomy

◆ ◆ ◆

A. Introduction
The thymus gland is a bilobate mass of lymphoid tissue located deep to the sternum in the anterior region of the mediastinum.
Thymectomy involves two surgical approaches: median sternotomy or transcervical.

The thymus gland is believed to play a role in myasthenia gravis. This is a neuromuscular disorder in which postsynaptic acetylcholine receptors are attacked, inducing rapid receptor destruction.

B. Preoperative assessment and patient preparation
1. History and physical examination
    a. *Respiratory (based on the myasthenia gravis patient)*
        (1) Weakness of pharyngeal and laryngeal muscles with a high risk of aspiration. Assess patient's ability to cough and handle secretions.
        (2) "Myasthenic crisis" an exacerbation involving respiratory muscles to the point of inadequate ventilation
    b. Cardiac: *potential cardiomyopathy*
    c. *Neurologic*
        (1) Fatiguability and fluctuating motor weakness of voluntary skeletal muscles that worsens with repetitive use and improves with rest
        (2) Ptosis and diplopia are initial symptoms
    d. Endocrine: *potential hypothyroidism*
2. Diagnostic tests
    a. *Pulmonary function studies need not be performed on all patients, but proper knowledge of the prothrombin time, tidal volume, vital capacity, and forced expiratory volume enables one to anticipate problems*
    b. *Laboratory tests include electrolytes, complete blood count, type and screen*
3. Preoperative medications and intravenous therapy
    a. Cholinesterase incubators *retard the enzymatic hydrolysis of acetylcholine at cholinergic synapses, causing acetylcholine to accumulate at the neuromuscular junction. Continue up to the morning of scheduled surgery.*
    b. *Immunosuppressive drugs*
        (1) Interfere with production of antibodies that are responsible for degradation of cholinergic receptors
        (2) Patients who have been on these drugs for more than 1 month in the past 6 to 12 months need supplementary steroids
    c. Antisialogogues and H_2 (histamine$_2$ receptor) blockers—*patients with bulbar involvement should be evaluated to determine the safety of these drugs*
    d. Sedatives and narcotics—*use with caution in patients with poor respiratory reserve*
    e. *Antibiotics*
    f. *18-gauge intravenous tube with moderate fluid replacement*
C. Room preparations
1. Monitoring equipment
    a. *Peripheral nerve stimulator*
    b. *Arterial line*
        (1) If arterial blood gas monitoring is deemed necessary
        (2) Some suggest placing the catheter in the left radial artery for continuous monitoring in case the innominate artery is damaged
2. Pharmacologic agents
    a. *Standard*

  b. *Depolarizing muscle relaxants are not to be used with myasthenia gravis patients*
  c. *Nondepolarizing muscle relaxant: myasthenia gravis patients have varying responses. A small dose of atracurium 3 to 5 mg per 70 kg or vecuronium 1 to 2 kg per 70 kg can be given, but anticipate prolonged weakness*
 3. *Position:* supine

D. Anesthetic techniques
  General anesthesia—endotracheal intubation is required.

E. Perioperative management
 1. Induction
  a. *When anesthetizing myasthenia gravis patients, avoidance of all muscle relaxants is preferred*
  b. *An inhaled anesthetic by itself should provide sufficient relaxation of skeletal muscle for intubation of the trachea*
 2. Maintenance
  a. *Ability to dissipate the effects of inhaled drugs at the conclusion of anesthesia is important for evaluation of muscle strength*
  b. *Prolonged effects of narcotics, especially on ventilation, detracts from the use of these drugs for maintenance*
 3. Emergence
  a. *Before extubating the patient, it is important to know that respiratory ability is adequate*
  b. *Minimal extubation criteria*
   (1) Vital capacity of 15 mL/kg
   (2) Head lift for at least 5 seconds
   (3) Tidal volume greater than 10 mL/kg
   (4) Ability to follow commands
   (5) Negative inspired force greater than -25 mm Hg
  c. *Reversal of neuromuscular blockade is controversial—the additional anticholinesterase may increase weakness and precipitate a cholinergic crisis*

F. Postoperative considerations
 1. Patients may need to be observed in an intensive care unit
 2. Anesthesia and surgery often decrease the need for anticholinesterase drugs in the postoperative period

F. Bronchoscopy

◆   ◆   ◆

A. Introduction
 The procedure permits direct inspection of the larynx, trachea, and bronchi. Indications include collection of secretions for cytologic or

bacteriologic examination, tissue biopsy, location of bleeding and tumors, removal of a foreign body, and implantation of radioactive gold seeds for tumor treatment.

B. Preoperative assessment
1. History and physical examination
   a. Respiratory: *evaluate for chronic lung disease, wheezing, atelectasis, hemoptysis, cough, unresolved pneumonia, diffuse lung disease, and smoking history*
   b. Cardiac: *question underlying dysrhythmias because they may arise with stimulation of the scope, or they could be a sign of hypoxemia during the procedure*
   c. Gastrointestinal: *access drinking history and nutritional intake*
2. Diagnostic tests
   a. *Chest radiography*
   b. *Computed tomography*
   c. *Pulmonary function test with lung disease*
   d. *Laboratory tests include complete blood count, electrolytes, glucose, prothrombin times, partial thromboplastin time*
3. Preoperative medications and intravenous therapy
   a. *The patient may already be on sympathomimetic bronchodilators and aminophylline*
   b. *Sedatives and narcotics are to be used with caution in patients with poor respiratory reserve*
   ROBINALOZINC. *Cholinergic blocking agents reduce saluation, tracheobronchial and pharyngeal secretions*
   d. *Intravenous lidocaine: 0.5 to 1.5 mg/kg decreases airway reflexes*
   e. *Topical anesthesia: 4% lidocaine using a nebulizer to anesthetize the airway by spraying the palate, pharynx, larynx, vocal cords, and trachea*
   f. *One 18-gauge peripheral intravenous with minimal fluid replacement*

C. Room preparation
1. Monitoring equipment
   a. *Oxygen saturation monitors hypoxemia secondary to intermittent and uneven ventilation*
   b. Electrocardiogram: *higher incidence of ventricular arrhythmias— best treated with increasing ventilation, administering lidocaine, or both*
   c. *End-tidal carbon dioxide (EtCO's) assess for hypercarbia secondary to inadequate ventilation*
   d. Peripheral nerve stimulation: *in patients suspected of malignancy, consider the possibility of a myasthenic syndrome. These patients are sensitive to nondepolarizers*
   e. *Dental guard prevents damage*
   f. *Bacterial filters protect the anesthesia machine from contamination and respiratory secretions*
   g. *Arterial line—if thoracotomy is planned or the patient is unstable*
2. *Pharmacologic agents:* propranolol, lidocaine, and cardiac drugs
3. *Position:* supine—table may be turned. One must manage an upper airway that is shared with the surgeon.
   SHOULDER ROLL IF RIGID BRONCHOSCOPY

D. Anesthetic techniques
1. Local infiltration or general anesthesia
2. Technique of choice is general anesthesia
   Must discuss with the surgeon if a rigid or flexible fiberoptic bronchoscopy will be performed
3. Nerve blocks
   a. Transtracheal: *2 mL of 2% plain lidocaine through the cricothyroid membrane using a 22-gauge needle attached to a small syringe*
   b. Superior laryngeal: *25-gauge needle anterior to the superior cornu of the thyroid cartilage*
      If topical anesthesia is employed, consider total dosage of local anesthetic and be prepared to treat local anesthetic toxicity

E. Perioperative management *FLEXIBLE OR RIGID?*
1. Induction
   a. Flexible bronchoscopy   *— HOLD TUBE DURING PROCEDURE*
                                    — CUT TUBE AT 26 cm
      (1) Endotracheal tube must be long enough (8.0 to 8.5 mm) to permit endoscope to pass easily
      (2) Do not administer O_2 through the suction channel of the flexible bronchoscope to avoid gas trapping and inducing barotrauma
   b. Rigid bronchoscopy
      (1) Conventional ventilation
         (a) Ventilation through the side port requires high gas-flow rates and an intact glass eyepiece
         (b) Suction, biopsy, and foreign-body manipulation require removal of the glass and loss of ventilation
      (2) Jet ventilation
         (a) Give patients high inspired oxygen and hyperventilate them before apneic oxygenation
         (b) Perform jet ventilation through the side port of a catheter alongside the bronchoscope
         (c) Place the tracheal tube to the left side of the mouth because the surgeon will insert the scope down the right side
         (d) The endotracheal tube must be smaller in diameter to allow surgical access
   c. *After preoxygenation, general anesthesia is induced with the insertion of an oral endotracheal tube*
   d. *Succinylcholine may be contraindicated if the patient has severe muscle-spasm wasting or complains of myalgia*
2. Maintenance   *JAFFE   PAIN* ⅒
   a. *General anesthesia must provide good muscle relaxation without patient movement: coughing, laryngospasm, or bronchospasm*
   b. *Cardiac dysrhythmia may be a problem (i.e., supraventricular tachyarrhythmia, premature ventricular contraction, and atrial dysrhythmias). Plan appropriate treatment modalities.*
   c. *Volatile anesthetics are useful to provide adequate suppression of upper-airway reflexes and permit high inhaled concentrations of oxygen*

COMMON PROCEDURES

    d. *Air leaks around the bronchoscope may be minimized by having an assistant externally compress the hypopharynx*

    e. *Spontaneous ventilation is preferred in cases of foreign body removal—positive airway pressures could push the foreign body deeper into the bronchial tree*

  3. Emergence – CAN BE "STORMY"

    a. *The patient should be awakened rapidly with complete return of airway reflexes prior to extubation*

    b. *Patient needs to have a cough to clear secretions and blood from the airway*

F. Postoperative implications

  1. If nerve blocks are administered, keep the patient from eating or drinking for several hours postoperatively—the blocks cause depression of airway reflexes

  2. Subglottic edema may be treated with aerosolized racemic epinephrine and intravenous dexamethasone (0.1 mg/kg)

  3. Chest radiographs to detect atelectasis or pneumothorax

G. Breast Biopsy

◆ ◆ ◆

A. Introduction

Breast cancer is diagnosed via excisional biopsy (by needle aspiration or open excision), followed later by a more definitive surgical procedure designed to decrease tumor bulk and thus enhance effectiveness of systemic therapy (chemotherapy, hormonal therapy, or radiation). Carcinoma of the breast is an uncontrolled growth of anaplastic cells. Types include ductal, lobular, and nipple adenocarcinomas.

B. Preoperative assessment and patient preparation

  1. History and physical examination

    a. *Most common initial sign of carcinoma of the breast is a painless mass*

    b. *Bloody discharge is more indicative of cancer than spontaneous unilateral serous nipple discharge*

    c. *Signs of advanced breast cancer include dimpling of skin, nipple retraction, change in breast contour, edema, and erythema of the breast skin*

  2. Diagnostic tests

    a. *Mammography, thermography, ultrasonography*

    b. *Metastases to bone are frequent; therefore, bone scan and measurement of the alkaline phosphatase may be indicated*

    c. *Laboratory tests include hemoglobin, hematocrit, electrolytes, glucose*

  3. Preoperative medications and intravenous therapy

    a. *The patient may be on hormone therapy*

b. Use light sedation and short-acting narcotics preoperatively because the procedure lasts less than 1 hour

c. Metoclopramide (Reglan)—outpatients have an increased gastric volume and there may be insufflation of air into the stomach if one is using a mask technique

d. One 18-gauge intravenous tube with minimal fluid replacement

C. Room preparation

1. Monitoring equipment

a. Standard

b. Noninvasive blood pressure cuff on the side opposite of surgery

2. Pharmacologic agents: standard

3. Position: supine—may need to tuck the surgical arm to the side

D. Anesthetic techniques

1. Local infiltration and general anesthesia

2. Technique of choice is general anesthesia with mask technique

E. Perioperative management

1. Induction: consider rapid sequence induction and endotracheal intubation with a patient who is obese or on a full stomach

2. Maintenance: no indications

3. Emergence: if rapid sequence induction is used, perform an awake extubation

F. Postoperative implications—none

H. Mastectomy

♦   ♦   ♦

A. Introduction

A total mastectomy (simple or complete mastectomy) removes only the breast. No axillary node dissection is involved. It is used for the treatment of duct carcinoma in situ. A radical mastectomy involves removal of the breast, underlying pectoral muscles, and axillary lymph nodes. There are two major alternatives to radical mastectomy. They are modified radical mastectomy and wide local excision of the tumor (partial mastectomy or lumpectomy) with axillary dissection. This treatment is followed by postoperative radiation therapy to the remaining breast.

B. Preoperative assessment

Patients often have no other underlying medical problems. One should consider the anesthetic implications of metastatic spread to bone, brain, liver, lung, and other areas. Preoperative assessment should be routine, with special consideration to the following:

1. Cardiac: cardiomyopathies may result from chemotherapeutic agents (e.g., doxorubicin at doses > 75 mg/m^2). Patients exposed to this type of drug may experience cardiac dysfunction, and a cardiac consultation may be needed to determine ventricular function.

COMMON PROCEDURES

2. *Respiratory:* if the patient has undergone radiation therapy, there may be some respiratory compromise. Drugs such as bleomycin (greater than 200 mg/m^2) can cause pulmonary toxicity and necessitate administration of low fractional inspiration of oxygen (≤ 0.30).

3. *Neurologic:* breast cancer often metastasizes to the central nervous system, and there could be signs of focal neurologic deficits, altered mental status, or increased intracranial pressure. If mental status is altered, full medical work-up should be undertaken without delay: postpone surgery until the cause is found.

4. *Hematologic:* the patient may be anemic secondary to chronic disease or chemotherapeutic agents.

C. Room preparation

Monitors and equipment are routine. If the procedure is for a superficial biopsy, one can use monitored anesthesia care with sedation. Be sure to place the blood pressure cuff on the arm opposite the operative site.

The patient is placed in the supine position during the procedure.

D. Perioperative management and anesthesia techniques

1. Routine induction and maintenance

2. Pressure dressings are often applied with the patient anesthetized and "sitting up" at the conclusion of the procedure. Communicate with the surgeon if this type of dressing will be used in order to time emergence more appropriately. If there are no further considerations, the patient may be extubated in the operating room.

E. Considerations

1. Deep surgical exploration may inadvertently cause a pneumothorax. The patient should be monitored for signs and symptoms of pneumothorax, which include increased peak inspiratory pressures, decreased arterial carbon dioxide pressure, asymmetric breath sounds, hemodynamic instability, and hyper-resonance to percussion over the affected side.

2. Diagnosis is concluded by a chest radiograph.

3. Treatment includes placing the patient on a fractional inspired oxygen of 100% and insertion of a chest tube.

F. Postoperative implications

1. If the patient is unstable hemodynamically (which may suggest a tension pneumothorax), place a 14-gauge angiocatheter in the second intercostal space while the surgeons set up for a chest tube.

2. A postoperative chest radiograph may be needed if a pneumothorax is possible.

I. Axillary Node Dissection

♦ ♦ ♦

This procedure is the same as a mastectomy except that the incision is over the breast or previous biopsy site. A separate transverse incision is made in the axilla using different instruments. Prior to closure, an axillary drain is placed.

J. Chest Tube Insertion

◆   ◆   ◆

A. Introduction

Chest tubes with attached drainage systems are placed in the pleural cavity to drain fluid, blood, or air from the pleural cavity and to reestablish a negative pressure that will facilitate expansion of the lung.

Pneumothorax:	2nd and 3rd intercostal spaces, anterior
Hemothorax:	7th, 8th, or 9th intercostal space, posterior
Thoracotomy:	one tube in the 2nd or 3rd intercostal space anterior and another in the lower posterior axillary line

B. Preoperative assessment and patient preparation

1. History and physical examination: *Respiratory:* rate and quality, evidence of dyspnea, labored breathing, tachypnea, tachycardia, quality and distribution of breath sounds, mediastinal shift, subcutaneous emphysema, and crepitus
2. Diagnostic tests
   a. *Chest radiograph*
   b. *Auscultation of lung sounds*
3. Preoperative medication and intravenous therapy
   a. *Sedatives and narcotics—use with caution in patients with poor respiratory reserve*
   b. *One 18-gauge peripheral intravenous with* minimal *fluid replacement*

C. Room preparation

1. *Monitoring equipment:* standard—procedure may be performed away from the main operating room (intensive care unit). All anesthetizing equipment must be available.
2. *Pharmacologic agents:* standard
3. *Position:* supine

D. Anesthetic techniques

1. Local infiltration and sedation
2. Local infiltration—administered by surgeon
3. Intravenous sedation with midazolam, brevital, or propofol in sedative doses

E. Perioperative management

1. *Induction:* no specific indications
2. *Maintenance:* no specific indications
3. *Emergence:* support the airway and maintain ventilation

COMMON PROCEDURES

F. Postoperative implications
1. Portable chest radiographs to confirm placement and rule out complications
2. Chest tubes, to be terminated when radiography reveals the lung has re-expanded and when drainage has slowed to less than 75 mL/day

CARDIAC SURGERY

A. Coronary Artery Bypass Grafting

♦ ♦ ♦

Methods have been devised to promote coronary blood flow since it has been determined that thrombosis causes the development of myocardial infraction. Some of these methods involve shunting collateral pericardial blood to epicardial arteries and implantation of the internal mammary artery to the left ventricle without ligating side-branches. Saphenous veins can also be anastomosed to the epicardial coronary arteries. The technique of coronary artery bypass involves bypass to a narrowed or occluded epicardial coronary greater than 1 mm in diameter with a small-diameter conduit distal to the narrowed segment. The proximal arterial inflow source is the ascending aorta.

The surgeon approaches the heart via a median sternotomy, and the patient is supported on full coronary artery bypass. The most common strategy used is for all distal (epicardial) anastomoses to be performed during a period of aortic cross-clamping and cardiac arrest. Myocardial protection is achieved by hypothermia and occasional repercussion via anterograde or retrograde cardioplegia. Cardiac standstill and a bloodless field are mandatory when these small-diameter anastomoses are constructed with an obstruction to flow in a minimal amount of time.

The cross clamp is removed, and the heart is allowed to resume beating. A partially occluding aortic cross-clamp can be applied to allow for the construction of the proximal aortic anastomoses. After an adequate period of resuscitation, the patient is weaned from cardiopulmonary bypass (CPB). And decannulation is performed, heparin is reversed, and the chest is closed.

Typical target arteries requiring CPB include the distal right coronary artery (RCA) and its major terminal branch, the posterior descending artery. Typical target arteries on the left include the left anterior descending (LAD) with its diagonal and septal branches. This coronary artery courses in the posterior atrioventricular groove and is not easily accessible for bypass. Therefore, this procedure is usually performed to its obtuse marginal or posterolateral branches.

The choice of the vein graft depends on its availability and durability. The internal mammary artery appears to have superior long-term performance with patency rates of 90% after 10 years. On the other hand, the saphenous vein graft has a 50% patency rate at 10 years.

The usual preoperative diagnosis of these patients is coronary artery disease with class 3 or 4 angina. This type of angina occurs with minimal exertion or at rest.

A. Preoperative assessment and patient preparation

Patients are divided into two main groups: those with good left-ventricular (LV) function and those with poor LV function. The latter are considered to be at high risk. These patients are usually in cardiac failure: ejection fraction below 40%, LV end-diastolic pressure over 18 mm Hg, cardiac index less than 2.0 L/m^2 per min, ventricular dyskinesias, three-vessel disease, occlusion of the LAD or left main equivalent, valvular disease, recent myocardial infarction (MI) (or one in progress), ventricular aneurysm, ventricular septal defect (VSD), old age.

1. History and physical examination

   a. *Cardiac*

      (1) *Check:* history of angina (stable, unstable at rest, and precipitating factors); exercise tolerance; congestive heart failure—symptoms are shortness of breath, orthopnea, pulmonary edema; jugular venous distention; 3rd heart sound; recent MI (within 6 months); dysrhythmia; hypertension; vascular disease (carotid stenosis, aortic disease); valvular disease (aortic stenosis or mitral regurgitation). VSD or LV aneurysm may increase the risk of perioperative complications.

      (2) *Tests:* 12-lead electrocardiogram, stress test, thallium scan (to check for irreversible ischemia), echocardiogram, cardiac catheter

      (3) *Postinfarction VSD:* postinfarction VSD is associated with high operative morbidity and mortality rates. This is because of the difficulty in repairing the friable tissue lesion. These patients are considered to be at high risk and often require support, including the intra-aortic balloon pump during induction and before and after bypass.

      (4) *LV aneurysm:* usually a late complication of the infarction, although it can occur early when it is associated with cardiac rupture. Cardiac rupture carries a high mortality rate. These patients usually have poor myocardial function and should be anesthetized with full monitoring, including pulmonary arterial catheterization. Following bypass, the LV cavity is smaller and less compliant. Adequate cardiac output requires an adequate preload, a higher-than-normal heart rate and sinus rhythm, and possibly the use of inotropics. Hemostasis is often difficult to obtain, and treatment usually includes the use of blood and blood products.

      (5) *Emergency revascularization:* usually occurs with an acute MI. Sometimes occurs with acute LV failure or after failed percutaneous transluminal coronary angioplasty. The patient may be stable, suffering acute ischemia, hemodynamically unstable, or in full cardiac arrest.

      (6) *Considerations:* full-stomach precautions and the need for rapid sequence induction in lieu of ischemia (*this is determined by the guidelines of your institution*). Prior use of fibrinolytic agents increases the possibility of hemorrhage. Consider the

use of antifibrinolytic agents (e.g., aminocaproic acid) and the need for inotropes and antiarrhythmics. Morbidity and mortality in these patients are increased.

b. Respiratory: *assess for any smoking history, chronic obstructive pulmonary disease (COPD). Encourage the patient to stop smoking 2 weeks before surgery, if possible. Treat COPD to optimize therapy prior to surgery. Tests include chest radiography and pulmonary function tests (if available).*

c. Neurologic: *assess for previous stroke or carotid artery disease; signs and symptoms should be documented and evaluated*

d. Renal: CPB *places the patient at risk for renal failure—check the baseline renal function*

e. Endocrine: *diabetes is common, and perioperative control of blood glucose is highly important*

f. Hematologic: *patients are often on aspirin or dipyridamole therapy, which could cause intraoperative hemorrhaging; therefore these agents should be stopped 5 to 10 days before surgery, if possible. Heparin should be stopped 2 to 4 hours preoperatively (in some patients, heparin infusion is continued into the operating room).*

2. *Laboratory tests:* hemoglobin and hematocrit; type and cross-match for 8 units of packed red blood cells; other tests per the history and physical examination (e.g., electrolytes, blood urea nitrogen, creatinine, glucose, arterial blood gases, bleeding time, prothrombin time, partial thromboplastin time, platelet count)

3. *Premedication:* nitrates, beta-blockers and Ca^{2+} channel blockers, antidysrhythmics, and antihypertensives should be continued prior to surgery. Diuretics usually are excluded on the day of surgery. Anxiolytics aid in the placement of preinduction lines. Preoperative sedation could include diazepam (10 mg orally) or lorazepam (1 to 2 mg orally) the night before and 1 to 2 hours prior to arrival in the operating room, with the addition of morphine (0.1 mg/kg IM) and scopolamine (0.3 mg IM). Severely compromised patients require less premedication.

B. Room preparation

1. Standard monitoring equipment and invasive monitors are placed prior to induction. An arterial line is placed in the right radial artery if a left internal mammary artery (LIMA) graft is to be obtained. Retraction of the sternum may compress the left subclavian vein and dampen the arterial line waveform. (In some institutions, the arterial line is placed in the left radial artery to monitor the circulation to the left upper extremity. If the waveform is dampened, the surgeon is requested to release some of the tension while harvesting the LIMA graft, or the surgeon is requested to quickly obtain the graft to provide the necessary circulation to the left upper extremity.)

2. Central venous pressure or pulmonary arterial catheter. In the low-risk group of patients, the central venous pressure catheter is adequate; with high-risk patients, the pulmonary arterial catheter is useful in monitoring hemodynamics when weaning from bypass and

COMMON PROCEDURES

during vasoactive therapy. Pulmonary arterial catheters usually are routinely monitored for all patients undergoing CABG.

3. The electrocardiogram is monitored in leads II and V (or in areas most at risk for ischemia). Transesophageal echocardiography is used to monitor wall-motion abnormalities, papillary muscle dysfunction, and mitral regurgitation.

4. *Intravenous therapy:* two large-bore tubes, 16-gauge, cordis right internal jugular vein and Swan-Ganz catheter. Normal saline or lactated Ringer's solution is infused at 6 to 8 mL/kg per hour. Warm all fluids and humidify all gases.

5. *Drugs:*
   a. *Standard drips of nitroglycerin, phenylephrine, nitroprusside (Nipride) should be available*
   b. *Beta-blockers (esmolol, labetalol) should be available*
   c. *Muscle relaxant should be available (vecuronium, rocuronium, or pancuronium—whichever the patient can tolerate)*
   d. *Heparin is given at 300 units/kg*
   e. *Syringes are needed for laboratory test draws, including arterial blood gases and activated clotting time*
   f. *Fentanyl 20 to 100 µg/kg or sufentanil 5 to 20 µg/kg*
   g. *Midazolam 50 to 350 µg/kg*

C. Perioperative management and anesthetic technique

1. Induction
   a. *Use a high-dose narcotic technique with fentanyl and midazolam; this can be supplemented with etomidate (0.1 to 0.3 mg/kg).*
   b. *Muscle relaxation is with pancuronium (0.1 mg/kg) pushed slowly to prevent tachycardia or vecuronium (0.1 mg/kg).*
   c. *The sympathetic response to laryngoscopy must be blocked. High-dose narcotics (esmolol, 0.1 to 0.5 mg/kg over 1 minute with an infusion of 40 to 100 µg/kg per minute; sodium nitroprusside, 0.5 to 3.0 µg/kg per minute; lidocaine 1.0 to 2.0 mg/kg; or a combination of these agents) may decrease or abolish the sympathetic response.*

2. Maintenance
   a. *High-dose narcotics (total: fentanyl 50 to 10 µg/kg or sufentanil 10 to 20 µg/kg with midazolam 50 to 350 µg/kg for amnesia)*
   b. *Patients with good LV function may benefit from the use of volatile agents.*
   c. *Nitrous oxide is generally avoided*
   d. *Position: the patient is supine throughout most of the case. The arms are tucked at both sides, so ensure that all peripheral lines are patent and functioning well. Be sure there is enough extension tubing on the peripheral lines. Before the aorta is decannulated, the patient is placed into the Trendelenburg position.*
   e. Important: *the patient undergoing CABG requires extensive preparation and draping. Before performing the median sternotomy, the surgeon tests the saw. At that point, the lungs must be deflated. Disconnect the breathing circuit from the inspiratory limb and turn off your ventilator until the sternotomy is complete. Deflating the lung will prevent accidental injury to the lung. After the sternotomy is*

complete you may resume the patient's ventilation with smaller tidal volumes and faster rates. The surgeon will be able to access the LIMA without the lungs interfering in the field.

f. Prebypass anticoagulation: *Normal baseline activated coagulation time (ACT) is 90 to 130 seconds. Heparin (3 mg = 300 U/kg) is given via central venous access. Aspirate to make sure the heparin is in the central line. Check the ACT 3 minutes after the infusion of heparin. The ACT must be greater than 400 seconds (check with your institution).*

g. Cannulation of the aorta: *keep the mean arterial pressure at approximately 70 mm Hg prior to cannulation to prevent extension of the aortotomy*

h. Venous cannulation: *blood loss can be excessive with venous cannulation. Atrial dysrhythmias also are possible.*

i. Transition to CPB: *this is a dangerous period for the patient because of the many hemodynamic changes*

   (1) Once there is no pulmonary blood, ventilation is discontinued

   (2) Withdraw the pulmonary arterial catheter 4 to 6 cm

   (3) Stop intravenous drugs and decrease fluids to keep vein open

   (4) After 5 minutes on CPB recheck an ACT to ensure anticoagulation and check arterial blood gases to verify oxygenation

   (5) Check for adequate venous drainage. The central venous pressure will fall to a low level.

   (6) Initial arterial pressures may be very low but will usually increase

   (7) Anesthetics (e.g., fentanyl and midazolam) may be needed. A repeat dose of muscle relaxant should be used to prevent movement or shivering.

   (8) Unilateral dilation of the pupils may indicate arterial inflow into the innominate artery (unilateral carotid perfusion)

   (9) Most cardiac operations are performed under mild hypothermia (i.e., 28°C). If profound hypothermic circulatory arrest is to be utilized then 18°C is the target temperature

j. Bypass period

   (1) Check ACT levels every 20 to 30 minutes and keep above 400 seconds. Add heparin 5000 to 10,000 units if needed.

   (2) Keep mean arterial pressure at around 50 to 60 mm Hg for cerebral perfusion.

   (3) The hematocrit will fall approximately 20%, which is acceptable in most patients

   (4) Keep urine output above 1 mL/kg per hour. If needed, give mannitol, furosemide, or both, assuming pump flow is appropriate

k. Termination of bypass

   (1) Prior to discontinuation of CPB, the core temperature of the patient should be at least 36.5°C

(2) During rewarming, patient awareness may pose a problem. If using inhalation agents, discontinue them and give benzodiazepine with or without a narcotic to prevent awareness.

(3) Muscle relaxant should also be given at this time

(4) Correct any acidosis, check serum K^+ and make sure it is 4.5 to 5.5 mEq/L. The hematocrit should be greater than or equal to 20%

l. *Air maneuvers are used to remove intracardiac and intra-aortic air. Air maneuvers are performed. Ventilation is resumed once pulmonary blood flow is adequate. This will aid the removal of air.*

m. *Weaning from bypass*

(1) The aortic cross-clamp is off for 30 minutes prior to weaning from CPB. This will allow for rewarming and reperfusion of the heart.

(2) Normal sinus rhythm or atrioventricular pacing is preferred. Have vasoactive drugs available.

(3) The heart is gradually volume-loaded and transfused from the oxygenator. Assess cardiac output and blood pressure and adjust vascular resistance as necessary. Inotropes are usually needed at this stage.

n. *Reversal of anticoagulation*

(1) Once the patient is off CPB, anticoagulation must be reversed with protamine (1.0 to 1.3 mg/100 U). Protamine must be given slowly over 10 to 30 minutes.

(2) The ACT is checked again to ensure that it has returned to control values

o. Blood pressure: *measured to ensure patency of the grafts and the aortotomy site. Keep the systolic blood pressure at less than 120 mm Hg.*

p. Post-CPB bleeding: *if the patient continues to bleed following CPB, and the ACT is normal, and there is no surgical cause for bleeding, then infuse 10 units of platelets.*

3. *Emergence:* The patient remains ventilated postoperatively for 12 to 24 hours (depending on the institution). Postoperative pain is controlled with narcotics, and sedation is usually provided with benzodiazepines.

D. Postoperative complications

Postoperative complications include infarction, ischemia, tamponade, dysrhythmias, cardiac failure, coagulopathy, and hemorrhage.

B. Aortic Valve Replacement

◆ ◆ ◆

A. Introduction

Disease of the aortic valve may present as valvular stenosis, insufficiency, or a combination of both. Valvular disease is usually caused by rheumatic disease, but it may also occur secondary to calcific degeneration in the elderly. Endocarditis and congenitally bicuspid valve account for most of the remainder. It is rarely possible to repair the aortic valve; therefore, most conditions require valve replacement.

There are three commonly used prostheses. They include the porcine bioprostheses, mechanical prostheses, and the cryopreserved homograft. The last is expensive and in short supply.

After routine bicaval and aortic cannulation, the patient is placed in full cardiopulmonary bypass. The left side of the heart is drained through a pulmonary artery vent, and the left atrial vent is inserted through the right superior pulmonary vein or through a left-ventricular vent inserted via the left ventricular apex.

Once the heart is arrested, the aorta is opened to expose the aortic valve. The stenotic valve is usually heavily calcified, and all calcium must be debrided for the prosthesis to be properly seated.

To prevent perivalve leaks or impingement on the coronary ostia, proper sizing and positioning are mandatory.

Systemic rewarming is initiated during the final stages of the valve insertion, and the left ventricle is allowed to fill during aortic closure. With the patient in the head-down position, air is vented from the left side of the heart and aorta, and the cross-clamp is removed to allow for myocardial perfusion.

Vasodilators are almost always used because of the excessive vasospasm in both the coronary and the pulmonary circulations after the period of hypothermia.

B. Preoperative assessment

1. *Cardiovascular:* symptoms of aortic stenosis include those of angina pectoris, syncope, and congestive heart failure (indicates severe disease with a 2-year life expectancy). The ejection murmur is best auscultated at the 2nd right interspace. The electrocardiogram will exhibit left-ventricular hypertrophy. Aortic orifice sizes are as follows:

$$\text{Normal} = 2.6\text{--}3.5 \text{ cm}^2$$
$$\text{Moderate aortic stenosis} = 0.7\text{--}0.9 \text{ cm}^2$$
$$\text{Critical aortic stenosis} = <0.5 \text{ cm}^2$$

Tests include electrocardiography, echocardiography, and angiography.

2. Respiratory
   a. *Pulmonary congestion may cause respiratory compromise*
   b. *Tests include chest radiography*

3. Neurologic
   a. *Syncopal episodes may have resulted in neurologic deficits*
   b. *This should be well documented*

4. Renal: pre-renal failure is frequently related to aortic regurgitation secondary to a decreased cardiac output

5. Hepatic
   a. *Congestive heart failure may result in passive liver congestion. Coagulopathy may result from decreased liver function.*
   b. *Tests: liver function tests, prothrombin time, partial thromboplastin time*

6. *Hematologic:* hemoglobin and hematocrit, clotting profile. Type and cross-match for 8 units of packed red blood cells.
7. *Laboratory:* routine chemistry and digoxin level if indicated
8. *Premedication:* low blood pressure in a patient with aortic stenosis could be harmful. Be careful with sedation.

C. Room preparation
1. Routine monitoring equipment. Special equipment would include transesophageal echocardiography, hemodynamic monitoring (arterial line, central venous pressure, pulmonary arterial catheter), and cardiopulmonary bypass. Two large-bore intravenous tubes, 16-gauge. Central line with a pulmonary arterial catheter. *Fluids:* normal saline or lactated Ringer's at 6 to 8 mL/h.
2. Warm all fluids
3. Humidify gases
4. Drugs
   a. *Fentanyl 20 to 100 μg/kg, etomidate 0.1 to 0.3 mg/kg, midazolam 50 to 350 μg/kg. Muscle relaxation with vecuronium or pancuronium (if there is no tachycardia), 0.1 mg/kg.*
   b. Vasopressors: *phenylephrine 50 to 100 μg bolus or 0.1 to 4 μg/kg per minute infusion*
   c. *Atrial fibrillation or supraventricular tachyarrythmia should be treated with cardioversion. Negative inotropes and beta-blockers are contraindicated.*
   d. *Be cautious of vasodilators, including nitroglycerin*
   e. *Heparin 300 units/kg will be needed for prebypass*

D. Perioperative management and anesthetic technique
Anesthetic technique is general anesthesia.
1. Induction:
   a. *Usually a high-dose narcotic with oxygen, fentanyl, etomidate, and muscle relaxation as stated earlier. Induction is a critical period. Surgeons and cardiopulmonary bypass should be available and ready to proceed.*
   b. *The danger is hypotension with a cycle of ischemia and further hypotension and more ischemia. Avoid drugs that cause tachycardia.*
2. *Maintenance:* high-dose narcotic, low-dose inhalation oxygen and air. Consider the same methods for cardiopulmonary bypass.
3. *Postbypass:* these patients may be hyperdynamic and may require vasodilators for hypertension—inotropes may also be needed. Because of the hypertrophied, noncompliant ventricle, filling pressures may be higher than normally required.
4. *Emergence:* transport these patients to the intensive care unit sedated, intubated, and ventilated.

E. Postoperative implications
1. Postop ventilation is required for approximately 12 to 24 hours, depending on the institution. Inotropic and vasodilator therapy is usually continued postoperatively. Later, the patient is weaned from the inotropic support.
2. Complications
   a. *Hemorrhage*
   b. *Tamponade*
   c. *Cardiac failure*
   d. *Dysrhythmias*
   e. *Ischemia*

3. Pain management includes the use of opioids for analgesia and benzodiazepines for sedation
4. Postoperative tests
   a. *Electrocardiography*
   b. *Chest radiography*
   c. *Electrolytes*
   d. *Hemoglobin and hematocrit*
   e. *Coagulation profile*
5. *Note:* review the procedure for coronary artery bypass grafting (Chapter A in this section) for more information on management of the patient on cardiopulmonary bypass

MITRAL VALVE REPAIR OR REPLACEMENT

This procedure is performed for correction of postrheumatic mitral valvular stenosis or insufficiency, as well as for mitral prolapse and degenerative mitral insufficiency or repair following endocarditis. For severe rheumatic calcific mitral stenosis, mitral valve replacement with preservation of subannular structures may be needed. Mitral regurgitation secondary to posterior leaflet abnormalities or annular dilatation can be repaired.

The technique for mitral valve repair or replacement is similar regardless of the mitral pathology. Cardiopulmonary bypass is established after aortic and bicaval venous cannulation. The left side of the heart is vented through the pulmonary artery. The aorta is cross-clamped, and diastole is arrested with cardioplegia given through the aortic root, augmented with a topical cooling with a continuous pericardial saline infusion or a cooling jacket. A vertical incision in the left atrium just posterior to the atrial septum provides exposure. With suitable exposure, one can decide whether to replace or to repair the valve.

Preoperative and postoperative evaluation is facilitated with transesophageal echocardiography. After filling the left ventricle and left atrium with blood, the atrium is closed, air is evacuated from the left side of the heart, the cross-clamp is removed, and coronary perfusion is resumed. After a satisfactory period of resuscitation and all the air has been evacuated from circulation, cardiopulmonary bypass may be discontinued with the assistance of an inhalation agent.

Preoperative assessment, room preparation, perioperative management, and postoperative implications are the same as for aortic valve replacement.

COMMON PROCEDURES

C. Pericardial Window

♦ ♦ ♦

A. Introduction

The draining of fluid into the left hemothorax to relieve tamponade may be attempted but it does not benefit a true constrictive process.

A pericardial window or pericardiocentesis could be managed under local anesthesia prior to induction. Drainage of a small amount of fluid may dramatically improve the patient's status.

B. Preoperative assessment and patient preparation

1. History and physical examination
   a. *Respiratory*
      (1) Oxygenation may be impaired if the patient has a restrictive disease. If the effusions are significant, venous return may be decreased, which will cause a decrease in the cardiac output.
      (2) *Tests:* chest radiographs; check for active disease, fibrosis, effusions, pericardial calcification; arterial blood gases and pulmonary function tests (if time permits)
   b. *Cardiovascular*
      (1) A large pericardial effusion, which can develop slowly, may cause few or no symptoms. A small and rapidly forming effusion may lead to cardiac tamponade. Right ventricular pressure waveforms are unchanged during tamponade but show a dip and a prominent Y-descent in constrictive pericarditis.
      (2) The severity of the physical symptoms is determined by the degree of tachycardia, hypotension, and filling pressures
      (3) *Tests:* electrocardiography, echocardiography
   c. Gastrointestinal: *chronic hepatic congestion may cause decreases in procoagulants. Ascites may cause an increase in intra-abdominal pressure. Therefore, consider these patients to be on a full stomach.*
   d. Renal: *pericarditis may cause renal failure, and renal failure may cause pericarditis. Test blood urea nitrogen, creatinine, creatinine clearance, and electrolytes.*
   e. Hematologic: *routine laboratory tests with a coagulation profile. If possible, correct coagulopathy with fresh frozen plasma, platelets, or both.*

2. *Premedication:* little or no premedication is indicated. Benzodiazepines may be used (midazolam 0.05 to 0.2 mg/kg IM). Consider the full-stomach status of the patient. Other drugs include ranitidine (50 mg IV), metoclopramide (10 mg IV), and sodium citrate (30 mL by mouth).

C. Room preparation

1. Standard monitoring equipment and full hemodynamic monitoring (transesophageal echocardiography and cardiopulmonary bypass on standby for pericardiectomy)
2. *Position:* supine or supine with the left hemithorax elevated
3. *Intravenous therapy:* one large-bore tube with a central line

D. Perioperative management and anesthetic technique

1. Induction
   a. *Ketamine 1 to 2 mg/kg or etomidate 0.2 to 0.3 mg/kg, with or without narcotics (fentanyl 12 to 30 μg/kg), depending on the patient's status. Consider maintaining spontaneous ventilation in tamponade patients until drainage is complete. Intermittent positive-pressure ventilation may cause rapid decompensation and cardiac arrest (due to decreased venous return).*

  b. For full-stomach precautions, use rapid sequence induction with
     succinylcholine and cricoid pressure
2. Maintenance: narcotic and low-dose inhalation agent. Cardiac output
   depends on a high preload. Inotropes (dobutamine, epinephrine) may be
   needed.
3. Emergence: extubate in the operating room

E. Postoperative implications
  1. Following pericardial window, patients improve with the relief of
     the tamponade.
  2. Complications
     a. Hemorrhage
     b. Coagulopathy
     c. Ventricular hypofunction
     d. Dysrhythmias
     e. Ischemia
  3. Pain management: consider opioids for pain relief and
     benzodiazepines for sedation. Consider insertion of an intrathoracic
     or a thoracic epidural catheter.

D. Cardiac Surgery Plan of Care*

♦ ♦ ♦

RISK FACTORS

1. Age: Increased risk with increased age
2. Sex: Males > females
3. Hyperlipidemia: High levels of low-density and intermediate-density
   lipoproteins are associated with atherosclerosis. Apoproteins are polar lipids.
4. Hypertension: Increased risk with high blood pressure (BP), especially
   diastolic BP
5. Smoking: The risk of those who smoke ≥1 pack per day is 70- to 200-
   fold that of nonsmokers.
6. Diabetes mellitus (DM): DM increases risk for myocardial infarction
   (MI) by twofold.

PATIENT ASSESSMENT

Cardiac output distribution: heart, 5%; kidneys, 20%; muscles, 22%; liver,
24%; intestines, 8%; brain, 12%.

A. Cardiac evaluation
  1. Hypertension, heart disease (coronary artery disease [CAD];
     angina, MI, congestive heart failure [CHF], smoking, chronic

*Courtesy of Ronald Manningham, CRNA.

COMMON PROCEDURES

obstructive pulmonary disease [COPD], carotid artery stenosis, transient ischemic attack/cardiovascular accident, diabetes, renal disease, age > 70 years, male sex)

2. Electrocardiogram (ECG), previous history of MI, angina, causes, symptoms, treatment, number of laboratory tests performed (abnormalities always indicate increased perioperative risks)

3. Cardiac catheterization report:
   a. *Degree of vessel occlusion, presence of collaterals*
   b. *Chamber pressures, pulmonary artery (PA) pressures*
   c. *Ventricular function: left ventricular (LV) function, ejection fraction (EF) > 55% (EF < 35% indicates increased risk of postoperative MI)*
   d. *Cardiac output and index*
   e. *Unbypassable vessels that may increase the chance of perioperative ischemia.*

4. Chest radiography (heart size, pulmonary vascular flow), exercise tolerance tests (dysrhythmias, ischemic threshold, location of ischemia, ventricular dysfunction) induced ischemia, arrhythmias, and hemodynamic changes (ambulatory)

5. ECG (Holter 12–48 hours, with symptoms diary; dysrhythmias, ST depression)

6. Echocardiography (EF, valvular function, congenital defects, segmental wall motion)

7. Pharmacologic stress perfusion imaging (diphyidamole thallium scan, a vasodilator [dipyridamole] is administered to cause maximal dilation of coronary arteries; vessels with fixed stenoses will not dilate, allowing less perfusion agent to reach the myocardium; avoid if patient has heart block, asthma, theophylline, caffeine, COPD)

8. Dobutamine echocardiography (abnormally contracting muscle segments seen on resting echocardiography are classified as ischemic or infarcted, good for patients on theophylline or caffeine or with COPD)

9. Good heart function if EF > 55%, left ventricular end-diastolic pressure (LVEDP) < 12, cardiac index (CI) 2.5 or better, and no areas of ventricular dyskinesia

10. Impaired heart function if EF < 40%, LVEDP > 18, CI .20

11. Calculate and record body surface area

B. Pulmonary evaluation

1. Asthma, emphysema, smoking history (to decrease carboxyhemoglobin and nicotine tachycardia, quit at least 2 days prior)

2. Pulmonary function tests for increased operative risk, with forced vital capacity (FVC) < 50% predicted, forced expiratory volume in 1 second (FEV_1) < 2.0 L, FEV_1/FVC < 50%

3. Room air arterial blood gases Pa_{CO_2} > 45 mm Hg on room air

4. Assess lung sounds; relieve bronchospasm with B_2 adrenergic agents (terbutaline sulfate, albuterol), phosphodiesterase inhibitors

(aminophyline), parasympatholytics (atropine), steroids, mast cell stabilizers (cromolyn sodium)
5. Chest radiography
C. Neurologic evaluation: carotid stenosis, TIA/CVA
D. Renal evaluation: chronic end-stage renal diagnosis
E. Laboratory tests: arterial blood gases, electrolytes, complete blood count (CBC), platelet count, coagulation tests, activated clotting time (ACT), type and crossmatch with blood available (2 units packed red blood cells [PRBCs] in room for redos)
F. Medications: aspirin, digoxin, beta-blockers

ROOM PREPARATION

A. Monitors: 5-lead ECG, A-line/central venous pressure/PA transducers, CO setup, zero all lines.
B. D_5W 250 mL on macrodrip tubing for CO with 10 mL syringe.
C. LR 1000 mL on minidrip and manifold for cordis line.
D. LR 1000 mL setup on Omni-Flow pump, NTG, and sodium nitroprusside on secondary lines.
E. LR 1000 mL on blood tubing for one 14-g or 16-g IV [2 IV sites for redos].
F. Two units of PRBCs in room, and ensure availability of platelets for redos.
G. Oxygen tank and Ambu bag for transport to the surgical intensive care unit (SICU).
H. Transesophageal electrocardiography (TEE) in room for valves (TEE 2D Echo permits on-line evaluation of regional wall motion and global ventricular function).
I. OET 8.0/9.0 on stylet, laryngoscope blade and handle, oral airway, and tongue blade.
J. Cordis kit and Swan-Ganz catheter with VIP port; lidocaine, 10 mg/mL; A-line setup and 10-mL flush; I.V. materials, sterile gloves, and gown.
K. Drips
1. NTG, 50 mg/500 mL (100 μg/mL) on Omni-Flow
2. Sodium nitroprusside, 50 mg/250 mL (200 μg/mL) on Omni-Flow
3. Neo-Synephrine, 25 mg/250 mL (100 μg/mL)
4. Epinephrine 2 mg/250 mL (8 μg/mL)
5. Have dobutamine and dopamine available
L. Syringes: Obtain drips, cardiac pack, and other drugs from pharmacy
1. NTG, 20 μg/mL (2 mL from bottle diluted with 8 mL normal saline [NS])
2. Sodium nitroprusside, 20 μg/mL (1 mL from bottle diluted with 9 mL NS)
3. Neo-Synephrine, 100 μg/mL (10 mL from bag)
4. Epinephrine, 8 μg/mL (10 mL from bag)
5. Atropine, 0.4 mg/mL (2 mL)
6. Lidocaine, 20 mg/mL (5 mL)
7. Ephedrine, 10 mg/mL (50 mg diluted in 40 mL NS)

8. Propranolol HCl, 0.2 mg/mL (1 mg diluted in 4 mL NS)
9. CaCl, 100 mg/mL (10 mL)
10. Heparin, 1000 units/mL (20 mL)
11. Sufentanil citrate, 50 μg/mL (20 mL)
12. Pancuronium bromide, 1 mg/mL (10 mL)
13. Pancuronium bromide, 5 mg + vecuronium bromide, 10 mg (2 mg/mL) in 10 mL syringe
14. Protamine, 250 mg + 1 g CaCl in 40-mL syringe.
15. Aminocaproic acid, 5 g/bottle, 4 bottles for redos
16. Have propofol and etomidate available

PATIENT PREPARATION

A. Rarely will patient be sedated (check with CRNA/Anesthesiologist); apply O_2, pulse oximetry, ECG.
B. Peripheral IV, 14-g or 16-g (2 IVs if redo).
C. Right radial A-line (left becomes dampened with chest retraction).
D. Second case right internal jugular cordis in preop.
E. Transport to operating room. Attach to monitoring equipment. Wide-tape all electrodes. Two Bovie pads on back. Zero and calibrate lines. Check all connections.
F. Insert right internal jugular cordis and float Swan-Ganz catheter, monitor pressures and shoot preinduction cardiac output.
G. Preinduction laboratory tests: hematocrit, coagulation tests, ACT, K^+, room air arterial blood gases, random blood sugar, then place on 100% O_2 via mask.

INDUCTION

Goal: Slow induction to optimize oxygenation and prevent hypoxia. Half of all intraoperative ischemic events occur before bypass.

A. 100% O_2 via mask; avoid using N_2O if possible.
B. NTG, 20–25 μg/min as needed ischemia (note ST segment changes with induction).
C. Muscle relaxant priming dose, 1 mL (helps decrease chest wall rigidity while the vagolytic effect of pancaronium bromide offsets the bradycardia of sufentanil citrate).
D. Benzodiazepine: lorazepam, 2–4 mg; midazolam HCl, 2–5 mg; clonidine, 0.3 mg PO; or diphenhydramine, 25 mg IV ×2; diazepam, 0.4 mg/kg.
E. Have NTG, Neo-Synephrine, atropine, and lidocaine ready.
F. Sufentanil citrate, 3 μg/kg in incremental doses (sufentanil citrate is 7–10 times more potent than fentanyl, with the highest mu receptor specificity [90%], no histamine release, and lowest incident of breakthrough hypertension). Manage bradycardia, chest wall rigidity, and long duration of action.
G. Muscle relaxant, 9 mL. Assist, then control ventilation.
H. Aortic and mitral valve stenosis anesthesia goals; AVOID ↓ systemic vascular resistance (SVR) and tachycardia (keep heart rate [HR] ≈ 60 bpm).

I. Aortic and mitral valve regurgitation anesthesia goals; AVOID ↑ SVR and bradycardia (keep HR ≈ 90 bpm).
J. While waiting for the full muscle relaxation, the saphenous veins may be drained by elevation of legs, and the Foley catheter with thermistor may be inserted.
K. Laryngoscopy, intubation, note patient response; confirm endotracheal tube placement.
L. Check and pad pressure points (ulnar nerve, radial nerves, occiput, and heels).
M. Postinduction: ether screen, esophageal, TEE if valve, shoot postinduction CO, draw labs (arterial blood gases), and give antibiotics; start sufentanil drip at 2–5 mL/hr.

INTRAOPERATIVE

A. High levels of patient stimulation occur at the following times: (1) Induction/intubation, (2) incision, (3) sternal split and spread, (4) sympathetic nerve dissection, and (5) cardiotomy. Maintain adequate levels of anesthesia to avoid increasing catecholamine levels (treat with sufentanil citrate, 2–5 mL as necessary), which can precipitate hypertension, ischemia, and heart failure. Treat hypertension with NTG or sodium nitroprusside (SNP).
B. Low levels of stimulation occur preincision, during mammary dissection, cardiopulmonary bypass (CPB) cannulation. Deep levels of anesthesia may cause hypotension, bradycardia, and ischemia.
C. Skin incision: sufentanil, 2–5 mL (10–20 μg/kg) as needed, to avoid tachycardia and breakthrough hypertension.
D. Sternotomy: sufentanil, 2–5 mL (10–20 μg/kg), as needed. Lungs must be deflated during sternal sawing by disconnecting exhalation limb and providing adequate muscle relaxation (redos need NOT drop lungs, decrease tidal volume, and increase respiratory rate because a different saw is used and is a slower process). Confirm equal inflation of lungs after chest is open. This is the most common period for awareness and recall. (Redo hearts must have aminocaproic acid infusing, and 2 units PRBCs checked and ready in room because vein grafts, right atrium, right ventricle, or greater vessels may be cut or torn. The femoral vein should be identified and prepped by team).
E. Harvesting left internal mammary artery/right internal mammary artery and/or saphenous vein: Decrease tidal volume and increase respiratory rate while surgeon is dissecting mammary artery. The chest is retracted to one side, with the table up and rotated away from surgeon. Keep BP up to prevent vasospasm, which leads to ischemia. Surgeon sprays NTG or SNP over vessel to prevent vasospasm (watch for decreasing BP and maintain normotensive state).

F. Pericardiotomy: Ensure adequate anesthetic depth. Observe wall motion and myocardial contractility. A pericardial sling is made prior to heparinization and cannulation. This provides a dam for the cardioplegia solution and iced normal saline slush. The sling can also serve to lift the heart. After the pericardium is opened, the postganglionic sympathetic nerves are dissected from the aorta to allow insertion of arotic cannula. This is a period of high-level stimulation because of sympathetic discharge with nerve manipulation. Attenuate with beta-blockers and vasodilators.

G. Heparinization: Activate antithrombin III (stops blood clotting during CPB)
   1. Onset: immediate; duration (T1/2 β): 2 hours; metabolism by heparinases in liver.
   2. Aspirate back on central line to ensure venous access.
   3. Dose: 3 mg/kg (300 units/kg), or body surface area ×100 mg (10,000 units/kg [1 mg = 100 units]).
   4. Give prior to aortic cannulation. Surgeon can also administer heparin directly into the heart. (Decreases viscosity; watch for decreased BP and reflex increase in HR).
   5. Check ACT 3 minutes after heparin given. Must be >400 seconds prior to initiation of CPB (normal ACT, 70–110 seconds). Keep surgeon aware of all ACTs.
   6. If ACT is NOT adequate, then one third of original dose should be given (if necessary, up to 3 times until original dose is doubled). Check ACT every 5 minutes until >400 seconds. If a double dose is given and ACT is still low, consider heparin resistance or low antithrombin III. Replace antithrombin III with fresh frozen plasma.
   7. Turn off IVs once on CPB to minimize fluid intake.

H. Aortic cannulation: Done first in case something goes wrong. Bypass by cutting a hole in right atrium and inserting two pump suckers (suction bypass). Purse string sutures are used to keep the cannula in place and to close the incision after cannulas are removed. Keep systolic BP at 100 mm Hg to avoid blood spray or aortic dissection. The cannula is placed in the ascending aorta proximal to the innominate artery and distal to the sites of saphenous vein graft, if used. Pay attention to perfusionist and surgeon communication about cannula pressure readings. (Complications include entering innominate, carotid, or subclavian arteries, embolism [air or plaque], dysrhythmias, aortic dissection [aortic and radial pulsatile pressures should correlate]). Check lines for air bubbles after filling with normal saline.

I. Venous cannulation: Placed in right atrium (through the appendage, but this is only a partial bypass because some of the blood is not removed from the heart (done in coronary artery bypass grafting) or superior vena cava and inferior vena cava (bicaval decreases rewarming and venous return to the heart and allows caval snares to be placed so that the right atrium can be opened without introducing air into the venous return). Can result in hypotension due to volume depletion or mechanical compression, especially, if the inferior vena cava is cannulated. Dysrhythmias, mainly atrial, can occur due to surgical manipulation. Purse string sutures are used to keep the cannulas in place and to close the incision after the cannulas are removed. Bypass can be started immediately if patient is hemodynamically unstable.

J. Cardiopulmonary bypass: CPB sustains systemic blood flow, oxygenation, and ventilation during periods when heart and lungs are arrested.

1. Ensure adequate level of muscle relaxation/amnesia with extra doses of pancuronium. Surgeon notifies purfusionist to go on bypass (record time and maintain mean arterial pressure (MAP) at 50–70 mm Hg to maintain coronary perfusion before cross-clamping; treat with Neo-Synephrine).

2. When pulmonary blood flow ceases, stop ventilation, disconnect exhalation limb of circuit to deflate lung (increases surgeon visibility), and turn off vent, gas analyzer, and pulse oximeter. Continue O_2 flow at 2 L/min. Reset timer on Foley.

3. Pressure = flow × resistance. Venous cannula carries blood passively away from right atrium to reservoir. Pump oxygenates, removes CO_2, and cools/warms blood. (Membrane oxygenator is less traumatic to RBCs and is made of polypropylene, whereas bubble oxygenator is cheaper but traumatic to RBCs.) Roller pumps cause positive displacement of blood, which causes damage to blood components. Aortic cannula carries oxygenated blood back to the aorta.

4. Hypotension is associated with CPB due to the 2 L of prime solution, which causes hemodilution, decreases blood viscosity, dilutes circulating catecholamines, contains a small amount of NTG, and contains no O_2; thus, hypoxic vasodilation occurs. Prime solution can contain electrolyes, buffer, mannitol, lidocaine, and heparin. PRBCs can be added to prevent hemodilution and hypoxic effects.

5. Patient assessment: 30–60 seconds after initiation of CPB.
   a. *Check pupils. Examine conjuctiva for chemosis and reassess pupils size and for unilateral dilation, which may indicate arterial inflow into innominate artery (unilateral carotid perfusion).*
   b. *Examine face for color, symmetry, temperature, and edema.*
   c. *Check carotid pulses, which should feel like trills because of nonpulsatile flow.*
   d. *Examine heart for distention and contractility.*
   e. *Examine pump lines for arteriovenous color differences.*

6. Hypothermia
   a. *Patient is cooled to 28–32°C, which decreases O_2 demands of tissues and allows for lower CPB flows. Shifts autoregulation to left to 25–125 mm Hg. Each 1°C decrease in temperature leads to an 8% decrease in metabolic rate. A 10°C decrease in temperature leads to a decrease in metabolism by ½. Carbon dioxide and O_2 are more soluble; thus, expect lower $PaCO_2$ on arterial blood gas testing.*
   b. *Iced saline around heart cools it to 8–15°C.*

   c. Watch for ventricular fibrillation, which causes increased utilization of
      O_2 and requires immediate cardioplegia to arrest heart.
   d. Placement of aortic vent and cardioplegia line.

K. Cardioplegia
   Goal is to obtain a motionless heart and a clean dry operative field.
   1. Aorta is cross-clamped. (Record time of CPB on/off and cross-clamp on/off.) Pay attention to perfusionist and surgeon communication in regards to "flow up/flow down" accompanying clamping/unclamping.
   2. *Cardioplegia* is the application of a cold solution (4°C) high in K^+ (20–40 mEq) that produces electromechanical quiescence. Arrests heart in diastole and produces energy conservation. (If arrested in systole, as seen with calcium, tetany results.)
   3. This solution causes the myocardial cells to depolarize; contraction occurs, calcium goes into the cells, the myocardium relaxes, but membrane repolarization is prevented.
   4. Four parts blood for one part of cardioplegic solution. Components of the cardioplegia solution may include: K^+, Na^+, Ca^{2+}, Mg^{2+}, mannitol and/or albumin (osmotic), NTG (coronary dilator), HCO_3 (buffer), Ca^{2+} channel blockers, propranolol HCl, glucose (cellular energy), hemoglobin (oxygen-carrying), and lidocaine or procaine (membrane stabilization).
   5. Repeat application of solution every 20–30 minutes, or if heart temperature is >18°C to maintain hypothermia, prevent lactic acid accumulation, and deliver some minimal available O_2.
   6. Keep MAP between 30 and 60 mm Hg. Patients with carotid stenosis may require higher pressures. Cerebral perfusion pressure (CPP), = MAP. LVEDP = 0. PA pressures should be < 15 mm Hg; central venous pressure < 5 mm Hg.
   7. K^+ can cause systemic hyperkalemia. Treat with 10 units of regular insulin I.V., 50 g of glucose, hyperventilation, HCO_3, calcium, and furosemide.

L. EGG: ventricular fibrillation usually occurs twice during CPB: during cooling and during warming. Inform surgeon.

M. Urine output
   Should be maintained above 1 mL/kg (notify surgeon if less). Large outputs of 300–1000 mL/hr can be seen if mannitol is used in priming solution. Low urine outputs can be attributed to absent pulsatile flow, hypothermia, and decreased renal blood flow, and increased catecholamines cause release of ADH. Treat low urine outputs with mannitol, furosemide, adequate perfusion, and renal dose dopamine.

N. Hemodynamics during CPB
   1. Maintain MAP between 30 and 70 mm Hg with a venous saturation >60%. If cerebral circulation is impaired, keep MAP at 60 mm Hg. Low MAP causes decreased peripheral perfusion. High MAP damages blood components, increases blood in operative field, and increases warmed blood to heart. Treat low SVR with Neo-Synephrine, high SVR with NTG or SNP.

2. Reasons for decreased venous saturation: increased O_2 consumption with light anesthesia, low CPB flows, decreased O_2 delivery from oxygenator, or decreased O_2 carrying capacity of hemoglobin secondary to hemodilution.

O. Physiologic response to CPB

1. Platelets: clumping, degranulation occur after contact with nonendothelial surfaces. Leads to reduction in numbers, inhibits adhesiveness and aggregation.

2. Proteins: denaturation of oncotic and carrier proteins (albumin, lipoproteins, and gamma-globulin). Leads to increased viscosity, clumping of RBCs, fat embolism. Amplification of "humoral system" proteins. Factor XII stimulation of coagulation and fibrinolytic cascade. Complement system activation releases kallikrein and bradykinin; generalized inflamatory response that increases capillary permeability. Altered enzymic function.

3. Blood: RBCs become stiffer and less distensible, which leads to lysis and hemoglobinuria, which leads to impaired renal tubular function. Leukocyte damage and activation leads to degranulation. Complement activation causes pulmonary sequestration of neutrophils leading to inflammatory response and lung injury.

4. Endocrine: Elevated epinephrine levels during hypothermia cause peripheral vasoconstriction and impair release of insulin (hyperglycemia and release of free fatty acids). Norepinephrine levels rise early during CPB in patients, leading to postoperative hypertension. Renin and aldosterone levels are increased, promoting sodium retention and potassium excretion. Increased vasopressin produces increased sodium and water diuresis. Angiotensin elevation leads to vasoconstriction.

5. Hemodilution: Reduces requirements for homologous blood transfusion. Reduces blood viscosity and improves tissue perfusion. Counteracts negative effects of hypothermia on tissue perfusion (vasoconstriction and impaired O_2 release from hemoglobin). Dilutes coagulation factors and platelets, contributing to coagulopathy. May increase interstitial edema.

6. Hypothermia: Reduces tissue metabolism and O_2 consumption. Improves myocardial protection. Provides end-organ (brain, kidney) protection in case of low-flow negative effects. Decreases intraoperative awareness. Increases SVR. Shifts the oxyhemoglobin curve to the LEFT, impairing tissue O_2 release. This effect is offset by increased O_2 solubility at lower temperatures and lower metabolic demand. Contributes to decreased platelets and platelet function.

7. Renal: Renin-angiotensin-aldosterone system alterations promote increased renal vascular resistance and sodium and water retention. Lead to decreased renal blood flow, glomerular filtration rate, and tubular function. Hemodilution protects kidneys by increasing cortical plasma flow. Hemaglobinuria may result from long bypass runs (>4 hr).

8. Liver/Intestines: Jaundice may occur in up to 23% of patients following CPB. Mucosal ischemia may occur due to splanchnic vasoconstriction induced by elevated angiotensin, as well as to microembolism of platelets and leukocytes.

9. Changes in cerebral autoregulation from 50–100 mm Hg to lower values. Embolic phenomena from fat, thrombi, platelets, foreign substances, and air embolism. Important to keep blood glucose levels between 100 and 200 mg/dL to prevent cerebral ischemic episodes.

10. Pulmonary: Lungs inactivate catecholamines under normal circumstances. This lack of degradation during CPB may contribute to increased catecholamines seen during CPB. May contribute to high PVR. The lungs have a high affinity for narcotics, especially fentanyl. May see decreased pulmonary blood flow post-CPB due to embolism (ventilation-perfusion mismatch and edema), as well as localized vasoconstriction due to elevated catecholamines.

P. Potential bypass catastrophies

1. Aortic dissection (cannula placed within arterial wall cannulation): Cannula should always be transduced; ensure that the pulsation correlates with arterial line. Treatment is repositioning of aortic cannula by surgeon.

2. Carotid or innominate artery hyperperfusion (see H and J.5); reposition catheter.

3. Stone heart

4. Reversed cannulation: Blood is drained from aorta, causing hypotension, and is infused into vena cava at high pressures. Execute gas embolism protocol.

5. Massive gas embolism (from oxygenator reservoir vortexing or clotting, opened beating heart, or leak or kink in lines): Vigilance is the prevention. Treatment includes

   a. *Stopping CPB and placing patient in Trendelenburg's position.*

   b. *Remove aortic cannula, vent air for cannulation site, and institute retrograde SVC perfusion for 2–4 minutes.*

   c. *Carotid compression is performed during (b) to allow purging of air from vertebral bodies.*

   d. *When no additional air can be expelled, resume anterograde CPB, maintaining hypothermia for 40–50°minutes. (Lower temperatures increase gas solubility and help reabsorption of gas bubbles.)*

   e. *Express coronary air by massaging and needle aspiration. Induce hypertension because hydrostatic pressure shrinks bubbles and "pushes" them through the vessels.*

   f. *Steroids and wean from CPB. Ventilate patient with 100% O_2 for at least 6 hours to maximize the blood-alveolar gradient for elimination of N_2. Hyperbaric chambers may accelerate reabsorption of residual bubbles.*

Q. Preparing end of CPB
  1. Draw up protamine/calcium.
  2. Gather ORAL gastric tube and large dressing.
  3. O₂ tank, Ambu bag, drugs in bag on Omni-Flow, prepare intensive care unit report.
  4. Valve replacements "de-air" heart to decrease risk of air embolism, which can be observed with TEE.

REWARMING

A. **Rewarming is sensed as hyperthermia by hypothalamus. Awareness is possible. Supplemental doses of pancuronium, lorazepam, and sufentanil may be required. Watch for the return of electrical activity of heart (treat ventricular fibrillation with lidocaine and defibrillation). Consider lidocaine drip if ventricular fibrillation is refractory.**
B. **Check TRIPLE**
  1. T = temperature (Increase operating room temperature. Patient is rewarmed to core temperature of 37°C, 20 minutes prior to termination of CPB. When temperature rises close to 32°C, the SVR and MAP may decrease [treat with Neo-Synephrine]. Rewarming accelerates metabolism of drugs given.)
  2. R = rate and rhythm (For adequate cardiac output, patient requires sinus rhythm with HR of 70–100 bpm. Use pacer, atropine, or cardioversion, if needed.)
  3. I = Inhalation (FIO₂ = 100%. Re-expand lungs with 2–4 breaths at 30–40 cm H_2O to resolve atelectasis. Observe field to ensure that you are not affecting grafts. Resume mechanical ventilation.)
  4. P = Pressure (Support as needed. High BP places stress on new grafts; low BP can cause ischemia.)
  5. L = Laboratory test results (Check test results: prothrombin time, partial thromboplastin time, ACT, fibrinogen, Sonoclot, arterial blood gases, hematocrit, electrolytes, glucose.) If K⁺ is trending <4.0 mEq at separation, supplement).
  6. E = Everything else (Level table, zero all lines.)
C. **Unclamping of aorta: Observe the heart for volume, rate, and contractility. The perfusionist may give/take 50 to 100-mL increments of blood. Monitor filling pressures, distention, or hypotension as indicators that the heart cannot handle the volume. Consider treatment with calcium chloride, epinephrine, or dobutamine for support.**

DISCONTINUING CPB

A. **Flow is decreased by 50%; the heart is visually inspected for distention of chambers and wall motion abnormalities. Observe ECG for dysrhythmias.**

B. Ensure adequate hemodynamic parameters; use inotropes and pressors as needed. Pulmonary capillary wedge pressure is a poor indicator of left atrial function after CPB.

C. Venous line is removed first.

D. Protamine is administered, 1 mg per 1 mg of heparin. Calcium chloride, 1 g, is mixed with protamine to counteract depressed contractility, decreased pH, decreased Ca^{2+} levels. (EXTREME CAUTION in digitalized patient may lead to stone heart.)

   1. Protamine is a base that combines with acidic heparin to form a stable salt and inactivates the anticoagulant effect.

   2. Administered slowly, over 5–10 minutes, into a peripheral venous site. Notify surgeon when ½ is administered so that pump suckers can be turned off to prevent coagulation in pump. Observe for hypotension, increased pulmonary artery pressure (PAP).

   3. Reactions can include: histamine release; anaphylactic/anaphylactoid reactions (IgE-mediated venodilation, decreased cardiac filling, and decreased SVR); and pulmonary vasoconstriction (increased airway pressures). Increased risk of allergic reactions in patients allergic to fish, in patients who have been treated with protamine-containing insulin, or in the presence of antiprotamine antibodies in serum of infertile or vasectomized men. Treat reaction with diphenhydramine and/or epinephrine, 0.1–0.3 mg.

E. Check hemoglobin, hematocrit, K^+, ACT, and arterial blood gases. Begin infusing cardiotomy blood because patient will require volume. ACT goal is to return to preoperative level. Hematocrit of 15% or less may be acceptable without transfusion. Patient will slowly hemoconcentrate.

F. Aortic line is removed, chest tubes are inserted, hemostasis is obtained, and incision is closed. Chest closure causes a transient increase in intramediastinal pressure, which may depress systemic venous return.

G. Check cardiac output when sternal wires closed and patient is stabilized.

H. Transport to SICU when hemodynamically stable. Lifepak, Ambu bag with O_2 tank, Omni-Flow, and tabletop drugs. Ventilation settings: respiratory rate, 8–12 bpm (for $PaCO_2$ of 35–45 mm Hg); FIO_2, 100%; tidal volumes, 10 mL/kg; PEEP, 5 cm H_2O.

POSTOPERATIVE COMPLICATIONS

A. Hypokalemia

B. MI and acute graft closure

C. Ischemia

D. Tamponade

E. Hemorrhage

F. Prosthetic valve failure

Agent	Dosage	Onset	Duration	Action
Nitroprusside	0.5–10 μg/kg per min	30–60 s	1–5 min	Direct arterial and venous vascular smooth muscle relaxation
Nitroglycerin	5–100 μg per min	1 min	3–5 min	Direct venous dilation
Esmolol	0.5 mg/kg over 1 min	1 min	12–20 min	Direct beta$_1$ antagonist
Labetalol	2.5–20 mg	1–2 min	4–8 hr	Direct alpha$_1$, beta$_1$, and beta$_2$ antagonist
Propranolol	0.2–3 mg	1–2 min	4–8 hr	Direct beta$_1$ antagonist
Hydralazine	2.5–20 mg	5–20 min	4–8 hr	Direct vascular smooth muscle relaxation
Nifedipine	10 mg	5–10 min	4 hr	Direct vascular smooth muscle relaxation
Epinephrine	8–32 μg	30–60 s	1–5 min	Direct alpha$_1$, alpha$_2$, beta$_1$, and beta$_2$ agonist
Ephedrine	2.5–10 mg	30–60 s	1–5 min	Mixed alpha$_1$, alpha$_2$, beta$_1$, and beta$_2$ agonist
Aminocaproic acid	10 g loading; 1 g/hr	30–60 s	3–5 hr	Coagulant
Protamine	1 mg per mg heparin	30–60 s	2 hr	Heparin antagonist
Phenylephrine	10–200 μg/min	30–60 s	15–30 min	Pure alpha
Norepinephrine	2–20 μg/min	30–60 s	10 min	Alpha$_2$, beta$_2$

COMMON PROCEDURES

IMPORTANT CONCEPTS

A. **Bernoulli's principle:** Small opening causes rapid blood flow (nozzle effect).

B. **Bainbridge's reflex:** Stretch receptors in right atrium sense change in venous return and elicit a corresponding change in HR.

C. **Frank-Starling mechanism:** The intrinsic ability of the heart to adjust to changes in venous return (stretch receptors). Venous return is affected by blood volume, blood distribution (sepsis), pericardial pressure (tamponade), venous tone (vasodilation with spinal anesthesia), HR, and rhythm.

D. **Baroreceptor reflex:** Stretch receptors in walls of major blood vessels sense increases in BP, cause reflex decrease in HR, contractility, and arterial and venous tone.

E. Chemoreceptors: aortic bodies (vagus nerve) and carotid bodies (glossopharyngeal nerve) detect decrease in O_2 and/or increase in CO_2 and H^+, sending a message to vasomotor center to increase respiration and decrease HR. Mechanism to protect heart.

F. CPP = DPP − LVEDP. Coronary blood flow is almost entirely controlled locally.
   Vasoconstriction: epinephrine, norepinephrine, Ca^{2+}, angiotensin II, vasopressin.
   Vasodilation: $\downarrow O_2$, $\uparrow CO_2$ H^+, K^+, Mg^{2+}, bradykinin, histamine, adenosine, and prostaglandins.

G. Sympathetic nervous system: → Norepinephrine → $\uparrow$ HR, $\uparrow$ Force, $\uparrow$ Excitability + Vasoconstriction, and $\downarrow$ Conduction time.
   Parasympathetic nervous system: →Acetylcholine → $\downarrow$ HR, $\downarrow$ Force, $\downarrow$ Excitability, and $\uparrow$ Conduction time.

H. Cardiac muscle has the highest O_2 consumption rate of entire body (8 mL O_2/100 g per minute)
   1. Decreased myocardial O_2 supply with tachycardia, diastolic hypotension, increased preload, hypocapnia, coronary vasospasm, anemia, hypoxia, and decreased 2,3-diphosphoglycerate.
   2. Increased myocardial O_2 demand with tachycardia, increased preload, increased afterload, increased contractility.
   3. $\dot{V}_{O_2}$ = (Arterial O_2 − Venous O_2 content) × CO
      Ca_{O_2} = (1.39 × Hgb × Sa_{O_2}) + (0.003 × Pa_{O_2})
      Cv_{O_2} = (1.39 × Hgb × Sv_{O_2}) + (0.003 × Pv_{O_2})
      Normal extraction is 25%.

I. SVR = MAP − CVP/CO × 80
   PVR = PAP − LAP/CO × 80

J. MAP = DBP + Pulse Pressure/3

K. Ohm's law: Q = ΔP/R (Q = blood flow; P = pressure; R = resistance)

L. Poiseuille's law: Q = $\pi\Delta Pr^4/8\eta L$
   1. Q = rate of blood flow; ΔP = change in pressure; r = radius; l = length; η = viscosity.
   2. $\uparrow$ Diameter → $\uparrow$ flow (diameter of a vessel plays the greatest role in blood flow).
      $\uparrow$ Diameter by ¼, $\uparrow$ flow by 68%.
      $\uparrow$ Diameter by ⅓, $\uparrow$ flow by 80%.
      $\uparrow$ Diameter by ½, $\uparrow$ flow by 94%.
   3. $\uparrow$ Length → $\downarrow$ flow ($\downarrow$ Length by ½, $\uparrow$ flow 2 times)
   4. $\uparrow$ Pressure → $\uparrow$ flow
   5. $\uparrow$ Viscosity → $\downarrow$ flow (viscosity is a temperature-dependent physical property of a substance—that is, it is dependent on the friction of its component molecules as they slide by one another).

M. EF = SV/EDV; normally, 65% of blood in ventricles is ejected in each SV.

N. CO = SV × HR; normal ≈ 5.6 L/min; RCO = LCO. Stroke work of RV is ⅐ that of LV because PVR is much less than SVR.

O. Cardiac muscle metabolism: 60% of energy from FFA.

VASCULAR SURGERY

A. Abdominal Aortic Aneurysm

SEE ALSO p. ??

◆ ◆ ◆

A. Introduction

Abdominal aortic surgery may be required for atherosclerotic occlusive disease or aneurysmal dilatation. These processes can involve the aorta and any of its major branches, leading to ischemia or rupture and exsanguination. Elective surgery is indicated when the aneurysm diameter is greater than 5 cm; each centimeter greater than 5 increases the chances of rupture.

Surgical repair involves proximal and distal clamping of the aorta, opening of the aneurysm, evacuation of the thrombus, and placement of a synthetic graft. A midline transabdominal surgical approach or retroperitoneal left thoracoabdominal approach may be used.

The aorta is the main artery arising out of the left ventricle of the heart. It supplies oxygenated blood to all tissues and organs of the body except the alveoli of the lung. The aorta is subdivided into the ascending aorta, the aortic arch, and the descending aorta, which has thoracic and abdominal portions. The abdominal aorta is the second portion of the descending aorta. It descends through the aortic hiatus of the diaphragm, enters the abdominal pelvic cavity and travels down the ventral surface of the vertebral column. The abdominal aorta terminates at the fourth lumbar vertebra by dividing into the right and left common iliac arteries.

B. Preoperative assessment

1. History and physical examination

   a. *Respiratory*

      (1) Assess for pulmonary disease: chronic obstructive pulmonary disease, chronic bronchitis, asthma, and emphysema

      (2) These patients have varying degrees of hypoxemia, hypercapnia, hypoventilation, ventilation-perfusion abnormalities, increased mucous secretions, bronchospasms, or small airway obstruction

   b. Cardiac: *evaluate coronary artery disease, angina, hypertension, dysrhythmias, congestive heart failure, and left ventricular dysfunction*

   c. Renal: *assess baseline status because the kidneys may be affected with cross-clamping*

     d. *Neurologic*
       (1) Spinal cord ischemia may occur with repair of the distal descending thoracic aorta
       (2) Assess for transient ischemic attacks, strokes, carotid bruits
     e. Endocrine: *this patient population is prone to diabetes mellitus*
     f. Other: *Back or flank pain may indicate expanding or leaking abdominal aortic aneurysm*
  2. Diagnostic tests
     a. *Chest radiography*
     b. *Echocardiogram with ejection fraction*
     c. *12-lead electrocardiogram*
     d. *Pulmonary function test with abnormal pulmonary histories*
     e. Angiograms: *estimate the difficulty of the procedure and relationship of cross-clamping to the renal arteries*
     f. Laboratory tests: *complete blood count, electrolytes, glucose, blood urea nitrogen, creatinine, urinalysis, prothrombin time, partial thromboplastin time, type and cross-match*
  3. Perioperative medications and intravenous therapy
     a. Antihypertensives: *usually need 24 to 48 hours prior to surgery*
     b. Antianginals: *nitrates, calcium channel blockers, and beta-blockers; continue until the day of the procedure*
     c. *Digoxin*
       (1) Assess serum level prior to procedure
       (2) Hypokalemia following intraoperative diuresis will increase the likelihood of digoxin toxicity
     d. Antiarrhythmics: *continue until day of surgery*
     e. Anticoagulants: *warfarin should be substituted with heparin postoperatively, allowing the patient's level to normalize. Plan to hold heparin 4 hours prior to surgery.*
     f. Bronchodilators: *continue until surgery*
     g. *Antibiotic*
     h. Epidural catheter (for postoperative pain management): *perform test dose on the awake patient. There is a remote risk of epidural hematoma formation from anticoagulation during surgery.*
     i. *Preoperative sedatives and narcotics*
       (1) Use with caution in patients with poor respiratory reserve
       (2) Onset of intravenous medications may be delayed because of low cardiac outputs
     j. *Two peripheral, large-bore (16- to 18-gauge) intravenous lines with variable fluid management*

C. Room preparation

  1. Monitoring equipment
     a. *Pulmonary artery catheter monitors cardiac function and adequacy of fluid and blood replacement*
     b. *Arterial line*
       (1) Right radial artery or left radial artery if the aneurysm involves the innominate artery
       (2) Maintain mean arterial pressure close to 100 mm Hg in the upper body and greater than 50 mm Hg distal to the aneurysm

    c. *Somatosensory evoked potential or electroencephalogram evaluates central nervous system viability during aortic cross-clamping*

    d. *Transesophageal echocardiography monitors left-ventricular function during cross-clamping*

    e. *Foley catheter assesses global renal function*

    f. *Warming modalities*

    g. *Electrocardiogram—leads V5 and II—detects myocardial ischemia*

  2. Pharmacologic agents

    a. *Prepare infusions of nitroglycerin, nitroprusside, phenylephrine, and dopamine*

    b. Drugs: *mannitol, furosemide, sodium bicarbonate, heparin, protamine, calcium*

    c. *Volume*

      (1) Intravascular volume is depleted by hemorrhage, third-spacing into the bowel and peritoneal cavity, and insensible losses associated with a large abdominal incision

      (2) Greatest blood loss occurs when aneurysm is opened and the arteries are back-bleeding

    d. Crystalloids: *use if electrolytes, glucose, and osmolarity are within normal limits*

    e. *Colloids*

      (1) Albumin, hetastarch (Hespan), blood

      (2) Maintain hematocrit in 3-cm range for oxygen-carrying capacity

    f. Autotransfusion: *blood is obtained from the operative field*

  3. *Position:* supine

D. Anesthetic techniques

  1. Regional blockade with general anesthesia or general aesthesia

  2. Technique of choice is general anesthesia with endotracheal intubation because hemodynamic changes are significant

  3. *Regional blockade:* epidural catheter placement and test dose preoperatively; analgesia to T4–T5

  4. With general anesthesia, an endotracheal tube is needed

E. Perioperative management

  1. Induction

    a. *If the patient is hypotensive with a rupturing abdominal aortic aneurysm, perform an awake intubation or rapid sequence induction with ketamine and succinylcholine*

    b. *A slow, "controlled" induction is preferred with the use of an opioid and nondepolarizing muscle relaxant*

    c. *Omit thiopental and other cardiac depressors in the patient with poor left-ventricular function*

    d. *Anticipate exaggerated blood-pressure changes; maintain within 20% of baseline*

    e. *Minimize pressor response during intubation of trachea by limiting duration of laryngoscopy to less than 15 seconds*

  2. Maintenance

    a. *O_2 air, opioid, and volatile anesthetic*

    b. *Cross-clamping of the thoracic aorta at the suprarenal or supraceliac level is not necessary for surgery*

COMMON PROCEDURES

Clamping Stage	Goals	Drugs to Prepare
Preclamping	Maintain blood pressure 20% baseline (low-normal)	• Volatile anesthetic • Nitroglycerin, nitroprusside (Nipride) • If pulmonary capillary wedge pressure (PCWP) is increased and cardiac output is decreased, inotropic support (dopamine, epinephrine) may be needed
	Maximize urinary output	Mannitol, furosemide (Lasix)
	Minimize fluids	Monitor crystalloid administration
	Prevent thrombosis	Heparin—monitor activated clotting times
Cross-Clamping	Prevent myocardial infarction	• Decrease afterload C; nitroglycerin and nitroprusside • Monitor electrocardiogram for ischemia • Monitor the cardiac output—expect a decline
	Maintain oxygenation	• Oxygen/air or 100% oxygen • Monitor oxygen saturation and arterial blood gases
	Maintain urinary output (0.5 mL/kg per hour)	• Anuria is rare • Dopamine (1–5 mg/kg)
Pre-Release	Prevent myocardial infarction, declamping, hypotension	• Monitor electrocardiogram • Ask surgeon for a 10-minute warning before aortic clamp is removed • Lighten anesthesia depth • Discontinue vasodilating agents (nitroglycerin and nitroprusside) • Increase central venous pressure and PCWP 4–6 mm Hg with fluids (and blood if needed) • Have vasodepressors ready
Post-Release	Maintain blood pressure and vital signs	Use vasodepressors (dopamine, epinephrine, phenylephrine)
	Correct acidoses	• Mechanical ventilation • Bicarbonate administration (pH < 7.25) • Calcium chloride ($CaCl_2$) administration
	Correct coagulation profile	Protamine
	Maintain urine output	Volume—crystalloids and colloids, dopamine

3. Emergence
   a. *Recommended that these patients should remain intubated and taken to an intensive care unit because there are major fluid shifts, probably increased blood loss, and stress from surgery*
   b. *Unless the patient is stable, do not reverse muscle relaxants or try to awaken the patient*
   c. *Consider initiating regional blockade through the epidural catheter for postoperative analgesia*

F. Postoperative implications
   1. Consider ventilatory support for several hours or overnight
   2. Potential complications include myocardial ischemia/infarction, renal failure, peripheral vascular insufficiency, stroke, intestinal ischemia/infarction, paraplegia/monoparesis, fluid shifts, electrolyte imbalance, and coagulopathies

B. Peripheral Vascular Procedures

♦ ♦ ♦

A. Introduction
   These procedures include femoral-femoral, femoral-popliteal, femoral-tibial, illeofemoral, axillofemoral, and embolectomies. Obstruction most often is in the superficial femoral artery, followed by common iliac claudication in the gastrocnemius muscle, whereas rest pain and ischemic ulceration gangrene occur with severe occlusion.
   Procedures are classified as inflow or outflow vascular reconstruction. The inflow reconstruction procedures bypass the obstruction in the aortoiliac segment (aortoiliac endarterectomy or aortofemoral bypass). These are more stressful procedures requiring cross-clamping of the aorta. Outflow procedures are performed distal to the inguinal ligament to bypass the femoropopliteal or distal obstruction.

B. Preoperative assessment
   1. History and physical examination
      a. Respiratory: *assess for pulmonary disease: chronic obstructive pulmonary disease, chronic bronchitis, asthma, and emphysema*
      b. Cardiac: *evaluate for coronary artery disease, angina, hypertension, dysrhythmia, congestive heart failure, and left ventricular dysfunction*
      c. Endocrine: *this patient population is prone to diabetes mellitus*
      d. Musculoskeletal: *decreased or absent popliteal and pedal pulses, delayed capillary reflexes, blanching or elevation of the leg followed by dependent edema after lowering it, and pain with walking relieved by rest*

2. Diagnostic tests
   a. *Chest radiography*
   b. *Echocardiogram with ejection fraction*
   c. *12-lead electrocardiogram*
   d. *Pulmonary function test with abnormal pulmonary histories*
   e. *Doppler studies*
      (1) Determinations of systolic blood pressure at level of ankle compared with brachial
      (2) Assess the severity of ischemia, urgency of revascularization, and baseline values for evaluation of operative results
   f. Angiography: *determine the precise site of the actual lesion*
   g. Laboratory tests: *complete blood count, electrolytes, glucose, blood urea nitrogen, creatinine, urinalysis, prothrombin time, partial thromboplastin time, type and cross-matching*
3. Preoperative medications and intravenous therapy
   a. *Elderly population with coexisting medical disease requiring pharmacologic support (i.e., antihypertensives, antianginals, antiarrhythmics, digoxin). These medications may be continued up to the day of the operation*
   b. *Sedatives and narcotics*
      (1) Use with caution in patients with poor respiratory reserve
      (2) Onset of intravenous medications may be delayed because of potentially low cardiac output
   c. *Two peripheral large-bore (16- to 18-gauge) intravenous tubes with moderate fluid management*
   d. Epidural catheter: *test dose on the awake patient; there is a risk of epidural hematoma from anticoagulation during surgery*

C. Room preparation
   1. Monitoring equipment
      a. *Electrocardiogram—leads V5 and II to detect myocardial ischemia and diagnose tachyarrhythmias*
      b. *Warming modalities*
      c. *Foley catheter*
      d. *Arterial line and central venous pressure monitoring may be necessary*
   2. Pharmacologic agents
      a. *Have nitroglycerin, nitroprusside drugs within quick access*
      b. *Drugs: vasopressors, heparin, beta-blockers*
      c. *May be asked to administer dextran solution*
   3. *Position:* supine

D. Anesthetic techniques
   1. Regional blockade, general anesthesia, or a combination technique of choice—regional anesthesia avoids airway problems and sequelae, provides greater hemodynamic stability with coexisting diseases, provides sympathetic blockade that increases circulation in the lower extremity, reduces the incidence of intravascular clotting, facilitates postoperative pain relief, suppresses the endocrine stress response, and decreases blood loss in selected cases
   2. Regional blockade—analgesia to T10; epidural or spinal
      a. *The elderly population is more sensitive to local anesthetics; reduce dose by 50%*

      b. Some practitioners administer ephedrine prophylactically to prevent
      hypertension
      (1) 25 mg IM prior to block
      (2) 5 mg IV immediately post block
   c. Tetracaine (1% hyperbaric) is recommended for spinal anesthesia
      (1) Procedures rarely are short enough to use lidocaine
      (2) Vasoconstrictors may be added to solution (to a nondiabetic
      patient) if a block of longer duration is desired
   d. Level is slightly above the skin dermatome necessary for usual incisions
      (T12) but sympathetic innervation of lower extremities, which
      contains visceral afferent fibers, is believed to occur at T10–L2

E. Perioperative management

  1. Induction
    a. General anesthesia
      (1) Goal is smooth transition from awake state to surgical
      anesthesia and the maintenance of cardiovascular stability
      (2) A slow "controlled" induction is preferred with the use of an
      opioid and nondepolarizing muscle relaxant
      (3) Muscle relaxation may be chosen on the basis of
      cardiovascular effect
        (a) Pancuronium—if the heart rate is slowed during
        induction
        (b) Vecuronium—if the heart rate is in the desired range
      (4) Onset of drugs may be delayed with low cardiac output
      (5) Omit thiopental and other cardiac depressors in patients with
      poor left-ventricular function
      (6) Anticipate exaggerated blood-pressure changes—maintain
      within 20% of baseline
      (7) Minimize pressure response during intubation of trachea by
      limiting duration of laryngoscopy to less than 15 seconds
    b. Regional anesthesia
      (1) Review the principles of sympathetic block
      (2) Consider administering blockade with the operative side
      down so that the onset of sympathetic and sensory blockade
      is more rapid on the dependent site. Theoretically, the level
      will be higher on the dependent side. The total volume of
      anesthetic requirements may be decreased.
  2. Maintenance
    a. Surgeon will ask that heparin be administered via intravenous
    push—ensure the patency of the port prior to injection
    b. One may perform intraoperative angiography
      (1) Allergic reactions may occur with dye
      (2) Level of surgical stimulation changes, blood pressure decreases
      when surgical activity stops in preparation for angiography.
      Blood pressure and heart rate may increase when dye is
      injected.
      (3) Repeat injection of contrast dye during multiple attempts at
      angiography may cause osmotic diuresis
    c. Hyperkalemia and acidosis due to ischemic extremities are possible,
    and myoglobin can be released into the circulation

COMMON PROCEDURES

d. *Maintain the hematocrit above 30 to maximize the oxygen-carrying capacity—do not give too many red cells or too few crystalloids: there is an increase in blood viscosity and the possibility of graft thrombosis*
e. *Unclamping of femoral artery rarely affects hemodynamics significantly. The lower extremity receives arterial blood through collateral vessels even when the femoral artery is occluded.*
f. *Regional anesthesia*
(1) Attention to patient comfort is important
(2) Sedation is aimed at reducing patient anxiety without producing respiratory depression or unresponsiveness

3. Emergence
a. *Initiate regional blockade through the epidural catheter for postoperative analysis prior to the end of the case*
b. *Base extubation on the patient's general health, amount of blood loss, and overall status after the procedure*

F. Postoperative implications
1. Obtain hemoglobin and hematocrit
2. Assess the musculoskeletal status of the operative extremity

Reference

Barash PG, Cullen BF, Stoelting RK. Clinical Anesthesia. Philadelphia, PA: J.B. Lippincott Co., 1992.

C. Thoracic Aortic Aneurysm

• • •

A. Introduction
Aneurysms that effect the thoracic aorta include ascending and arch defects (60% to 70%) or descending lesions (30%). These dissections are sometimes classified (Crawford) into the segments and arteries that are involved (types 1 to 4). Surgery is performed to prevent rupture, repair leaking or expansion of the aneurysm, and possibly for acute or chronic dissections. Diseases of the thoracic aorta may be associated with atherosclerosis, connective tissue disorders (Marfan's syndrome), congenital abnormalities, trauma, infection (syphilis), hypertension, and inflammatory processes.

B. Preoperative assessment and patient preparation
1. History and physical examination
a. Cardiac: *coexisting disorders may include hypertension (70% to 90% of patients), angina, coronary artery disease, congestive heart failure, myocardial ischemia, and peripheral vascular disease*
b. Respiratory: *manifestations may include hemoptysis, stridor, hoarseness, dyspnea, or pleural effusion*
c. Neurologic: *assess for any pre-existing condition*

d. Renal: *kidneys may be affected secondary to coexisting diseases*

e. Gastrointestinal: *Bowel ischemia has been associated with descending aneurysms.*

2. Patient preparation

a. Laboratory tests: *complete blood count, electrolytes, blood urea nitrogen, creatinine, prothrombin time, partial thromboplastin time, urinalysis, and arterial blood gases*

b. Diagnostic tests: *electrocardiography, echocardiography, Doppler, magnetic resonance imaging, chest and abdominal radiography*

c. Preoperative medications: *anxiolytics and analgesics as indicated*

d. Intravenous therapy: *central line, two 14- to 16-gauge intravenous tubes; consider pulmonary arterial catheter.*

C. Room preparation

1. *Monitoring equipment:* standard with arterial line, pulmonary arterial catheter, and Foley catheter

2. *Additional equipment:* fluid warmers, cardiopulmonary bypass, cell saver, and transesophageal echocardiography

3. Drugs

a. Miscellaneous pharmacologic agents: *heparin, diuretics, vasodilators/constrictors, inotropes, adrenergic antagonists, opioids, nondepolarizing muscle relaxant, and antibiotic*

b. Intravenous fluids: *calculate for major blood loss. Crystalloids at 6 to 8 mL/kg per hour. Estimated blood loss is 200 to 800 mL.*

c. Blood: *Type and cross-match for 8 to 10 units of packed red blood cells*

d. Tabletop: *standard*

D. Perioperative management and anesthetic technique

Anesthetic technique is general anesthesia.

1. *Induction:* smooth induction to maintain hemodynamic stability can be accomplished with etomidate (0.1 to 0.3 mg/kg) or thiopental (4 to 6 mg/kg), high-dose fentanyl (20 to 100 μg/kg) or sufentanil (5 to 20 μg/kg), pretreatment with lidocaine (1.5 mg/kg), and vecuronium (0.1 mg/kg). Consider midazolam (50 to 350 μg/kg) and esmolol as indicated. A double-lumen endotracheal tube may be required.

2. *Maintenance:* maintain the mean arterial pressure at 60 to 80 mm Hg and urinary output at 0.5 to 1.0 mL/kg per hour. Inhalational agent/O_2 narcotic is used. The aorta is cross-clamped for 25 to 120 minutes, and cardiopulmonary bypass may be instituted for 30 to 150 minutes. The position is supine or lateral decubitus.

3. *Emergence:* The patient is transported to an intensive care unit intubated and remains ventilated for 24 to 48 hours.

E. Postoperative implications

1. *Complications:* cardiac, respiratory, and renal failure are immediate postoperative risks. Other complications include hemorrhage, hypertension, coagulopathy, myocardial ischemia, and arrhythmias.

2. *Postoperative pain management:* consider an epidural catheter

COMMON PROCEDURES

D. Aorta-Bifemoral Bypass Grafting

◆ ◆ ◆

A. Introduction
Aorto-bifemoral bypass grafting is commonly performed to correct symptomatic unilateral iliac occlusive disease, which generally occurs in males older than 55 years.

B. Preoperative assessment and patient preparation
1. History and physical examination
   a. Cardiovascular: *30% to 50% of patients have coexisting coronary artery disease. Other common risk factors are myocardial infarction, hypertension, angina, valvular disease, congestive heart failure, and arrhythmias.*
   b. Respiratory: *most patients have a significant history of smoking and possibly chronic obstructive pulmonary disease*
   c. Neurologic: *check for coexisting cerebrovascular disease*
   d. Renal: *chronic renal insufficiency is common*
   e. Endocrine: *many patients have diabetes and its associated complications*
2. Patient preparation
   a. Laboratory tests: *complete blood count, prothrombin time, partial thromboplastin time, bleeding time, electrolytes, blood urea nitrogen, creatinine, creatinine clearance, and urinalysis*
   b. Diagnostic tests: *12-lead electrocardiography, pulmonary function tests, arterial blood gases, chest radiography, magnetic resonance imaging, computed tomography, and arteriography*
   c. Preoperative medications: *knowledge of daily medications is essential. Cardiac medications are continued, and anticoagulant therapy is sometimes held for 4 hours prior to surgery. Anxiolytics, sedatives, and analgesics are used as indicated.*
   d. Intravenous therapy: *central line, two 14- to 16-gauge intravenous tubes. Estimated blood loss is 500 mL.*

C. Room preparation
1. *Monitoring equipment:* standard with arterial line and central venous pressure catheter, pulmonary arterial catheter, or both. ST-segment analysis and transesophageal echocardiography are beneficial.
2. *Additional equipment:* fluid warmer; consider cell saver
3. Drugs
   a. Miscellaneous pharmacologic agents: *osmotic and loop diuretics, local anesthetics, antibiotic, adrenergic antagonists, inotropic agents, vasodilators/constrictors, and heparin*
   b. Intravenous fluids: *calculate for major blood loss. Consider rapid infusion of crystalloids, colloids, or both to treat hypovolemic states.*
   c. Blood: *type and cross-match for 4 units of packed red blood cells*
   d. Tabletop: *standard*

D. Anesthetic technique
General anesthesia, epidural anesthesia, or a combination of general and regional anesthesia.

E. **Perioperative management**
1. *Induction:* use smooth induction to preserve cerebral perfusion and to maintain hemodynamic stability. For general anesthesia, consider etomidate, fentanyl, lidocaine, and muscle relaxants to decrease episodes of tachycardia and hypotension. For regional anesthesia, consider placing an epidural catheter prior to beginning anticoagulation.
2. *Maintenance:* for general anesthesia, consider oxygen/air, volatile agent/narcotic. For regional anesthesia, use local anesthetic/narcotic/anxiolytic. Maintain blood pressure within the high-normal range.
3. *Emergence:* maintain hemodynamic stability, prevent hypertension and tachycardia. For general anesthesia, use full reversal of muscle relaxants and smooth extubation.

F. **Postoperative implications**
Complications include hemodynamic instability, myocardial ischemia, hemorrhage, respiratory failure, renal failure, and neurologic changes.

E. Carotid Endarterectomy

♦ ♦ ♦

A. **Introduction**
Surgical excision of fibrous atherosclerotic plaque at or near the bifurcation of the common carotid artery is performed for the treatment of transient ischemic attacks. It is reserved for patients with lesions of greater than 80% blockade in the carotid artery. Cerebral angiography is used to determine the location and severity of stenosis. The operative mortality rate is 1% to 2% and is due to myocardial infarction; the operative morbidity rate is 4% to 10% and is due to stroke.

B. **Preoperative assessment and patient preparation**
1. History and physical examination
   a. Cardiac: *assess normal range of blood pressure and heart rate and note asymmetries in blood pressure between arms. Obtain a detailed history of cardiovascular function.*
   b. Neurologic: *assess and document pre-existing neurologic deficits to distinguish new deficits*
   c. Respiratory: *obtain preoperative blood gases if pulmonary disease is suspected. Preoperative arterial carbon dioxide pressure dictates this value during anesthesia.*

COMMON PROCEDURES

    d. General: *optimal control of hypertension, diabetes, chronic obstructive pulmonary disease, and chronic renal failure is imperative prior to surgery*

  2. *Diagnostic tests:* electrocardiogram, complete blood count, blood urea nitrogen, blood sugar, chest radiography, creatinine, electrolytes, typing and cross-matching, arterial blood gases, other cardiac tests as needed according to history

  3. Preoperative medication and intravenous therapy

    a. *Continue all cardiac medications until time of surgery*

    b. *Two 16- to 18-gauge intravenous tubes with moderate fluid replacement*

    c. *Premedication is minimal*

C. Room preparation

  1. Monitoring equipment

    a. *Standard with arterial line, electrocardiogram with lead V5 and ST-segment monitoring*

    b. *Hemodynamic monitoring*

    c. *Electroencephalogram, somatosensory evoked potential; carotid stump pressure monitoring may be used to assess cerebral ischemia*

  2. *Pharmacologic agents:* standard tabletop setup with ephedrine, phenylephrine, esmolol, nitroglycerin, labetalol, heparin, and protamine available

  3. *Position:* supine; arms may be treated at side. A roll may be placed under the shoulder blades to extend the neck. The head may be placed on a doughnut. Determine if the table will be turned and attach monitors accordingly.

D. Anesthetic techniques

  1. Regional blockade or general anesthesia

  2. Technique of choice is general anesthesia

    a. Regional blockade: *cervical plexus block at the transverse process of C3–C4 and along the inferior border of the sternocleidomastoid muscle—offers advantage of an awake patient, allowing for continuous neurologic monitoring*

    b. General anesthesia: *allows for control of ventilation, oxygenation, and lash of patient movement. General anesthetics protect the brain by depressing the level of cerebral metabolism and the cerebral metabolic rate of oxygen.*

E. Perioperative management

  1. Introduction

    a. *A slow, controlled induction is preferred with the use of an opioid and nondepolarizing relaxant*

    b. *Anticipate exaggerated blood-pressure changes with induction. Adequate hydration is imperative. Use of lidocaine and esmolol will attenuate the response to laryngoscopy.*

  2. Maintenance

    a. *Maintain arterial blood pressure in the patient's normal range*

    b. *Prior to cross-clamping, increase blood pressure by 20 to 30 mm Hg. Document the cross-clamping time.*

    c. *If a shunt is used, document shunt insertion and removal*

      d. *Maintain arterial carbon dioxide pressure in the patient's normal range*

      e. *If the surgeon stretches the baroreceptor nerve endings, ask the surgeon to inject the area of bifurcation with 1% lidocaine 10 to 15 minutes prior to carotid artery occlusion*

  3. Emergence

      a. *Smooth emergence is important—use lidocaine to blunt reflexes*

      b. *The patient may need to be awake at the end of the procedure so the surgeon can assess for neurologic deficits*

F. Postoperative considerations

Hypertension is common. Other complications include carotid body damage, hemorrhage with compromise of the airway, myocardial infarction, stroke, and dysfunction of cranial nerves VII, IX, X, and XII.

F. Portasystemic Shunts

◆ ◆ ◆

A. Introduction

Portasystemic shunt procedures are performed to prevent or cease variceal hemorrhage due to portal hypertension in patients with liver disease, cirrhosis, ascites, and hypersplenism. The redistribution of blood from the portal vein to the inferior vena cava causes variations in flow and resistance of the liver, intestine, and spleen. This hemodynamic alteration aids portal perfusion and oxygenation with net effects of increased venous return and cardiac output. Variations in procedures include portacaval, end-to-end, end-to-side, mesocaval, mesorenal, or splenorenal shunts.

B. Preoperative assessment and patient preparation

  1. History and physical examination

      a. Cardiac: *associated disorders include increased heart rate, circulating blood volume, and intrathoracic pressure. Variations of cardiac output, cardiomyopathy, congestive heart failure, coronary artery disease, and decreased response to catecholamines and systemic vascular resistance may be present.*

      b. Respiratory: *hypoxemia may be related to ventilation-perfusion mismatch, increased closing volume, increased functional reserve capacity, atelectasis, right-to-left pulmonary shunting, increased disphosphoglycerate, pulmonary infections, and impaired hypoxic pulmonary vasoconstriction.*

      c. Neurologic: *manifestations may include hepatic encephalopathy with associated confusion and obtundation*

      d. Renal: *renal impairment and failure, with electrolyte imbalance is frequently observed*

      e. Gastrointestinal: *gastric or esophageal varices with gastrointestinal bleeding is common*

COMMON PROCEDURES

      f. Endocrine: *abnormal glucose utilization, increased growth hormone, intolerance to carbohydrates, and irregular sex hormone metabolism may be observed*

  2. Patient preparation

     a. Laboratory tests: *arterial blood gases, complete blood count, prothrombin time, partial thromboplastin time, bleeding time, electrolytes, blood urea nitrogen, creatinine, creatinine clearance, urinalysis, diffuse intravascular coagulation profile, albumin, bilirubin, serum glutamic-oxalo-acetic transaminase, serum glutamic-pyruvic transaminase, ammonia, alkaline phosphatase, lactate*

     b. Diagnostic tests: *electrocardiography, echocardiography, pulmonary functions tests, chest radiography*

     c. Preoperative medications: *avoid intramuscular injections. Anxiolytics are administered in small doses as indicated. Consider metoclopramide (10 mg) and ranitidine (50 mg).*

     d. Intravenous therapy: *central line, two 14- to 16-gauge intravenous tubes. Consider a pulmonary arterial catheter.*

C. Room preparation

  1. *Monitoring equipment:* standard with arterial line, central venous pressure catheter, and urinary catheter

  2. *Additional equipment:* fluid warmer, cell saver, Bair-Hugger, and rapid infuser

  3. Drugs

     a. Miscellaneous pharmacologic agents: *opioid (fentanyl), midazolam, vasodilators and vasoconstrictors, inotropes, nondepolarizing muscle relaxants (atracurium), and antibiotics*

     b. Intravenous fluids: *calculate for major blood loss. Estimated blood loss is 1000 to 2000 mL.*

     c. Blood: *type and cross-match for 8 to 10 units of packed red blood cells, platelets, fresh frozen plasma, and cryoprecipitate*

     d. Tabletop: *standard*

D. Anesthetic technique

General anesthesia, epidural anesthesia, or a combination of general and regional anesthesia.

E. Perioperative management and anesthetic technique

  1. General anesthetic is the technique of choice

  2. *Induction:* rapid sequence induction with thiopental (3 to 5 mg/kg), succinylcholine (1 to 2 mg/kg). Consider etomidate (0.2 mg/kg) or ketamine (1 mg/kg).

  3. *Maintenance:* inhalational agent/oxygen/fentanyl/midazolam and nondepolarizing muscle relaxant of choice—position is supine

  4. *Emergence:* patient generally is transported to the intensive care unit

F. Postoperative implications

  1. *Complications:* coagulopathy, renal failure, hypothermia, encephalopathy, jaundice, and anemia

  2. *Postoperative pain management:* passive cutaneous anaphylaxis

ORTHOPEDICS
A. Arthroplasty

❖   ❖   ❖

HIP

A. Introduction

Replacement of joint surfaces is required primarily in inflammatory or degenerative conditions within the joint, such as those accompanying rheumatoid arthritis or osteoarthritis from degeneration of the synovium or cartilage. As one or more of the normal joint tissues deteriorate or degenerate, the bone ends are exposed, causing pain and limitation of joint movements. Joint stiffness and muscle atrophy follow further increasing pain, limiting movement and mobility. Exposed bone surfaces will lead to bone growth that may eventually adhere to the opposing bone ends, causing bony ankylosis and loss of joint movement. Therefore, replacement of the deteriorated or degenerated tissues and bones restores movement and relieves pain.

Total joint replacement involves removal of some or all of the synovium, cartilage, and bone in both sides of the joint. One of the joint bone surfaces is then replaced with a metallic prosthesis, whereas the other surface is replaced with a ceramic or plastic, silicone-lined prosthesis. The metallic-plastic material is necessary to prevent metal-to-metal wear, friction, and possible electrolytic reactions from the interactions and intermingling of joint fluids.

B. Preoperative assessment and patient preparation

1. History and physical examination
   a. *With this elderly population, assess for coexisting medical diseases*
   b. *Carefully assess blood volume, central venous pressure, and orthostatic hypotension, because dehydration may mask hemoglobin changes due to hematoma formation*
2. Diagnostic tests
   a. Radiographs: *hip and chest film*
   b. Laboratory tests: *complete blood count, electrolytes, glucose, blood urea nitrogen, creatinine, urinalysis, prothrombin time, partial thromboplastin time, bleeding time of the patient on aspirin, and typing and cross-matching*
3. Preoperative medications and intravenous therapy
   a. *Anticoagulants—heparin*
   b. *Antirheumatic or anti-inflammatory medications*
   c. *Antibiotics*
   d. *Sedatives and narcotics—use with caution in the elderly population*

  e. Two peripheral, large-bore (16- to 18-gauge) intravenous tubes with moderate fluid replacement
  f. Epidural catheter placement—perform test dose on awake patient

C. Room preparation
 1. Monitoring equipment
  a. Standard
  b. Indwelling urinary catheter—controversial
   (1) Absence of bladder drainage can cause overdistension, affecting bladder function
   (2) Insertion may cause urinary tract infection
  c. Central venous pressure—trend volume status
  d. Warning modalities
  e. Electrocardiography—leads V5 and II—detect myocardial ischemia and diagnose tachyarrhythmias in the elderly population
  f. Transesophageal echocardiography—assess fat and bone deposits when acetabulum is reamed and curetted
  g. X-ray shields for self protection
  h. Arterial line—monitoring of hypotensive techniques
 2. Pharmacologic agents
  a. Within access, sodium nitroprusside drip
  b. Vasopressors
 3. *Position:* lateral; special orthopedic table may be used

D. Anesthetic techniques
 1. *Considerations:* regional blockade, general anesthesia, a combination of both
 2. Technique of choice
  a. Regional anesthesia
  b. Reduced blood loss and postoperative deep venous thrombosis/pulmonary embolism
 3. *Regional blockade:* either of the following
  a. Epidural catheter placement and preoperative test dose
  b. One-time spinal for analgesia to T10
 4. General anesthesia
  a. Endotracheal tube must be inserted
  b. Combination with regional anesthetic allows reduced dosages of agents, control of airway
 5. Induction
  a. General anesthesia
   (1) Thorough airway assessment with arthritic population
   (2) Induction performed on stretcher
   (3) Succinylcholine may be contraindicated with crush injuries if large amounts of muscle tissue are devitalized
  b. Regional anesthesia—spinal/epidural: review principles of sympathetic blocks
 6. Maintenance
  a. Laminar flow is used to minimize infections and can increase evaporative fluid and heat losses from the operative site
  b. Controlled hypotensive techniques facilitate surgical exposure and decrease blood loss
   (1) Blood pressure parameters need to be individualized
   (2) Maintain mean blood pressure of 50 to 70 mm Hg

(3) Deepen anesthesia with volatile anesthetic

(4) Initiate nitroprusside drip

c. *Methylmethacrylate administration is used as a space-filling mortar and may cause hypotensive effects*

(1) High-risk group—arteriosclerotic patients (who compensate poorly for sudden cardiovascular dynamic changes) and those whose fluid and blood replacement was inadequate

(2) Causes—heat production during cement mixing and the resultant vasodilatation that decreases the systemic vascular resistance

(3) Occurs within 30 to 60 seconds after application up to 10 minutes post prosthesis insertion

(4) Prevent complications—communicate with the surgeon regarding application

(5) Use 100% oxygen, decrease vasodilating agent, maximize fluid status, and have vasopressor support available

7. Emergence

a. *If general anesthetic is implemented, patients are usually repositioned onto the stretcher prior to emergence*

b. *Base extubation on the patient's status*

c. *Initiate regional blockade through the epidural catheter for postoperative analysis prior to the end of the case*

E. Postoperative implications

1. Obtain laboratory results—hemoglobin and hematocrit; watch for hidden bleeding

2. Fat embolism typically appears 12 to 48 hours after a long bone fracture

a. *Signs and symptoms*

(1) Arterial hypoxemia

(2) Adult respiratory distress syndrome

(3) Central nervous system dysfunction (confusion, coma, seizures)

(4) Petechial (neck, shoulders, and chest)

(5) Coagulopathy

(6) Fever

b. *Treatment*

(1) Supportive

(2) Oxygenation

(3) Corticosteroids

(4) Immobilization of long bone fractures

3. Other potential complications include deep venous thrombosis and pulmonary embolism

KNEE (TOTAL KNEE REPLACEMENT)

A. Introduction

Arthrotomy of the knee joint is performed when metallic and plastic components are used for replacement of knee joint surfaces. The femur, patella, and tibia are exposed, and cartilage and a small

COMMON PROCEDURES

amount of bone are removed with a saw. The new components may
or may not be cemented.

B. Preoperative assessment

Routine, including history and physical examination. These patients
have been diagnosed with arthritis of the knee.

1. *Respiratory:* these patients may have rheumatoid arthritis and
   associated pulmonary conditions. Pulmonary effusions may be
   present. Rheumatoid arthritis involving the cricoarytenoid joints
   may exhibit itself by hoarseness. A narrow glottic opening may lead
   to a difficult intubation. Arthritic involvement of the cervical spine
   and temporomandibular joint may also complicate airway
   management.

2. *Cardiovascular:* depending on the severity of the arthritis, the
   patient may have a lowered exercise tolerance. Rheumatoid arthritis
   is associated with pericardial effusion. Cardiac valve fibrosis and
   cardiac conduction abnormalities can occur with possible aortic
   regurgitation. Test electrocardiogram and, if possible,
   echocardiogram and dipyridamole thallium imaging.

3. *Neurologic:* a thorough preoperative neurologic examination may
   yield evidence of cervical nerve root compression. If indicated,
   obtain lateral neck films for the determination of stability of the
   atlanto-occipital joint.

4. *Musculoskeletal:* positioning may be difficult because of the pain and
   decreased mobility of the joint

5. *Hematologic/laboratory:* hemoglobin and hematocrit, other tests
   related to the history and physical examination

6. Premedication
   a. *Mostly determined by institution*
   b. *Valium 5 to 10 mg orally 1 hour preoperatively (or midazolam
      [Versed] 1 to 3 mg in the preoperative holding area)*
   c. *Consider a femoral nerve block if patellar pain is prominent*
   d. *Lidocaine, 10 mL of a 1.5% solution with epinephrine 1:200,000,
      could be used*

C. Room preparation

1. Standard monitoring equipment. A tourniquet may or may not be
   used. JAFFE PAIN 7/10

2. The patient should have one large-bore intravenous tube

3. Fluid requirements include normal saline or lactated Ringer's at
   6 mL/kg per hour

4. Standard drugs for general or regional anesthesia

D. Anesthetic technique

1. This procedure can be done under general or regional anesthesia.
   Regional anesthesia could be with a subarachnoid block or
   placement of an epidural catheter. T8 IF TOURNIQUET
   S2-T12 IF Ø TOURNIQUET

2. Spinal anesthesia can be accomplished with 15 mg of 0.75%
   bupivacaine (with morphine 0.2 mg)

3. Epidural anesthesia can be dosed with 15 to 20 mL of 2% lidocaine
   with epinephrine 1:200,000 (in 5-mL increments every 3 to 5
   minutes)

- LACTIC ACIDOSIS WHEN TOURNIQUET DEFLATED - ↑VENT.
- METHYLMETHACRYLATE

E. **Perioperative management**
1. *Induction:* standard induction with routine medications. Muscle relaxation will be needed for the placement of the prosthesis.
2. *Emergence:* these patients are usually extubated in the operating room unless there was preoperative respiratory compromise. Otherwise, extubate the patient in the operating room.

F. **Postoperative implications**
Watch for posterior tibial artery trauma, peroneal nerve palsy (foot drop), hemorrhage from the posterior tibial artery, and tourniquet nerve injury, if indicated.

SHOULDER (TOTAL SHOULDER)

A. **Introduction**
This procedure is usually done for end-stage arthritis or following trauma. Rheumatoid arthritis and psoriatic arthritis are inflammatory conditions that may require shoulder replacement for correction of pain relief. These conditions are often associated with massive rotator cuff tears.

The patients that present for shoulder arthroplasty are the healthy post-trauma patient, nonrheumatoid arthritic, and rheumatoid arthritic.

B. **Preoperative assessment**
1. *Respiratory*
   a. *Rheumatoid arthritic patients may show signs of pleural effusion or pulmonary fibrosis. Hoarseness may be due to cricoarytenoid joint involvement. This patient may be difficult to intubate.*
   b. *Tests: chest radiography, pulmonary function tests (if indicated); arterial blood gases in compromised patients*
2. *Cardiovascular:* patients with rheumatoid arthritis may suffer from chronic pericardial tamponade, valvular disease, and cardiac condition defects
3. *Neurologic*
   a. *Arthritics may have cervical or lumbar radiculopathies. Preoperative documentation of these conditions is essential. Head flexion may cause cervical cord compression.*
   b. *Tests: cervical spine films to rule out subluxations in rheumatoid patients with neck or upper-extremity radiculopathy*
4. *Musculoskeletal:* with the possibility of limited neck and jaw mobility, special intubation may be indicated. Special attention must be paid to positioning in patients with bony deformities or contractures.
5. *Hematologic:* almost all nontrauma patients will be on some type of nonsteroidal anti-inflammatory drug, which should be stopped approximately 5 days before the procedure
6. *Endocrine:* rheumatoid patients will most likely be on some type of corticosteroid and therefore should have a supplemental dose of steroids to treat adrenal suppression (e.g., hydrocortisone 100 mg, IV).

7. *Laboratory tests:* hemoglobin and hematocrit from healthy patients, otherwise tests as indicated from the history and physical examination
8. *Premedication:* if a regional block is done, moderate to heavy premedication is indicated

C. Room preparation
1. Standard routine monitoring equipment
2. The patient will be in a semi-sitting position. A precordial Doppler device may used to detect venous air embolism.
3. One large-bore intravenous tube will be needed on the nonoperative side.
4. If the patient is more hemodynamically compromised, hemodynamic monitoring may be indicated.
5. *Fluid replacement:* normal saline or lactated Ringer's at 6 mL/kg per hour

D. Anesthetic technique
This procedure could be performed under a general or regional anesthetic technique. The interscalene approach to the brachial plexus alone or combined with a general anesthetic could be used for this procedure.

E. Perioperative management
1. *Induction:* standard induction. If the patient has limited range of motion, awake fiberoptic intubation may be indicated.
2. *Maintenance:* standard maintenance with muscle relaxation; consider a continuous opioid infusion because of the length of the procedure
3. *Position:* Semi-sitting or lawn-chair position
4. *Considerations:* If using N_2O during placement of the humeral component, discontinue it because of the increase risk of a venous air embolism with moderate muscle relaxation at that time
5. *Emergence:* the patient can be extubated in the operating room. Reverse muscle relaxant after positioning the patient back to a supine position

F. Postoperative implications
Consider a patient-controlled anesthesia pump or regional block technique for postoperative pain.

B. External Fixator Placement and Open Reduction and Internal Fixation of Extremities

♦ ♦ ♦

A. Introduction
Tibial fractures are fixed with percutaneous pins that are clamped to an external frame. Pins made of stainless steel are drilled into the

proximal and distal fragments of the fracture through stab wounds through the skin and subcutaneous tissue.

Open reduction and internal fixation is performed under direct vision. The fractures are fixed and stabilized with pins, plates, or a combination thereof. Radiographs are taken intraoperatively to confirm placement of hardware. After the incisions are closed, a splint or cast is applied.

B. Preoperative assessment

1. History and physical examination
   a. Respiratory: *10% to 15% of patients with bone fractures will develop fat emboli. Symptoms include hypoxemia, tachycardia, tachypnea, respiratory alkalosis, mental status changes, and conjunctival petechiae. Urinalysis shows fat in the urine. These patients should be adequately hydrated and mechanically ventilated, and the hypoxemia should be corrected.*
   b. Cardiovascular: *if blunt chest trauma occurs during the injury, cardiac contusion or tamponade are possible. Tachycardia hypotension or orthostasis should be managed with crystalloids (10 to 40 mL/kg per hour) or blood accordingly. For patients with hemodynamic instability or blood loss, consider using a tourniquet on the thigh for induction. Electrocardiography, creatinine, enzymes, and echocardiography help to determine the presence of cardiac injury.*
   c. Neurologic: *a thorough evaluation including mental status and peripheral sensory examination is indicated*
   d. Musculoskeletal: *consider a cervical spine injury if the mechanism of injury included rapid deceleration or trauma to the head or neck*
2. *Laboratory tests:* routine and indicated tests should be performed, including hemoglobin and hematocrit
3. *Premedication:* for trauma patients, minimal or no premedication is given. If the patient has severe pain on movement, opiates can be titrated for pain relief.

C. Room preparation

1. Standard monitoring equipment
2. Lead apron for protection during radiography
3. One large-bore intravenous tube. If the patient is hemodynamically compromised, consider an arterial line and central venous pressure monitoring.
4. Fluid replacement of normal saline or lactated Ringer's at 4 to 8 mL/kg per hour
5. If blood loss has been significant, type and cross-match for appropriate blood replacement

D. Perioperative management and anesthetic technique

1. Same as for knee or shoulder replacement
2. This procedure may be performed under general or regional technique. If the patient has suffered trauma, use general anesthesia with rapid sequence induction and cricoid pressure.
3. *Maintenance:* routine maintenance for general or regional anesthetic
4. *Position:* supine
5. *Emergence:* if the procedure is performed under a general anesthetic, the patient should be extubated in the operating room

E. Postoperative implications
1. Complications of hypoxemia may develop secondary to a fat embolism
2. Pain management can be controlled under a continuous epidural infusion

C. Pelvic Reconstruction

◆ ◆ ◆

A. Introduction

Surgical procedure that involves the open reduction of pelvic fractures, which are then maintained by the application of plates and screws. Bone grafting may be used to repair any defects. The surgical time for the procedure is 3 to 6 hours. These fractures may be caused by minor trauma, especially in elderly persons, but most result from high-impact trauma (i.e., motor vehicle trauma). Evaluation of the patient for potential coexisting trauma should include a thorough neurologic, thoracic, and abdominal assessment. The extremities may also be involved.

B. Preoperative assessment

1. *History and physical examination:* Obtain a verbal history from the patient or family member. Note any pre-existing disease processes, social history, current medications, past surgical history, and allergies.
   a. Cardiac: *assess for cardiac contusion or aortic tear. Tests: 12-lead electrocardiography, creatinine, isoenzymes, chest radiography (wide mediastinal silhouette suggests aortic tear). Transesophageal echocardiography or angiography if aortic tear is suspected. Consult with a cardiologist if indicated.*
   b. Respiratory: *assess for possible hemothorax, pneumothorax, pulmonary contusion, fat embolism, or aspiration. The patient may require supplemental oxygen or mechanical ventilation to correct hypoxemia. Coexisting trauma to the head or cervical spine may require fiberoptic intubation. Tests: chest radiography, arterial blood gases.*
   c. Neurologic: *a thorough neurologic evaluation including mental status and peripheral sensory examination. Note any pre-existing deficits. Consult with a neurologist if necessary. Tests: Computed tomography of the head is indicated for patients who experience a loss of consciousness prior to anesthesia.*
   d. Renal: *renal injury is possible with high-impact trauma. Rule out urethral tear before the Foley catheter is placed. A suprapubic catheter may be necessary. Intraoperative monitoring of urine output is mandatory to assess adequate renal perfusion. Consult a urologist if*

necessary. Tests: *urinalysis, blood urea nitrogen, serum creatinine, hematuria, myoglobinuria.*

e. Musculoskeletal: *cervical spine clearance may be required prior to neck manipulation (i.e., laryngoscopy). Consider evaluating thoracic and lumbar radiographs to rule out any deformity or instability prior to anesthesia.* Tests: *cervical spine radiography, others as indicated from the history and physical examination.*

f. Hematologic: *large blood loss associated with traumatic injury may occur. The patient's hematocrit should be restored to greater than 25% prior to induction of anesthesia. Type and cross-match for 6 units of packed red blood cells. Consider the use of cell-saver intraoperatively.*

g. Gastrointestinal: *patients should be assessed for abdominal injury associated with trauma.* Tests: *diagnostic peritoneal lavage.*

2. Patient preparation

a. Laboratory tests: *hemoglobin, hematocrit, electrolytes, prothrombin time, partial thromboplastin time, others as indicated from the history and physical examination*

b. Medications: *anxyiolytics, narcotics, antibiotics, and others as indicated from the history and physical examination. The patient may also be on anticoagulant therapy for the prevention of deep venous thrombosis. A broad-spectrum antibiotic should be administered preoperatively.*

C. Room preparation

1. *Monitoring equipment:* electrocardiogram, oxygen saturation (SpO_2), noninvasive blood pressure monitoring, temperature, arterial line, central venous pressure, pulmonary arterial catheter if indicated from the history and physical examination, peripheral nerve stimulator, urinary catheter, two large peripheral intravenous tubes

2. Additional equipment

a. Positioning devices and operating table: *the patient may be placed in the supine, lateral, or prone position. A fracture table may be used. Meticulously pad the chest, axilla, pelvis, and extremities to prevent potential nerve injury and ischemia. Prevent pressure to down ear and eye if the patient is in the lateral position. Maintain the neck in neutral alignment.*

b. *Because of the length of the procedure and surgical exposure, warming devices should be implemented (i.e., fluid warmer, warming blanket)*

c. *A nasogastric tube should be used to decompress the stomach if a rapid sequence induction is performed*

3. Drugs

a. Continuous infusions: *consider the use of intravenous-narcotic infusion. If an epidural catheter is placed for postoperative pain control, consider an intraoperative continuous incision to decrease anesthetic requirements.*

b. Intravenous fluids and blood: *estimated blood loss is greater than 1000 mL. Type and cross-match the patient for 6 units of packed red blood cells. Blood loss is replaced 1:1 with blood products of colloid solutions or 3:1 if crystalloid solutions are used. Consider the intraoperative use of cell-saver. Maintain urine output at 0.5 mL/kg*

COMMON PROCEDURES

per hour. Consider the use of deliberate hypotension to control blood loss in those patients without cardiovascular disease or carotid stenosis. Isoflurane, esmolol, sodium nitroprusside, or a combination thereof, titrated to decrease mean arterial pressure by 30% (but not <60 mm Hg), is commonly used. Any fluid deficits must be replaced prior to the institution of deliberate hypotension.

    c. Tabletop: *standard*

D. Perioperative management and anesthetic technique

1. *Introduction and maintenance:* a rapid sequence induction must be used for trauma patients to decrease the risk of aspiration. A standard indication may be used if the procedure is performed electively. Because of the painful nature of the injury, induction is best performed on the patient's bed or stretcher before moving to the operating table. Drugs for induction and maintenance should reflect the patient's history and physical examination, accounting for any significant medical history, current physiologic states, and drug allergies. Consider the use of a nondepolarizing muscle relaxant (NDMR) during induction if there are no airway concerns. Anesthetic gases should be warmed and humidified. Continued muscle relaxation is optional and left to the discretion of the anesthetist or the request of the surgeon.

2. *Emergence:* regional anesthesia is usually inadequate because of the length of the procedure, patient positioning, or both. An epidural catheter may be placed for supplemental use intraoperatively and for postoperative pain control. Trauma patients undergoing a rapid sequence induction should be fully awake and reflexive prior to extubation. Patients who suffer pulmonary complications related to trauma or the surgical procedure (i.e., fat embolism, pulmonary contusion, or aspiration) should not be extubated. NDMR should be reversed if extubation is the goal. Discontinue N_2O and volatile anesthetic agents and administer 100% O_2. Thoroughly suction the oropharynx. Assess reflexes. Extubate. Administer 100% O_2 and re-evaluate the respiratory status. Trauma patients may require placement in the intensive care unit postoperatively.

3. *Fat embolization:* 30% to 90% of patients with fractures are reported to experience fat embolization. Most patients remain asymptomatic. The incidence of fat embolization is higher in patients with long bone or pelvic fractures. The anesthetist must be aware of the development of potentially life-threatening events. Signs and symptoms include hypoxemia; tachycardia; tachypnea; respiratory alkalosis; mental status changes; petechiae on the chest, upper extremities, axillae, and conjunctiva; fat bodies in the urine; and diffuse pulmonary infiltrates. Treatment is supportive and prophylactic: O_2 therapy and continuous positive air pressure via mask or endotracheal tube, judicious fluid management to help decrease the severity of pulmonary capillary leaks, heparin, alcohol (controversial), or high-dose corticosteroids may all be considered.

E. Postoperative implications

Consider the use of continuous epidural infusion or patient-controlled anesthesia for postoperative pain control. The L4–S5 nerve roots may be damaged from the primary traumatic event or the operation. The result is hemiplegia with bladder and bowel dysfunction.

Intraoperative pressure on the ilioinguinal ligament may cause neuropathy of the femoral genitofemoral or femoral cutaneous nerve. A marked postoperative decrease in blood pressure may be related to retroperitoneal hematoma formation. Deep venous thrombosis prophylaxis should be instituted postoperatively (i.e., support hose and deep vein thrombosis prophylaxis).

D. Hip Pinning (Open Reduction and Internal Fixation)

◆ ◆ ◆

A. Introduction
Surgical procedure that involves the open reduction of a hip fracture that is maintained by the application of plates and screws. Bone grafting may be used to repair any defects. The surgical time for the procedure is 3 to 6 hours.

Hip fractures may result from high-impact trauma, but most result from minor trauma in elderly persons. If the fracture is related to high-impact trauma, a coexisting trauma should be thoroughly evaluated.

B. Preoperative assessment and patient preparation
1. *History and physical examination:* obtain a verbal history from the patient or family member. Note any pre-existing disease processes, social history, current medications, past surgical history, and allergies.
   a. Cardiac: *interview the patient regarding exercise tolerance and any known history of cardiac disease, hypertension, or arrhythmias. Tests: 12-lead electrocardiography; cardiac involvement may necessitate consultation with a cardiologist prior to surgery and further preoperative studies.*
   b. Respiratory: *interview and assess the patient for any pre-existing respiratory disease. Obtain a smoking history and history of any occupational exposure to respiratory irritants. Arthritis of the temporomandibular joint or cervical spine may increase the difficulty of intubation in elderly persons. Tests: chest radiography (severe respiratory disease may necessitate consultation with a pulmonary specialist), further preoperative work-up and optimization of the patient's pulmonary status.*
   c. Neurologic: *interview the patient regarding a history of transient ischemic attacks, carotid artery disease, cerebrovascular accident, or*

diabetic neuropathy. Note any pre-exisitng deficits, confusion, or disorientation. Tests: consultation with a neurologist may be necessary prior to surgery, especially if the deficit is of recent onset.

   d. Renal: obtain a history of any renal impariment or prostatic obstruction. Note any use of diuretics. Tests: blood urea nitrogen, serum creatinine, urinalysis (serum creatinine should remain unchanged with increasing age, whereas blood urea nitrogen gradually increases 0.2 mg/dL per year).

   e. Gastrointestinal: obtain any history of liver disease, alcohol abuse, hiatal hernia, gastric reflux, or diabetes. Tests: prothrombin time, partial thromboplastin time, serum albumin, liver function studies.

C. Patient preparation

1. Laboratory tests: hemaglobin, hematocrit, complete blood count, prothrombin time, partial thromboplastin time, others as indicated by the history and physical examination

2. Diagnostic tests: 12-lead electrocardiography, chest radiography, others as indicated by the history and physical examination

3. Preoperative medications: in general, elderly persons require reduced doses of premedication. Albumin, which binds acidic drugs (barbiturates, benzodiazepines, opioid agonists), tends to decrease with age, leaving a larger free fraction, whereas alpha$_1$ acid glycoprotein, which binds basic drugs (local anesthetics), increases—thus increasing the duration of spinal anesthetics. Because of the atrophy of salivary glands related to aging, anticholinergics are rarely required. A broad-spectrum antibiotic should be administered preoperatively.

D. Room preparation

1. Monitoring equipment: electrocardiography, oxygen saturation (SpO_2), noninvasive blood pressure monitor, arterial line, central venous pressure catheter, pulmonary arterial catheter (as indicated by the history and physical examination), peripheral nerve stimulator, temperature, Foley catheter

2. Additional equipment

   a. Positioning devices and operating table. The patient is usually placed in a lateral position. Aging skin atrophies and is prone to trauma from adhesive tape, electrocautery pads, and electrocardiographic electrodes. Arthritic joints may interfere with positioning; when possible, the elderly patient should be positioned for comfort. Meticulous padding of the axilla and all bony prominences decreases the risk of nerve injury and ischemia. Prevent pressure to the ears and eyes. Maintain the neck in neutral alignment.

   b. Because of the length of the procedure, the patient's usual age, and surgical exposure, warming modalities should be implemented (fluid warmer, warming blankets)

3. Drugs

   a. Continuous infusion: consider the use of continuous epidural infusion intraoperatively or for postoperative pain control

   b. Intravenous fluids: estimated blood loss is greater than 1000 mL. Type and cross-match for units of packed red blood cells. Blood loss is replaced 1:1 with blood products or colloid solutions or 3:1 if crystalloid solutions are used. Maintain the urine output at 0.5 mL/kg per hour. Keep in mind any pre-existing disease processes that may easily place the elderly patient in a state of fluid overload. Consider the use of cell-saver intraoperatively.

c. Tabletop: *standard. All equipment needed to implement the anesthetic plan should be available.*

E. Perioperative management and anesthetic technique

1. Regional and general anesthesia are both options for the elderly patient. Hip pinning may be performed using subarachnoid block or continuous epidural infusion extending to the T8 sensory level. Keep in mind the expected length of the procedure, the patient's history and physical examination findings, and the patient's level of cooperation and ability to lie still. One major advantage of regional anesthesia is a decreased incidence of postoperative thromboembolism. This is thought to be due to peripheral vasodilation and maintenance of venous blood flow in the lower extremities. Local anesthetics also inhibit platelet aggregation and stabilize endothelial cells. Difficult patient positioning and altered landmarks related to degenerative changes of the spine may increase the technical difficulty of performing a regional block. Postpuncture headaches are not as prevalent in the elderly population.

   If a general anesthetic is the best choice for the patient, drugs for induction and maintenance should reflect findings from the patient's history and physical examination. Anesthetic gases should be warmed and humidified. The maximum allowable concentration for inhalational agents is reduced by 4% per decade of age over 40 years. One advantage of general anesthesia is that the anesthetic can be induced with the patient on the bed or stretcher before moving to the operating table, avoiding painful positioning. A disadvantage of general anesthesia is that the elderly patient cannot be positioned for maximal comfort. Consider the use of nondepolarizing muscle relaxants during induction if there are no airway concerns. Continued muscle relaxation is optional and left to the discretion of the anesthetist or the request of the surgeon. The effects of nondepolarizing muscle relaxants that are renally excreted may be slightly prolonged in elderly persons because of reduced drug clearance.

2. *Emergence:* an epidural catheter may be placed for supplemental use with general anesthesia or for postoperative pain control. Patients undergoing rapid sequence induction should be fully awake and reflexive prior to extubation. Patients who suffer respiratory complications from trauma or the surgical procedure (fat embolism, pulmonary contusion, or aspiration) should not be extubated. If a nondepolarizing muscle relaxant is used it should be reversed if extubation is the goal. Discontinue N_2O and volatile anesthetic agents and administer 100% O_2. Thoroughly suction the oropharynx. Assess reflexes and extubate. Administer 100% O_2 and re-evaluate respiratory status. Trauma patients may require postoperative placement in the intensive care unit.

3. *Fat embolization:* (see Chaper C, Pelvic Reconstruction, in this section).

F. Postoperative implications

Consider the use of continuous epidural infusion of patient-controlled anesthesia for postoperative pain control. A marked decrease in blood pressure postoperatively may be related to hematoma formation. Deep venous thrombosis prophylaxis should be instituted postoperatively (support hose and deep vein thrombosis prophylaxis).

E. Open Reduction and Internal Fixation of Extremities

◆   ◆   ◆

A. Introduction

A surgical procedure involving a longitudinal incision made over the fractured bone so that it may be reduced and realigned under direct visualization; the bone is then stabilized and fixed using pins, plates, screws, and a prosthesis when applicable. Intraoperative radiography is used to confirm reduction and placement of hardware. Bone grafting may be utilized for bone defects needing repair.

Trauma and falls in the elderly are common indications for these procedures. Trauma patients require aggressive fluid therapy, large-bore intravenous tubes, and invasive monitors (arterial line and central venous pressure). Elderly patients may present with different concurrent disease processes.

B. Preoperative assessment

1. *Cardiac:* blunt chest trauma can produce cardiac contusion, tamponade, or aortic tear. Electrocardiography, creatine enzyme levels, and echocardiography help evaluate cardiac injury. In elderly patients, baseline electrocardiography helps evaluate previous myocardial infarction. Rheumatoid arthritis is associated with pericardial effusion, cardiac valve fibrosis, cardiac conduction, and aortic regurgitation.

2. *Respiratory:* pulmonary fat embolus occurs in 10% to 15% of long bone fractures. Signs and symptoms are hypoxemia, increased heart rate, tachypnea, respiratory alkalosis, mental status changes, and conjunctival petechiae. If a hemothorax or pneumothorax is present, a chest tube should be placed. Supplemental O_2 must be applied with such manifestations. Chest radiography and urinalysis for fat bodies help diagnose pulmonary embolism. Rheumatoid arthritis involving the cricoarytenoid joints may manifest as hoarseness, glottic narrowing, and difficult intubation. Arthritic involvement of the temporomandibular joint and cervical spine may further compromise airway management.

3. *Neurologic:* the possibility of coexistent neurologic trauma warrants the thorough preoperative mental status and peripheral sensory examination. Patients with a loss of consciousness should undergo computed tomography of the head before anesthesia is initiated. In arthritic patients a thorough preoperative examination may show evidence of cervical nerve root compression. The full range of neck motion should be evaluated; if deficits exist, lateral neck films determine the stability of the atlanto-occipital joint.

4. *Renal:* renal injury results from trauma to the collecting system, myoglobinuria from rhabdomyolysis, and acute ischemic tubular necrosis from hypovolemia or aortic dissection. Monitoring of urinary output is mandatory to detect intraoperative compromise of the collecting system and the adequacy of renal perfusion. Urinalysis, blood urea nitrogen, and creatinine help determine the level of functioning of the kidneys in both elderly patients and those who have suffered trauma.

5. *Hematologic:* hemophiliacs and patients with cancer may be included in this patient population. Careful administration of blood products and evaluation of clotting factors may be required. A consulting hematologist guides factor replacement in the hemophiliac patient; leukocyte-poor packed red blood cells or red cells negative for a particular antigen may be used in the cancer patient.

6. *Gastrointestinal/endocrine:* unless a pathology is revealed in the history and physical, these systems have no special considerations.

7. *Patient preparation:* laboratory and diagnostic tests were listed earlier

8. *Premedication:* aspiration may be a concern for the trauma patient. Histamine$_2$ blockers may be indicated. Preoperative sedation should be held on patients with neurologic changes.

C. Room preparation

1. *Monitoring:* standard monitors, central venous pressure, arterial line, pulmonary artery pressure monitoring, Foley catheter. Invasive monitoring is used for trauma patients and those whose history reveals significant problems in the respiratory, cardiovascular, or genito-urinary systems. The length of the proposed surgery also helps determine monitoring.

2. *Additional equipment:* tourniquets are used for lower-extremity fractures. The fracture table is needed for repairs of the pelvis and hips.

3. *Drugs:* the patient's history helps determine the use of continuous drips (e.g., nitroglycerin)

4. *Fluid and blood replacement:* follow the standard replacement guidelines = replenish fluids secondary to NPO time in the first 2 hours of surgery, 1 mL blood loss = 3 mL crystalloid replacement, to 2 to 15 mL/kg maintenance depending on fracture site, blood loss, and history and physical examination results. Trauma patients should be hemodynamically stable prior to the induction of anesthesia, if possible. The table top must be set up for general anesthesia at all times.

COMMON PROCEDURES

D. Anesthetic technique

General anesthesia is indicated with hip and pelvis surgery because of the duration and varied positions necessary to accomplish pelvic fixation.

Regional anesthesia permits evaluation of mental status, provides intact airway reflexes, and decreases blood loss in trauma patients. With combative patients, those requiring multiple concurrent surgical procedures, or procedures lasting more than 2 hours, general anesthesia should be used. Regional anesthesia also has the advantage of decreased blood loss, decreased deep venous thrombosis, minimal respiratory impairment, and effective postoperative analgesia. Anesthesia extending from S2 to T8 (if tourniquets are used) is adequate for lower-extremity surgery. Subarachnoid block and epidural blocks are useful. Agents used most often are 0.75% bupivacaine, 15 mg for subarachnoid block; epidural = 15 to 20 mL of 2% lidocaine.

E. Perioperative management

1. *Induction:* trauma patients who are to receive general anesthesia should undergo rapid sequence induction with cricoid pressure to prevent aspiration. Otherwise, anesthesia may be initiated with any induction agent, volatile anesthetic, or muscle relaxant unless contraindicated by history and physical examination.

2. *Maintenance:* with regional anesthesia, a propofol infusion may be indicated. With general anesthesia, N_2O, volatile anesthetics, O_2, and narcotics may be used. Muscle relaxation is needed in procedures requiring prosthesis insertion so that a full range of motion (passive) may be performed. Pad all pressure points. Unless the fracture is pelvic the patient will be supine. Pelvic fractures may be treated with the patient in the lateral decubitus, supine, or prone position.

3. *Emergence:* trauma patients must be extubated fully awake and after airway reflexes have returned. Do not extubate patients with evolving pulmonary injuries (fat embolism, aspiration, or contusion). When a tourniquet is used, controlled ventilation should be continued for 3 to 5 minutes after deflation of the tourniquet to help facilitate the metabolism of the lactic acid that has developed in the leg—this is especially imperative in patients with moderate to severe lung disease who may be unable to increase ventilation to buffer this acid load.

F. Postoperative implications

1. Pain managment is the most prominent postoperative concern

2. Patient-controlled analgesia and epidural infusion are two modes of therapy used for pain relief

Nerve damage related to positioning or tourniquet placement is a potential problem. Post-tourniquet syndrome is a self-limiting condition in which the affected limb is edematous, pale, and weak.

HEAD AND NECK
A. Thyroidectomy

• • •

A. Introduction

Hyperthyroidism results from excess secretion of T_3 and T_4 by the thyroid gland. Subtotal thyroidectomy may be used in the treatment of hyperthyroidism as an alternative to prolonged medical therapy. Extensive but incomplete removal of the thyroid gland induces remission in most patients.

B. Preoperative assessment and patient preparation

1. History and physical examination
   a. Respiratory: *palpate the thyroid gland to determine its size and relationship to the trachea*
   b. Cardiac: *assess the heart rate, blood pressure, and electrocardiogram*
2. Diagnostic tests
   a. *Complete blood count, electrolytes, glucose, blood urea nitrogen, creatinine, Ca^{2+}, electrocardiography, chest radiography*
   b. *Radiographs may be needed to visualize the trachea and thyroid gland*
   c. *Tests specific to the thyroid gland: T_3, T_4, and thyroid-stimulating hormone levels*
3. Preoperative medication and intravenous therapy
   a. *Maintain euthyroid state and control hyperkinetic circulation. Propylthiouracil, methimazole, potassium iodide, and beta-adrenergic antagonists may be used.*
   b. *Continue all antithyroid medications*
   c. *Normal thyroid function tests and a resting heart rate of less than 85 bpm are recommended prior to surgery. If the systolic blood pressure is above 140 mm Hg and the heart rate is above 100 bpm, surgery may be canceled and more antithyroid medication given. With tachycardia associated with cardiac irregularities, surgery may be postponed.*
   d. *Give adequate premedication to prevent an increase in sympathetic activity. Avoid anticholinergic drugs (they increase the heart rate).*
   e. *Consider two 16- to 18-gauge intravenous tubes and proximity of surgery to vessels of the neck*

C. Room preparation

1. *Monitoring equipment:* standard
2. *Pharmacologic agents:* beta-adrenergic blockers
3. *Position:* supine with the arms tucked at the side; a small pad may be placed between the shoulder blades to hyperextend the neck

D. Anesthetic techniques
1. *General anesthesia:* endotracheal intubation is required
2. *Goal of anesthetic management:* to achieve a depth of anesthesia that prevents an exaggerated sympathetic response to surgical stimulation and to avoid the administration of medications that stimulate the sympathetic nervous system

E. Perioperative management
1. Induction
   a. *An awake fiberoptic intubation may be indicated if the gland impinges on the airway*
   b. *An anode tube may be used to decrease the risk of kinking and airway obstruction*
   c. *Lidocaine and narcotics may be used prior to laryngoscopy to blunt the sympathetic nervous system response to intubation. An inhalational agent may be used to increase the depth of anesthesia prior to intubation.*
   d. *Induction agent of choice is thiopental—avoid ketamine*
   e. *Administer muscle relaxants that lack effect on the cardiovascular system*
2. Maintenance
   a. *Inhalational agents or opiods combined with N_2O are recommended to blunt the sympathetic nervous system response to surgical stimulation*
   b. *If the patient is not euthyroid, maintenance of beta-blockade is highly desirable*
   c. *The incidence of myasthenia gravis is increased in hyperthyroid patients*
   d. *Treat hypertension with direct-acting agents*
   e. *Monitor breath sounds with an esophageal stethoscope—the endotracheal tube is concealed under the sterile field and out of view*
   f. *Patients with exophthalmus are susceptible to corneal ulceration and drying—protect the eyes*
   g. *Monitor temperature, which may indicate thyroid storm or a hypermetabolic state*
3. Emergence
   a. *Reverse muscle relaxation completely—use glycopyrrolate (Robinul) rather than atropine (less chronotropic effect)*
   b. *Extubate the patient wide awake with protective reflexes intact. Assess the vocal cords by direct visualization for bilateral or unilateral paralysis.*

F. Postoperative considerations
1. Complications include recurrent laryngeal nerve damage, tracheal compression, hematoma formation, hypoparathyroidism
2. Thyroid storm may occur intraoperatively but is more likely in the first 6 to 18 hours after surgery

B. Parathyroidectomy

• • •

A. Introduction
Primary hyperparathyroidism results from excessive secretion of parahormone due to benign parathyroid adenomas (90% of cases),

hyperplasia (9%), or parathyroid carcinoma (2%). Symptoms result from accompanying hypercalcemia. Definitive treatment requires surgical removal of the adenoma or malignant gland. Hyperplasia of all four glands is treated by excision of all parathyroid tissue except half of one gland. Parathyroidectomy may be indicated in some cases of secondary hyperparathyroidism.

B. Perioperative assessment and patient preparation

1. Assess for clinical manifestations of hypercalcemia. Renal, cardiac, and central nervous system abnormalities are associated with chronic hypercalcemia.
2. Laboratory tests should include a current CA^{2+} level. Consider hemoglobin and hematocrit, electrolytes, magnesium, phosphate, blood urea nitrogen, creatinine, electrocardiography, and radiography.
3. Correct volume status and electrolyte irregularities
4. Elevated Ca^{2+} levels may be lowered initially with intravenous normal saline and furosemide. Emergency treatment is necessary with levels greater than 15 mg/dL. Treatment includes intravenous phosphates, mithramycin, calcitonin, glucocorticoids, and dialysis.

C. Room preparation

1. Standard tabletop setup
2. Supine position with arms tucked at the side; a small pad may be placed between the shoulder blades to hyperextend the neck. The operating table may be tilted to elevate the head and decrease bleeding.
3. Consider two intravenous tubes—proximity of surgery to vessels of the neck. Vigorous fluid therapy is indicated to correct hypervolemia and dilute the hypercalcemia. Volume frequently is contracted.

D. Perioperative management and anesthetic techniques

General anesthesia—no special anesthetic drug or technique is indicated.

E. Considerations

1. Avoid hypoventilation—acidosis increases ionized Ca^{2+}
2. Renal dysfunction coexist—adjust anesthetic techniques accordingly
3. Somnolence before induction may decrease anesthetic requirements
4. The response to muscle relaxants may be altered. A nerve stimulator is important. The patient may be sensitive to succinylcholine and resistant to nondepolarizers. Use caution with long-acting muscle relaxants if the surgeon wants to test nerve function.
5. Osteoporosis predisposes patients to vertebral compression during laryngoscopy and to bone fractures during transport. Position the patient gently to avoid pathologic fractures.
6. Monitor the electrocardiogram for short QT interval and prolonged PR interval

F. Postoperative considerations

1. Complications include recurrent laryngeal nerve damage, bleeding, and transit or complete hypoparathyroidism

COMMON PROCEDURES

2. Patients with significant preoperative bone disease may develop decreased calcium (hungry bone syndrome)—monitor serum Ca^{2+}, magnesium, and phosphorous levels closely

C. Tracheotomy

◆   ◆   ◆

A. Introduction

A tracheotomy is an incision into the trachea to form a temporary or permanent opening, the latter of which is called a tracheostomy. The incision is made through the second, third, or fourth tracheal ring, and a tube is inserted through the opening to allow passage of air and the removal of tracheobronchial secretions. Except in cases of head, neck, and face trauma, a tracheotomy is rarely performed as an emergency procedure.

B. Preoperative assessment and patient preparation

1. History and physical examination: *Respiratory:* vent settings, including peak airway pressures, respiratory rate, amount and color of tracheal secretions; assess the need for and frequency of sectioning, lung sounds, arterial blood gases, chest radiography, and palm infections

2. Diagnostic tests
    a. *Electrocardiography, chest radiography*
    b. Laboratory tests: *complete blood count, prothrombin time, partial thromboplastin time, platelets, electrolytes, glucose, blood and sputum cultures*

3. Preoperative medication and intravenous therapy
    a. *No preoperative medication is recommended*
    b. *Only one intravenous access tube with minimal fluid replacement*

C. Room preparation

1. Monitoring
    a. *Central venous pressure or pulmonary arterial catheter (or both), as well as an arterial line*
    b. *Peripheral nerve stimulation*
    c. *If peak airway pressures are greater than 60 mm H_2O may need a vent from the intensive care unit*
    d. *6-inch connector to attach track to vent*
    e. *Consider a bronchial adaptor—patients frequently have a bronchoscopy adaptor after tracheotomy placement*
    f. *Warming modalities*

2. *Pharmacologic agents:* none

3. *Position:* supine with arms safely tucked to the side

D. Anesthetic technique

Use general anesthesia and skeletal muscle paralysis or local anesthesia with measured anesthesia control

E. Perioperative management

1. *Induction:* titrate anesthetic agents to the patient's need
2. Maintenance
   a. *Adjust the oxygen/air mixture to maintain saturation at greater than 95%*
   b. *If the patient is stable, N_2O, an inhalation agent, and a narcotic may be introduced*
   c. *Avoid 100% oxygen—increases the chance of airway fires*
   d. *If an airway fire occurs:*
      (1) Pour saline into the pharynx to absorb the heat
      (2) Temporarily discontinue the oxygen source
      (3) Extubate and reintubate with a new endotracheal tube
      (4) Follow-up with chest radiography, bronchoscopy, steroids, and blood gases
   e. *Maintain constant communication with the surgeon! Use a team approach. Use hand ventilation during insertion of the tracheotomy tube.*
3. Emergence •
   a. *The patient may be transferred to the intensive care unit post procedure. The nondepolarizing muscle relaxant may not have to be reversed if prolonged ventilation is planned.*
   b. *100% oxygen via ambubag—monitoring devices functioning, returned to unit*

F. Postoperative implications

1. Assess patients for any symptoms suggesting pneumothorax, pneumomediastinum, cardiac tamponade, hemorrhage, subcutaneous emphysema
2. Suction the airway as often as necessary to maintain airway and remove secretions

COMMON PROCEDURES

D. Laryngectomy

♦ ♦ ♦

A. Introduction

Most cancers of the upper respiratory tract are squamous cell carcinomas. When the laryngeal musculature or cartilage is invaded, a total laryngectomy is performed. Intractable aspiration, with resultant pneumonia that has been unresponsive to other treatments, is another indication for laryngectomy.

A total laryngectomy involves removal of the vallecula and includes the posterior third of the tongue if necessary. Surgical exposure is from the hyoid bone to the clavicle. A tracheostomy is performed and an anode tube placed. The larynx is usually transected just above the hyoid bone. The trachea is brought out to the skin as an end-tracheostomy without the need for an endotracheal tube or tracheostomy tube as the pharynx is closed.

A supraglottic laryngectomy leaves the true cords by resection of the larynx from the ventricle to the base of the tongue. Surgical exposure is similar to that for a total laryngectomy. The specimen includes the epiglottis, the false vocal cords, the supraglottic lesions, and a portion of the base of the tongue. The thyroid perichondrium is approximated to the base of the tongue along with the strap muscles for closure. A temporary tracheostomy is required.

A hemilaryngectomy or vertical partial laryngectomy retains the epiglottis but involves removal of a unilateral true and false cord. Surgical exposure is similar to that of supraglottic laryngectomy, and a tracheostomy is required.

A near-total laryngectomy involves removal of all of the larynx. One arytenoid is utilized to construct a phonatory shunt for speaking. A permanent or temporary tracheostomy is created, and the procedure may be combined with neck dissection and pharyngectomy with flap reconstruction.

B. Preoperative assessment

Most patients will be older and present with a long history of tobacco and alcohol abuse. Associated medical problems may include chronic obstructive pulmonary disease, hypertension, coronary artery disease, and alcohol withdrawal.

1. History and physical examination
   a. Cardiac: *assess for signs and symptoms of coronary artery disease (angina, hypertension, hypercholesteremia, obesity, smoking, family history) and congestive heart failure (paroxysmal nocturnal dyspnea, orthopnea, peripheral edema)*
   b. Respiratory: *smoking (>40 packs/year) is associated with bronchitis, pulmonary emphysema, and chronic obstructive pulmonary disease, which impair respiratory function. Arterial blood gases may reveal CO_2 retention and hypoxemia. Pulmonary function tests demonstrate decreased forced expiratory volume, forced vital capacity, and the ratio of forced expiratory volume to forced vital capacity. Preoperative airway assessment is imperative because edema may distort airway anatomy, and tumor and edema may cause airway compromise. Tracheal deviation must be considered. Fibrosis, edema, and scarring from prior radiation therapy may distort the airway as well.*
   c. Assess for signs of alcohol withdrawal *(altered mental status, tremulousness, increased sympathetic activity)*
   d. Gastrointestinal: *weight loss, malnutrition, dehydration, and electrolyte imbalance can be significant*
   e. Hematologic: *anemias or coagulopathies may be present*
2. Patient preparation
   a. Laboratory tests: *baseline arterial blood gases, electrolytes, hemoglobin, hematocrit, prothrombin time, partial thromboplastin time, and, if indicated from the history and physical examination, hepatic function tests*
   b. Diagnostic tests: *chest radiography, electrocardiography, pulmonary function test, echocardiography, treadmill stress test as indicated from the history and physical examination. Indirect and direct laryngoscopies*

preoperatively and review of computed tomography may help in planning intubation.

   c. Medications: *treatment with a long-acting hypnotic, such as chlordiazepoxide or diazepam, as a precaution for delirium tremens can be considered, unless sedation would be contraindicated because of concerns of airway compromise. An antisialagogue (glycopyrrolate 0.2 mg IV) facilitates endoscopy by the surgeon (consider contraindications in patients with coronary artery disease).*

C. Room preparation
1. Monitoring equipment
   a. Standard monitoring equipment
   b. Foley catheter
   c. Arterial line—useful for serial laboratory and arterial blood gas studies
   d. Central venous pressure—if indicated by coexisting disease (prefer basilic/cephalic vein)
2. Additional equipment
   a. Regular operating table—may be turned 180 degrees
   b. Extension tubes
   c. Fluid warmer and humidifier
   d. Fiberoptic laryngoscope with anticipated difficult airway or potential for airway obstruction
   e. Tracheostomy under local anesthesia occasionally is necessary for severe airway management
3. Drugs
   a. Standard emergency drugs
   b. Standard tabletop
   c. Intravenous fluids
   d. 16- to 18-gauge or larger intravenous tubes (two); normal saline/lactated Ringer's solution at 3 to 5 mL/kg per hour
   e. Sudden large blood losses do not occur; transfusion usually is not necessary

D. Perioperative management and anesthetic technique
1. General endotracheal anesthesia
2. *Induction:* standard intravenous induction is appropriate with a normal airway. The choice of an induction drug should be based on the patient's medical condition. If airway difficulty is possible, direct laryngoscopy can be performed while the patient is breathing spontaneously, and a muscle relaxant may be administered once the glottis is visualized. In more difficult cases, awake intubation or fiberoptic laryngoscopy may be required.
3. *Maintenance:* supine position, head elevated 30 degrees; standard maintenance, considering the patient's pre-existing medical problems, with an inhalation agent and supplemental narcotics benefits patients with reactive airway disease. Use of nondepolarizing muscle relaxants should be discussed with the surgeon, because nerve stimulation for facial nerve localization may be performed. With tracheostomy and laryngectomy, the patient should receive 100% oxygen to promote oxygen reserves and prevent hypoxia in the event of a lost airway. The trachea is transected while the oral endotracheal tube is slowly removed. A

sterile anode tube with breathing circuit is placed in the distal airway by the surgeon and connected to the anesthesia machine. Bilateral breath sounds, airway compliance, and end-tidal CO_2 waveforms should be verified. Manipulation of the carotid sinus during dissection can result in hypotension and cardiac dysrhythmias. Treatment includes cessation of manipulation and infiltration of surrounding tissues with a local anesthetic or administration of intravenous atropine, if necessary. Unexplained hypotension, dysrhythmia, or both may indicate venous air embolism via large open neck veins. *Treatment:* give 100% oxygen, notify the surgeon, flood the field with normal saline, place the head down, aspirate air through the central venous pressure line, increase venous pressure via positive-pressure ventilation, and administer circulatory support as required.

4. *Emergence:* many patients undergo tracheostomy. If no tracheostomy is performed, the amount of airway edema and distortion needs to be discussed with the surgeon prior to determining extubation. A gradual emergence with stable hemodynamic parameters is an important consideration in the patient with coronary artery disease.

E. Postoperative implications

1. Nerve injury—facial nerve injury can cause facial droop. Recurrent laryngeal nerve injury can result in vocal cord dysfunction; diaphragmatic paralysis may result from phrenic nerve injury.
2. Pneumothorax may occur with low neck dissection
3. Airway impingement is due to restrictive neck dressings or hematoma development
4. Communication difficulties following laryngectomy

E. Radical Neck Dissection

◆ ◆ ◆

A. Introduction

Neck dissection is often performed when there is local tumor extension. A radical neck dissection involves a complete cervical lymphadenectomy with resection of the sternocleidomastoid muscle, internal jugular vein, and select cranial nerves. A functional neck dissection is a complete cervical lymphadenectomy, preserving the sternocleidomastoid muscle, internal jugular vein, and select cranial nerves. A modified neck dissection is a variation between a radical neck dissection and a functional neck dissection. Neck dissections are usually combined with resection of the primary lesions, such as those of the tongue, pharynx, and larynx. In a composite resection, a radical neck dissection, normally done first, is followed by a partial mandibulectomy and possibly a partial glossectomy. A tracheostomy is almost always performed with these resections.

Usually, one or two neck incisions, occasionally extending vertically to expose the neck from the mandible to the clavicle, are performed. The accessory nerve (XI), hypoglossal nerve (XII), and lingual nerves are identified and preserved. The sternocleidomastoid muscle, internal jugular vein, and submental triangle may or may not be resected. Drains are placed posteriorly, and the wound is closed in layers.

B. Preoperative assessment

Most patients will be older and present with a long history of tobacco and alcohol abuse. Associated medical problems may include chronic obstructive pulmonary disease, hypertension, coronary artery disease, malnourishment, and alcohol withdrawal.

1. History and physical examination
   a. Cardiac: *assess for signs and symptoms of coronary artery disease (angina, hypertension, hypercholesteremia, obesity, smoking, family history) and congestive heart failure (paroxysmal nocturnal dyspnea, orthopnea, peripheral edema)*
   b. Respiratory: *smoking (>40 packs/year) is associated with bronchitis, pulmonary emphysema, and chronic obstructive pulmonary disease, which impair respiratory function. Arterial blood gases may reveal CO_2 retention and hypoxemia. Pulmonary function tests demonstrate decreased forced expiratory volume, forced vital capacity, and the ratio of forced expiratory volume to forced vital capacity. Preoperative airway assessment is imperative because tumor or edema may distort airway anatomy and cause airway compromise. Tracheal deviation must be considered. Fibrosis, edema, and scarring from prior radiation therapy may distort the airway as well.*
   c. Neurologic: *assess for signs of alcohol withdrawal (altered mental status, tremulousness, increased sympathetic activity)*
   d. Gastrointestinal: *weight loss, malnutrition, dehydration, and electrolyte imbalance can be significant*
   e. Hematologic: *anemia or coagulopathies may be present*
2. Patient preparation
   a. Laboratory tests: *baseline arterial blood gases, electrolytes, hemoglobin and hematocrit, prothrombin time, partial thromboplastin time, and, if indicated from the history and physical examination, hepatic function tests. Hypokalemia increases the chances of life-threatening dysrhythmia.*
   b. Diagnostic tests: *chest radiography, electrocardiography, pulmonary function test, echocardiography, treadmill stress test as indicated from the history and physical examination. Preoperative indirect and direct laryngoscopies and review of computed tomography may help in planning intubation.*
   c. Medications: *treatment with a long-acting hypnotic such as diazepam as a precaution for delirium tremens can be considered, unless sedation would be contraindicated because of concerns of airway compromise. An antisialagogue (glycopyrrolate 0.2 mg IV) facilitates panendoscopy by the surgeon (consider contraindications in patients with coronary artery disease)*

COMMON PROCEDURES

C. Room preparation

1. Monitoring equipment
   a. *Standard monitoring equipment*
   b. *Foley catheter*
   c. *Arterial line—useful for serial laboratory and arterial blood gas studies*
   d. *Central venous pressure line—if indicated by coexisting disease (prefer basilic/cephalic vein)*

2. Additional equipment
   a. *Regular operating table turned 180 degrees*
   b. *Extension tubes*
   c. *Fluid warmer and humidifier*
   d. *Fiberoptic laryngoscope with anticipated difficult airway or potential for airway obstruction*
   e. *Tracheostomy under local anesthesia occasionally is necessary for severe airway management*

3. Drugs
   a. *Standard emergency drugs*
   b. *Standard tabletop*
   c. *Intravenous fluids: two 16- to 18-gauge or larger, normal saline or lactated Ringer's solution at 3 to 5 mL/kg per hour. Uncontrolled bleeding of the internal jugular vein at the skull base is rare but can result in sudden significant blood losses.*

D. Perioperative management and anesthetic techniques

1. General endotracheal anesthesia

2. *Induction:* standard intravenous induction is appropriate with a normal airway. The choice of an induction drug should be based on the patient's medical condition. If airway difficulty is possible, direct laryngoscopy can be performed while the patient is breathing spontaneously, and a muscle relaxant may be administered once the glottis is visualized. In more difficult cases, awake intubation or fiberoptic laryngoscopy may be required.

3. *Maintenance:* supine position, head turned to the opposite side; pillow below the shoulders; standard maintenance, considering the patient's pre-existing medical problems, with an inhalation agent and supplemental narcotics benefits patients with reactive airway disease. Use of nondepolarizing muscle relaxants should be discussed with the surgeon, because nerve stimulation for cranial nerve XI localization may be done. With tracheostomy and laryngectomy, the patient should receive 100% oxygen to promote oxygen reserves and prevent hypoxia in the event of a lost airway. The trachea is transected, whereas the oral endotracheal tube is slowly removed. A sterile anode tube with a breathing circuit is placed in the distal airway by the surgeon and connected to the anesthesia machine. Bilateral breath sounds, airway compliance, and end-tidal CO_2 waveforms should be verified. With right radical neck dissection prolonged Q-T interval on the electrocardiogram can progress to ventricular dysrhythmia and even cardiac arrest. These changes are due to interruption of cervical sympathetic outflow to the heart via the right stellate ganglion. The left cardiac sympathetic fibers most likely have different effects on cardiac excitability because

prolongation of the Q-T interval does not occur after left radical neck dissection. Manipulation of the carotid sinus during dissection can result in hypotension and cardiac dysrhythmia. Treatment includes cessation of manipulation and, if necessary, infiltration of surrounding tissues with a local anesthetic or administration of intravenous atropine. Unexplained hypotension or dysrhythmia may indicate venous air embolism via large open neck veins. *Treatment:* give 100% oxygen, notify the surgeon, flood the field with normal saline, place the head down, aspirate air through the central venous pressure line, increase venous pressure via positive-pressure ventilation, and administer circulatory support as required.

4. *Emergence:* many patients undergo tracheostomy. If no tracheostomy is performed, the amount of airway edema and distortion needs to be discussed with the surgeon prior to determining extubation. A gradual emergence with stable hemodynamic parameters is an important consideration in the patient with coronary artery disease.

E. Postoperative implications

1. Nerve injury—facial nerve injury can cause facial droop. Recurrent laryngeal nerve injury can result in vocal cord dysfunction, and diaphragmatic paralysis may result from phrenic nerve injury.
2. Painful shoulder syndrome
3. Pneumothorax may occur with low neck dissection
4. Airway impingement is due to restrictive neck dressings or hematoma development
5. Communication difficulties after laryngectomy

F. Maxillofacial Trauma

♦ ♦ ♦

A. Introduction

Two common etiologies for facial fractures are fights and gunshot wounds. Because of the forces required to cause facial fractures, other traumas (e.g., subdural hematoma, pneumothorax, cervical spine injury, intra-abdominal bleeding) often occur with these fractures. Airway management can be difficult because of the soft tissue injury to the tongue or airway. A tracheostomy under local or awake intubation should be strongly considered if any doubt exists about securing the airway. Nasal intubation is usually indicated for mandible or maxillary fractures, because at the end of the procedure intermaxillary fixation is performed. The surgeon may require monitoring of the facial nerve—if so, muscle relaxants are contraindicated. Naturally the surgical approach depends on the type and complexity of the fracture. Approach can vary from reduction for nasal fractures to the Caldwell-Luc approach for extensive maxillary bone fractures. Intermaxillary fixation may be required for zygomatic and maxillary fractures. Mandibular fractures are usually reduced and fixed with wires or plates.

B. Preoperative assessment

1. *Respiratory/airway management:* the extent of fractures is evaluated to determine appropriate airway management. Midface fractures are not usually nasally intubated. Access to the oropharynx may be difficult with mandibular fractures. An urgent tracheostomy is indicated for massive facial trauma.
2. *Neurologic:* thorough documentation of any neurologic deficits. Potential for meningitis is possible postoperatively.
3. *Musculoskeletal:* careful positioning is imperative, with special consideration for other trauma-related injuries
4. *Laboratory tests:* hematocrit and others as indicated from the history and physical examination
5. Standard premedication for neurologically intact patients

C. Room preparation

1. *Monitoring equipment:* standard; invasive monitoring may be needed for intracranial or other trauma
2. *Additional equipment:* regular operating table; some surgeons like the table turned 90 or 180 degrees or to have extension tubings available for the circuit
3. Drugs
   a. *Standard emergency drugs*
   b. *Standard tabletop*
   c. Intravenous fluids: *16- to 18-gauge (the patient may have significant blood loss with maxillary repairs); normal saline/lactated Ringer's solution at 6 to 8 mL/kg per hour*

D. Perioperative management and anesthetic technique

1. General endotracheal anesthesia
2. *Induction:* awake fiberoptic laryngoscopy should be performed if any doubt exists concerning the ease of intubation. For patients with LeFort (mandibular or maxillary) fractures, nasal intubation is preferred. Patients with nasal, orbital, or zygomatic fractures are usually orally intubated. Standard induction is appropriate for patients with normal airways. Nasal or oral right-angle endotracheal tubes are used to optimize the surgical field.
3. *Maintenance:* muscle relaxation is usually required. An anti-emetic is helpful for patients who will have their jaws banded or wired together. Metoclopramide (10 mg/IV) or ondansetron (4 mg IV) is suggested.
   a. *Standard maintenance*
   b. Position: *supine; check and pad all pressure points, abduct arms less than 90 degrees to avoid overstretching of brachial plexus*
4. *Emergence:* suction oropharynx carefully to avoid aspiration. Verify that any packs are removed prior to emergence. Patients with difficult airways or wired jaws should be fully awake and have protective reflexes before extubation. Wire cutters should be at the bedside at all times. Depending on the amount of trauma and soft tissue swelling, the patient may require extended intubation and ventilation postoperatively.

E. Postoperative implications
   1. Airway obstruction—have wire cutters available at all times if necessary for airway management. A throat pack may be obstructing the airway.
   2. Aggressive treatment of nausea and vomiting is imperative
   3. Pain management—intravenous narcotics, antiemetics

G. Tonsillectomy and Adenoidectomy

♦ ♦ ♦

A. Introduction
Tonsil and adenoid surgery are among the most common surgical procedures performed in the United States. Such surgery is indicated for the treatment of hypertrophic tonsil and adenoids and recurrent or chronic upper-respiratory-tract and ear infection.

B. Preoperative patient assessment and patient preparation
   1. History and physical examination
      a. Upper airway: *externally inspect tonsilar and adenoid hypertrophy. Adenoid hypertrophy can be determined by having the patient breathe with the mouth closed and evaluate the degree of nasal airway obstruction.*
      b. Oral: *because most of these procedures are performed in children, careful inspection for loose or missing teeth is necessary*
   2. *Diagnostic tests:* routine laboratory tests including prothrombin time and partial thromboplastin time
   3. Preoperative medication and intravenous therapy
      a. *Light sedation with benzodiazepine*
      b. *Minimal blood loss is expected, but massive hemorrhage can occur. One large-bore intravenous catheter is suitable.*

C. Room preparation
   1. *Monitoring equipment:* standard
   2. Pharmacologic agents
      a. *Standard*
      b. *No need for muscle relaxants*
   3. *Position:* supine, arms tucked to the sides, table turned 90 degrees

D. Anesthetic technique—general anesthesia with orogastric intubation

E. Perioperative management
   1. Induction
      a. *Nonspecific intubation with an oral right-angle endotracheal tube is beneficial but not necessary.*
      b. *Confirm the surgeon's preference*

2. *Maintenance:* nonspecific; the use of short-acting agents is suggested. Close monitoring of breath sounds is essential. The tube can easily be dislodged during placement of a mouth gag or during manipulation of the patient's head.

3. Emergence

   a. *Awake extubation after careful suction of oral pharynx with tonsil suction. Never suction the nasopharynx after adenoidectomy. Gently suction the oropharynx.*

   b. *Maintain the patient in Sim's position*

F. **Postoperative implications**

Postoperative bleeding is the most significant complication. If this occurs, intravenous access must be established, if it is not still present. The extent of bleeding is often hidden because of swallowing of blood. Rehydration is imperative with rapid sequence induction if re-exploration is planned.

H. Nasal Surgery

♦ ♦ ♦

A. **Introduction**

Nasal surgery is performed for cosmetic reasons, to restore the caliber of the nasal airway, or sometimes for both reasons. Rhinoplasty, septoplasty, and septorhinoplasty differ, however. In all nasal surgery, the nasal cavity is cocainized with 4% cocaine-soaked pledgets for 5 to 10 minutes. To ensure vasoconstriction and minimize bleeding, the site is infiltrated with 1.0% lidocaine and 1:100,000 epinephrine.

An incision is made in the septum down to the cartilage, and a submucoperichondral flap is elevated. This may be repeated on the contralateral side. Bone and cartilaginous deformities are resected or weakened. In rhinoplasty, the nasal contours are remodeled by tip remodeling, hump reduction, bone osteotomies, or combinations thereof. After surgery, both nasal cavities are packed, and external splints may be used for all nasal procedures.

B. **Preoperative assessment and patient preparation**

Generally, these procedures are elective and can be performed on an outpatient basis. It is important to identify patients with obstructive apnea. These patients often have chronic airway obstruction, redundant pharyngeal tissues, or both. Such patients, as well as asthmatic patients, should undergo arterial blood gas and pulmonary function testing. Ketorolac and acetylsalicylic acid should be avoided in patients who also have nasal polyps, because they often are hypersensitive to acetylsalicylic acid, a condition that can precipitate bronchospasm.

1. *History and physical examination:* carefully evaluate cardiovascular status, because the use of local vasoconstrictors may cause dysrhythmia, coronary artery spasm, hypertension, and seizures

2. Patient preparation
   a. Laboratory tests: *as indicated by the history and physical examination*
   b. Diagnostic tests: *arterial blood gases, pulmonary function tests, electrocardiography if indicated by the history and physical examination*
   c. *Standard premedication*

C. Room preparation
1. *Monitoring equipment:* standard
2. *Additional equipment:* regular operating table; the table is turned 90 to 180 degrees. Have an anesthesia circuit extension available.
3. Drugs
   a. *Standard emergency*
   b. *Standard tabletop*
4. *Intravenous fluids:* two 18-gauge IVs, normal saline/lactated Ringer's solution at 4 to 6 mL/kg per hour

D. Perioperative management and anesthetic technique
Use general endotracheal or local anesthesia with sedation; the choice depends on the preferences of the surgeon and the patient, as well as on the acetylsalicylic acid status of the patient
1. *Induction:* routine induction. Use of an oral right-angle endotracheal tube is convenient for the surgeon but is not necessary. If sedation technique is chosen, short-acting agents are best because these procedures are usually minor and patients are usually sent home.
2. *Maintenance:* routine
3. *Emergence:* counsel patients that nose will be packed with bandaging and possibly splinted, so mouth breathing will be necessary upon awakening

E. Postoperative implications
Elevate head of bed. Nasal packing and swallowed blood may contribute to postoperative nausea and vomiting. Mild analgesics after discharge are usually sufficient.

COMMON PROCEDURES

I. LeFort Procedures

◆   ◆   ◆

A. Introduction
Maxillary fractures are grouped by the LeFort system:
- *Type 1:* horizontal fracture separating the teeth and maxillary components from the upper facial structures
- *Type 2 (pyramidal):* triangular fracture across the ethmoid and the nose through the intraorbital rims and extending to the entire maxillary structure
- *Type 3 (craniofacial dysfunction):* essentially, the cranium and face are dissociated. Common coexisting injuries include cerebral contusions, intracranial hemorrhage, and cervical spine trauma. LeFort fractures are frequently associated with skull fractures, zygoma fractures, and

possible intracranial fractures and thus with cerebrospinal fluid rhinorrhea. The usual preoperative diagnosis is facial trauma.

B. Preoperative assessment and patient preparation

The airway is a priority. If the airway cannot be managed, emergency intubation becomes necessary. Avoid blind nasal intubation in patients with cerebrospinal fluid rhinorrhea or other evidence of nasopharyngeal trauma.

1. *Neurologic:* document any neurologic deficit; intracranial trauma may require invasive monitoring
2. *Laboratory tests:* hematocrit and any other tests as indicated by the history and physical examination; type and cross-match for 2 units of packed red blood cells

C. Room preparation

1. *Monitoring equipment:* standard
2. *Additional equipment:* fiberoptic cart
3. Drugs
   a. *Standard emergency*
   b. *Standard tabletop*
4. *Intravenous fluids:* one 18-gauge tube, normal saline/lactated Ringer's solution at 6 to 8 mL/kg per hour

D. Perioperative management and anesthetic technique

1. Use general endotracheal anesthesia
2. *Induction:* fiberoptic laryngoscopy should be performed if there is any doubt about the ease of intubation. Patients with mandibular and maxillary (LeFort 1 and 2) fractures should undergo intubation. Patients with nasal orbital or zygomatic fractures usually are intubated orally. Consider using anode or right-angle endotracheal tubes. A LeFort type 3 fracture is a contraindication for nasal intubation.
3. *Maintenance:* muscle relaxation is usually required. Consider the prophylactic use of anti-emetics for patients with wired jaws.
4. *Position:* supine; check and pad pressure points. Avoid stretching the brachial plexus and limit abduction to 90 degrees. Protect eyes with ophthalmic ointment.
5. *Emergence:* extubation should be performed when the patient is fully awake in the case of difficult airway or wired jaws. A wire cutter should be available at all times. Verify that throat packing has been removed before extubating. Patients with facial or airway swelling and those involved in multiple trauma may need continued postoperative intubation and ventilation.

E. Postoperative implications

1. For airway obstruction, wire cutters must be available
2. Aggressive treatment of nausea and vomiting is important
3. Pain management narcotics: anti-emetics as needed
4. Cerebrospinal fluid leak

J. Uvulopalatopharyngoplasty

◆ ◆ ◆

A. Introduction

Uvulopalatopharyngoplasty is performed primarily for treatment of obstructive sleep apnea. Tonsillectomy is often performed concurrently. Nasopharyngeal airway obstruction is relieved by removing redundant and obstructing tissues of the posterior pharynx.

Inspiratory muscle tone is lost during rapid-eye-movement sleep, resulting in relaxation of the pharyngeal muscles, thus creating airway obstruction. Adults presenting with obstructive sleep apnea are often obese.

B. Preoperative assessment

1. History and physical examination
   a. Cardiac: *hypoxia and hypercapnia may lead to pulmonary hypertension, cor pulmonale, cardiac arrhythmias, and failure of the left side of the heart*
   b. Respiratory: *frequent nocturnal arousals (up to 50 times per hour) are common. Periods of apnea may last up to 2 to 3 minutes. These patients present with a long history of snoring.*
   c. Neurologic: *loss of rapid-eye-movement sleep results in excess daytime somnolence, fatigue, and impaired judgment*
2. *Patient preparation:* medical management includes weight reduction in obese patients, decreasing alcohol consumption, and nasal continuous positive airway pressure
   a. Laboratory tests: *as indicated by the history and physical examination*
      (1) Prothrombin time
      (2) Activated partial thromboplastin time
      (3) Platelet count or bleeding time
      (4) Hemoglobin and hematocrit
   b. *Diagnostic tests*
      (1) Chest radiography
      (2) Electrocardiography
      (3) Pulmonary function tests
   c. Medications: *use minimal preoperative narcotics or sedatives because these patients have heightened sensitivity to them. Anticholinergics are helpful.*

C. Room preparation

1. Standard monitoring equipment
2. Additional equipment—airway adjuncts (expect difficult airway intubation)
   a. *Fiberoptic laryngoscope*
   b. *Multiple different laryngoscope blades*
   c. *Short laryngoscope handle*
   d. *Variously sized oropharyngeal airways*
   e. *Variously sized right-angle endotracheal tubes*
   f. *Laryngeal mask airway*
   g. *Transtracheal jet ventilator*

3. Positioning devices
   a. *Bath blankets to assume "sniffing" position*
   b. *Shoulder roll*
   c. *Foam head rest*
   d. *Padding for extremities*
4. Operating room table—ensure appropriate weight limit
5. Drugs
   a. Intravenous fluids: *0.9% normal saline or lactated Ringer's solution, 10 mL/kg per hour via an 18-gauge intravenous tube*
   b. Blood: *type and screen. Estimated blood loss is usually 50 to 250 mL but may be up to 4 units.*
   c. Tabletop: *rapid sequence induction set-up*
      (1) Induction agent of choice
      (2) Succinylcholine 1.5 mg/kg
      (3) Nondepolarizing muscle relaxant
      (4) Vasopressor of choice
      (5) Fentanyl 1 to 2 μg/kg
      (6) Lidocaine 1 to 1.5 mg/kg

D. Perioperative management and anesthetic technique
   1. Induction
      a. *Awake fiberoptic laryngoscopy and intubation may be indicated*
      b. *Inhalation with maintenance of spontaneous respiration and succinylcholine only after visualization of the larynx*
      c. *Intravenous rapid sequence induction after 3 to 4 minutes of preoxygenation, cricoid pressure, and elevation of the head of the bed*
   2. Maintenance
      a. Inhalation agent: *isoflurane or desflurane*
      b. 50% O_2 *(may require high fractional inspired oxygen)*
      c. Rose position: *supine, shoulder roll, head extension*
      d. *Operating table turned 90 to 180 degrees*
   3. Emergence
      a. *Lidocaine 1 to 1.5 mg/kg before extubation*
      b. *Extubation criteria*
         (1) Is the patient awake, alert, and following verbal commands?
         (2) Adequate muscle relaxant reversal
         (3) Acceptable respiratory mechanics

E. Postoperative implications
   1. Head of the bed is elevated
   2. Humidified oxygen
   3. Hemoglobin and hematocrit if blood loss was excessive
   4. Careful titration of narcotics

K. Ocular Procedures

• • •

OPEN EYE

A. Introduction

Intraocular pressure (IOP) is determined by the balance between production and drainage of aqueous humor and by changes in choroidal blood volume. Resistance to outflow of aqueous humor in the trabecular tissue maintains IOP within physiologic range.

Normal IOP is 12 to 16 mm Hg in the upright posture and increases by 2 to 3 mm Hg in the supine position.

When the globe is open, the IOP is equal to ambient pressure. If the volume of choroid and vitreous should increase while the eye is opened, the vitreous may be lost. Any deformation of the eye by external pressure on the globe will cause an apparent increase in intraocular volume.

B. Preoperative assessment and patient preparation

1. *History and physical examination:* standard—the patient may come in as an emergency with full stomach; ensure no other injuries
2. *Diagnostic and laboratory tests:* complete blood count, electrolytes, glucose, blood urea nitrogen, creatinine, urinalysis, prothrombin time, and partial thromboplastin time
3. Preoperative medication and intravenous therapy
   a. Metoclopramide: *Facilitate gastric emptying and increase tone of cardiac sphincter*
   b. *Antacids and cimetidine reduce the risk of aspiration pneumonitis*
   c. *Atropine or glycopyrrolate reduces oral secretions and may inhibit the oculocardiac reflex*
   d. *Narcotics: avoid—may cause nausea and vomiting*
   e. *Sedatives in preoperative hold area, titrated to effect*
   f. *One peripheral, large-bore (18-gauge) with minimal fluid replacement*

C. Room preparation

1. *Mounting equipment:* standard
2. Pharmacologic agents
   a. *Lidocaine intravenous push*
   b. *Atropine intravenous push*
3. *Position:* supine—table may be turned for the surgeon's access

D. Anesthetic techniques

General anesthesia with endotracheal intubation because of a retrobulbar block causes a transient rise in IOP.

E. Perioperative management

1. Induction
   a. *The goal is to avoid increasing IOP*
   b. *When preoxygenating, avoid pressing face mask onto the eyeball*
   c. *Awake intubation is contraindicated because it may cause coughing and bucking*
   d. *Intravenous lidocaine, 1 mg/kg, may alternate coughing and bucking*

311

  e. Use of succinylcholine in open eye-globe injuries is controversial—many practitioners feel that when succinylcholine has been preceded by pretreatment with a nondepolarizing relaxant and a barbiturate for induction, it is a safe combination for rapid sequence induction in the open eye, full-stomach situation

  f. Induction may be with thiopental plus a large dose of a nondepolarizing muscle relaxant

  g. Use of ketamine is contraindicated—causes moderate increase in IOP and nystagmus or blepharospasm

 2. Maintenance

  a. Inhalation agents cause dose-related decreases in IOP; the degree of IOP reduction is proportional to the depth of anaesthesia

  b. Oculocardiac reflex

   (1) Caused by traction on the extraocular muscles (medial rectus), ocular manipulation, or manual pressure on the globe

   (2) Signs and symptoms are bradycardia and cardiac dysrhythmias

   (3) Treatment is to stop surgical stimulus, administer atropine

  c. If respiratory acidoses is allowed to develop, the IOP may increase

 3. Emergence

  a. The goal is smoothness

  b. Empty the stomach with a nasogastric tube and suction the pharynx while the patient is still paralyzed or deeply anesthetized

  c. Administer an antiemetic, droperidol 1.25 to 2.5 mg IV, 20 to 30 minutes prior to end of surgery

  d. Administer lidocaine, 1 mg/kg, to prevent coughing during emergence

  e. The trachea should be extubated before there is a tendency to cough

F. Postoperative implications

 1. Transport the patient to the recovery room with the head up 10 to 20 degrees to facilitate venous drainage from the eye

 2. The patient can be placed on the side with the operative side up

 3. Shivering and pain can increase IOP and should be prevented

Bibliography

Badrinath SK, Vaszeery A, McCarthy RJ, Ivankovich AD. The effect of different methods of inducing anesthesia on intraocular pressure. *Anesthesiology*. 1986; 65:431–435.

STRABISMUS REPAIR

A. Introduction

Strabismus repairs are performed to correct ocular malalignment. This malalignment may be esotropia (eyes deviate inward) or exotropia (eyes deviate outward). This procedure straightens the eyes cosmetically and allows the patient binocular vision by the lengthening or shortening of individual muscles or pairs of muscles. The specific muscles involved are the horizontal rectus and the oblique muscles.

A forced duction test is performed by the surgeon after induction and intubation by manipulating the sclera of the operative eye in order to aid the surgical plan. An incision is made through the conjuctiva in the area of the muscle to be manipulated. The muscle is then isolated and sewn back farther on the globe if the muscle tension is to be increased. If the muscle tension needs to be decreased, a segment of the muscle is removed.

B. Preoperative assessment

Strabismus repair is the most common ophthalmic surgical procedure performed on children. These children are usually otherwise healthy. There is, however, a higher incidence of strabismus in children with cerebral palsy and myelomeningocele with hydrocephalus. Malignant hyperthermia also is more common with children undergoing strabismus repair.

1. History and physical examination
   a. *A careful family history should be obtained preoperatively, including any history of family problems with anesthesia*
   b. Respiratory: *for patients presenting with signs and symptoms of an acute urinary infection, surgery should be postponed, because these children are at greater risk for laryngospasm and bronchospasm*
2. Patient preparation
   a. Laboratory tests: *as indicated by the history and physical examination. Caffeine and halothane contracture tests may be indicated if the patient is believed to be susceptible to malignant hyperthermia.*
   b. Diagnostic tests: *as indicated by the history and physical examination*
   c. Medications: *Midazolam 0.5 to 0.7 mg/kg orally may be given with 20 to 30 mL of apple juice as a premedication*

C. Room preparation

1. *Monitoring equipment:* standard monitors (noninvasive blood pressure monitoring, electrocardiography, end-tidal carbon dioxide [$EtCO_2$], precordial stethoscope, peripheral nerve stimulations, O_2 analyzer, oxygen saturation [SpO_2], temperature)
2. Additional equipment
   a. *Standard emergency drugs (including lidocaine and atropine)*
   b. *Pediatric standard tabletop*
   c. *Intravenous fluids: 20- or 22-gauge peripheral intravenous tube, normal saline or lactated Ringer's solution at 5 to 10 mL/kg per hour*

D. Perioperative management and anesthetic technique

1. *Induction:* general endotracheal anesthesia is the technique of choice. Nondepolarizing relaxants may be used after the forced duction test is performed by the surgeon. Bradycardia is common owing to the oculocardiac reflex, so atropine is commonly used.
2. *Maintenance:* routine. Watch for signs and symptoms of malignant hyperthermia.
3. *Emergence:* nausea and vomiting are very common.

E. Postoperative implications

Aggressive prophylaxis and treatment of postoperative nausea and vomiting is required. Minimal analgesia is necessary

COMMON PROCEDURES

INTRAOCULAR PROCEDURES

FISTULA FROM ANTERIOR CHAMBER TO SUBCONJUNCTIVAL SPACE. → ↓ IOP

TRABECULECTOMY

A. Introduction

Intraocular procedures may refer to vitrectomy, glaucoma drainage, corneal transplant, and open-eye injury. These procedures involve entry into the vitreous humor. It is crucial to avoid increases in IOP with all intraocular procedures.

The most common of these procedures, a vitrectomy, is performed by making three openings into the vitreous cavity. One of these openings is used to instill balanced salt solution, another is made for insertion of a fiberoptic light. The third opening is made for the insertion of various instruments used to remove abnormal tissue from the vitreous cavity. Frequently a gas bubble is introduced during vitrectomy to tamponade retinal tears.

Patients undergoing intraocular procedures are usually elderly. It is imperative to consider associated conditions in this population. Frequently these patients are diabetic or hypertensive, or they have a history of myocardial infarction.

B. Preoperative assessment

1. History and physical examination

   a. Cardiovascular: *inquire about history of myocardial infarction, hypertension, congestive heart failure, and coronary artery disease, because these are common in this population. Assess for the same. Be aware that mannitol is frequently given prior to or during surgery as ordered by the surgeon. Rapid infusions of large doses of mannitol have been shown to precipitate congestive heart failure, pulmonary edema, hypertension, electrolyte disturbances, and myocardial ischemia. Therefore, it is imperative to have full knowledge of the patient's cardiovascular status. Diabetic patients are at greater risk for silent myocardial ischemia. A preoperative blood sugar test should be performed and repeated intraoperatively.*

   b. Neurologic: *peripheral neuropathies are common in the diabetic patient. If present, special care should be taken in positioning and padding pressure points intraoperatively.*

   c. Renal: *patients on chronic acetazolamide (carbonic anhydrase inhibitor) may have excess loss of HCO_3, Na^+, K^+, and water. They may be prone to acidosis, hyponatremia, and hypokalemia.*

   d. Gastrointestinal: *diabetic patients have delayed gastric emptying and are at greater risk of aspiration*

2. Patient preparation

   a. Laboratory and diagnostic tests: *as indicated from the history and physical examination*

   b. Medications: *midazolam (1 to 2 mg IV) may be given in divided doses as a premedication. Be cautious with sedatives in the elderly population. Also, the anesthesia provider must be aware that ocular drugs applied topically can have systemic effects. These include hypertensions arrhythmias, nausea and vomiting, agitation, excitement, disorientation, seizures, hypotension, and metabolic acidosis.*

C. Room preparation

1. *Monitoring equipment:* standard (noninvasive blood pressure monitoring, electrocardiography, $EtCO_2$, precordial stethoscope, peripheral nerve stimulator, O_2 analyzer, SpO_2, temperature)
2. Additional equipment
    a. *Standard emergency drugs*
    b. *Long breathing circuit (table will be turned)*
    c. *Right-angle endotracheal tubes*
    d. Intravenous fluids: *18-gauge peripheral intravenous tube, normal saline or lactated Ringer's solution at 5 to 10 mL/kg per hour*
    e. *Glucometer (if available) for diabetic patients*
    f. *Foley catheter if mannitol is given*

D. Perioperative management and anesthetic technique

General endotracheal tube anesthesia is appropriate for some patients undergoing these procedures. For other patients, measured anesthesia care may be chosen, with the surgeon or anesthesia provider administering a retrobulbar block. If measured anesthesia care is used, it is important to determine the patient's response to sedatives/narcotics prior to administration of the block. Once the table is turned and the patient draped, it can be difficult to maintain an airway if necessary. Care must be taken to avoid oversedation, however. If oversedated, patients tend to be startled when they arouse and may be confused and move about. A short-acting hypnotic (propofol) may be useful immediately prior to administration of the block. The surgeon does need to have the patient's cooperation during the block, because the surgeon may ask the patient to look from side to side. General endotracheal tube anesthesia is also appropriate.

1. *Induction:* standard intravenous induction. Ketamine is not a drug of choice, because increased IOP is to be avoided. Care must be taken to avoid pressure on the eyes with the mask. Nondepolarizing muscle relaxants are used for intubation and continued throughout the procedure, titrated to patient response. It is imperative the patient does not move during the procedure. All connections in the breathing circuit should be secured.
2. *Maintenance:* continuous intravenous anesthesia is an option. Another option is the use of inhalational agents. N_2O may or may not be used. If used, however, and the surgeon performs a gas-fluid exchange, the N_2O should be discontinued 5 to 10 minutes prior to this exchange. Consider an antiemetic (metoclopramide, droperidol) because of the high incidence of postoperative nausea and vomiting.
3. *Emergence:* smooth emergence and extubation is important. Coughing, bucking, and straining should be avoided to prevent increasing the IOP. Consider deep extubation, although care must be taken not to place pressure on the operative eye with the face mask.

E. Postoperative implications

Again, coughing, straining, and bucking should be avoided. The patient may be positioned prone or to one side (as ordered by the surgeon) for correct positioning of the gas bubble. The patient's

COMMON PROCEDURES

respiratory status should be ensured before turning the patient postoperatively.

L. Orbital Fractures

♦   ♦   ♦

A. Introduction
Surgical access to the orbit may be needed to repair orbital fractures. The orbit may be divided into several compartments, including the peripheral surgical space, subperiosteal space, central surgical space, and sub-Tenon's space. The approach for orbital wall fractures depends on the location and the pathology involved. The common approach to these fractures is the transperiosteal or extraperiosteal approach. A skin incision is made in the desired quadrant just outside the orbital rim. The periosteum is identified and incised and then resected from the wall and orbital margin.

B. Preoperative assessment and patient preparation
1. *History and physical examination:* patients are usually healthy aside from the underlying trauma. Evaluation should focus on any coexisting disease and systemic manifestations of the trauma.
2. *Laboratory tests:* as indicated by the history and physical examination
3. *Diagnostic tests:* as indicated by the history and physical examination
4. *Premedication:* standard

C. Room preparation
1. *Monitoring equipment:* standard
2. *Additional equipment:* regular operating table, which will be turned 90 to 180 degrees; an anesthesia circuit extension must be available
3. Drugs
    a. *Standard emergency*
    b. *Standard tabletop*
4. *Intravenous fluids:* one 18-gauge tube, normal saline/lactated Ringer's solution at 4 to 6 mL/kg per hour

D. Perioperative management and anesthetic technique
1. Use general endotracheal anesthesia
2. *Induction:* standard. An oral right-angle endotracheal tube may be preferred.
3. *Maintenance:* standard, muscle relaxation is not required
4. *Position:* supine; check and pad pressure points. Table is turned 90 degrees; have extension tubes or long tubes for anesthesia circuit. Check the eyes and tape or use ointment (or do both).
5. *Potential complication:* oculocardiac reflex is triggered by pain, direct pressure on the eye, and pulling on the extrinsic muscle of the eye. It has both trigeminal afferent and vagal efferent pathways.

Bradycardia is usual with oculocardiac reflex, although junctional rhythm, atrioventricular block, ventricular premature contractions, ventricular tachycardia, and asystole also occur. To treat, tell the surgeon to stop the stimulus and administer atropine as needed. Lidocaine infiltration near the eye muscles may help to attenuate the reflex, which is self-limiting (i.e., it will tire itself with repeated manipulations).

E. Postoperative implications

1. For nausea and vomiting, begin prophylactic treatment with metoclopramide (10 mg IV), droperidol (0.625 mg IV), or ondansetron (4 mg IV)

2. *Pain management:* parenteral opiates

OBSTETRICS AND GYNECOLOGY

A. Cesarean Section

◆ ◆ ◆

A. Introduction

Cesarean section (C-section) is the surgical removal of a fetus via an abdominal/uterine incision. A low transverse incision is the most common; for an emergency, a rapid vertical midline incision may be used. Indications for a C-section are failure of labor to progress, previous C-section, fetal distress, malpresentation of the fetus or cord, placenta previa, and genital herpes or other local infections.

B. Perioperative assessment

In emergency cases, the time for assessment will be brief. Special attention should be paid to airway assessment, because failed intubation is a major cause of maternal morbidity and mortality.

1. *Cardiac:* full-term pregnancy causes an increase in cardiac output of 30%. Immediately post partum, there is another large increase in cardiac output. There is also, normally, a mild decrease in blood pressure and systemic vascular resistance. Evaluate for pregnancy-induced hypertension.

2. *Respiratory:* pregnancy causes a mild respiratory alkalosis, increased minute volume, and a greatly reduced functional residual capacity. Also, upper-airway edema and increased blood volumes make nasal intubation virtually contraindicated.

3. *Gastrointestinal:* all pregnant patients past 16 weeks of gestation are considered to be on a full stomach

4. *Other:* evaluate for a history of gestational diabetes, HELLP syndrome (hemolysis, elevated liver enzymes, low platelet count), placenta previa, seizures, and non–pregnancy-related illnesses and surgeries

C. Patient preparation

1. A nonparticular antacid (such as sodium citrate, 30 mL) is routinely administered at most institutions, regardless of the anesthetic technique chosen. Sedation is best avoided. Benzodiazapines have been implicated as possible teratogens, and it is best to avoid maternal amnesia during childbirth.

2. Laboratory tests should include a type and screen, complete blood count, electrolytes, blood urea nitrogen, creatinine, glucose, prothrombin time, and partial thromboplastin time. In emergency C-sections, there may not be time to complete these tests.

D. Room preparation

1. *Monitoring:* standard. If there is a history of pregnancy-induced hypertension, an arterial line is recommended. If there is severe pre-

eclampsia, a central line is also recommended, with a pulmonary catheter in cases of hemodynamic instability.

2. *Positioning:* supine with left lateral uterine displacement. This is accomplished by placing a wedge under the right hip. Failure to use left lateral uterine displacement can result in aortocaval compression.

3. *Drugs and tabletop:* tabletop should be set up for a general anesthetic. Set out a smaller endotracheal tube as well (because of the airway edema). Have ephedrine and oxytocin drawn up. Have difficult airway equipment available. Some practitioners have a short "stubby" handled laryngoscope. Unless there is maternal hypoglycemia, avoid giving intravenous solutions with glucose because they may lead to neonatal hypoglycemia.

E. **Perioperative management and anesthetic techniques**

Always be ready for general anesthesia. Thiopental/succinylcholine is the most common combination for induction. Ketamine is a useful adjunct in cases of instability or bleeding. Volatile agents can be used and then substituted with narcotics after the fetus is delivered. Begin at a 0.5 maximum allowable concentration because requirements for obstetrics are typically 30% to 50% reduced. Avoid hypotension because uterine flow is pressure-dependent. Extubation is always performed awake because the danger of aspiration will be high. Regional anesthesia is the most common technique used on C-section patients. For spinal anesthesia, 0.75% bupivicaine, 11 to 12 mg, is usually enough to provide a dense block to T4. Volume loading should be accomplished before performing a spinal block. Ephedrine is also commonly needed in addition to volume. Epidural is also an attractive regional anesthetic, especially if the parturient has a catheter in place for laboring. "Topping up" the epidural along with narcotic and perhaps ketamine just prior to delivery are two techniques. If the patient is in danger of losing consciousness or reflexes, the airway must be protected and general anesthesia induced.

F. **Postoperative considerations**

For pain relief, narcotics may be administered parenterally, with patient-controlled analgesia, orally when tolerated, or intrathecally/epidurally if a catheter is in place. Nausea and vomiting are common in the immediate postpartum period.

B. Gynecologic Laparoscopy

◆ ◆ ◆

A. **Introduction**

Laparoscopy is a common endoscopic technique in gynecologic procedures. It is frequently used to diagnose or treat pelvic etiologies that may include sterilization, adhesions, pain, endometriosis, ectopic pregnancies, ovarian cysts and tumors, infertility, and vaginal hysterectomy. A pneumoperitoneum is achieved by insertion of a trocar and insufflation of CO_2.

B. Preoperative assessment and patient preparation

1. History and physical examination

   a. Cardiac: *assess for pre-existing disorders. Dysrhythmias and alterations in cardiac output may occur with insufflation of CO_2.*

   b. Respiratory: *assess for pre/co-existing diseases. Hypercarbia, increased airway pressures, and pneumothorax are potential complications of a pneumoperitoneum.*

   c. Gastrointestinal: *increased nausea and vomiting are associated with these procedures*

2. Patient preparation

   a. Laboratory tests: *complete blood count and other tests as indicated*

   → b. Diagnostic tests: *pregnancy testing and as indicated*

   c. Preoperating medications: *urgent procedures should be treated as a full stomach. Consider nonparticulate antacid, metoclopramide (10 mg), and ranitidine (50 mg).*

   d. Intravenous therapy: *one or two 16- to 18-gauge intravenous tubes*

C. Room preparation

1. *Monitoring equipment:* standard. Consider an arterial line and urinary catheter, if indicated.

2. *Additional equipment:* fluid warmer and Bair-Hugger

3. Drugs

   a. Miscellaneous pharmacologic agents: *opioid, nondepolarizing muscle relaxants, and antibiotic*

   b. Intravenous fluids: *Depend on the procedure performed; calculate as indicated. Estimated blood loss is less than 50 mL to 1000 mL.*

   c. Blood: *type and screen*

   d. *Tabletop: standard*

D. Perioperative management and anesthetic technique

1. General anesthesia is preferred

2. *Induction:* standard induction, as indicated

3. *Maintenance:* inhalational agent/O_2/opioid and nondepolarizing agent as indicated. Consider droperidol (1 mg) and metoclopramide (10 mg). *Position:* lithotomy. Trendelenburg to improve pelvic exposure.

4. *Emergence:* standard emergence

E. Postoperative implications

Complications include nausea and vomiting, anemia

C. Hysterectomy—Vaginal or Total Abdominal

◆　◆　◆

A. Introduction

Hysterectomy is commonly performed to treat uncontrolled uterine bleeding, dysmenorrhea, uterine myoma, gynecologic cancer, adhesions, endometriosis, and pelvic relaxation syndrome. Frequently laparoscopy is utilized; for ovarian cancer prophylaxis, a bilateral salpingo-oophorectomy may be performed as well.

B. Preoperative assessment
1. History and physical examination
   a. Cardiac: *assess volume status; hypovolemia secondary to bleeding may be present*
   b. Respiratory: *assess for pre/co-existing disease*
   c. Renal: *electrolyte imbalance due to a bowel preparation is possible*
2. Patient preparation
   a. Laboratory tests: *complete blood count, electrolytes, blood urea nitrogen, creatinine, prothrombin time, partial thromboplastin time*
   b. Diagnostic tests: *chest radiography and arterial blood gases*
   c. Preoperative medications: *anxiolytics as indicated. Consider metoclopramide (10 mg) and droperidol (1 to 2.5 mg IV) for prophylaxis of nausea and vomiting.*
   d. Intravenous therapy: *two 16- to 18-gauge intravenous tubes; consider central line*

C. Room preparation
1. *Monitoring equipment:* standard with urinary catheter; consider an arterial line and central venous pressure catheter
2. *Additional equipment:* fluid warmer and Bair-Hugger
3. Drugs
   a. Miscellaneous pharmacologic agents: *opioid, anxiolytic, nondepolarizing muscle relaxant, local anesthetic, and antibiotic*
   b. Intravenous fluids: *vaginal; calculate for moderate blood loss, crystalloids at 4 to 6 mL/kg per hour. Estimated blood loss is 750 to 1000 mL. Abdominal; calculate for a moderate to large blood loss, crystalloids at 6 to 10 mL/kg per hour. Estimated blood loss is 1000 to 1500 mL.*
   c. Blood: *type and cross-match for 2 to 4 units of packed red blood cells*
   d. Tabletop: *standard*

D. Perioperative management and anesthetic technique
1. General or regional anesthesia; subarachnoid block or epidural with a sensory level of anesthesia of T6–T8
2. *Induction:* standard. Choice as indicated.
3. *Maintenance:* general anesthesia; inhalational agent/O_2/opioid/anxiolytic and nondepolarizing muscle relaxant. Regional; local anesthetic of choice, supplemental anxiolytic and sedation. *Position:* abdominal—supine. Vaginal—lithotomy.
4. *Emergence:* standard

E. Postoperative implications
1. *Complications:* nausea and vomiting, anemia
2. *Pain management:* patient-controlled anesthesia or epidural opiates

D. Loop Electrosurgical Excision Procedure

◆ ◆ ◆

A. **Introduction**

Loop electrosurgical excision procedure (LEEP) is performed for the diagnosis and treatment of cervical intraepithelial neoplasia. This form of electrosurgery utilizes a loop electrode for excision and fulguration to prevent cervical bleeding. Other types of therapy that may be used to ablate cervical lesions are cryosurgery and CO_2 laser surgery.

B. **Preoperative assessment and patient preparation**

1. *History and physical examination:* this procedure is generally done on young, healthy patients and is occasionally performed during pregnancy. Assessment should be thorough.
   a. Cardiac: *assess for pre-existing disease*
   b. Respiratory: *assess for history of smoking or other lung diseases*
   c. Neurologic: *assess for pre/co-existing diseases, evaluate, and document*
2. Patient preparation
   a. Laboratory tests: *pregnancy test, hemoglobin and hematocrit, urinalysis*
   b. Preoperative medications: *anxiolytics may be utilized if the patient is not pregnant*
   c. Intravenous therapy: *one 18-gauge intravenous tube*

C. **Room preparation**

1. *Monitoring equipment:* standard. If pregnancy is over 16 weeks, fetal monitoring may be utilized.
2. *Drugs:* standard tabletop
3. *Intravenous fluids:* calculate for minimal blood loss, 2 to 4 mL/kg per hour. Estimated blood loss is 50 to 200 mL.

D. **Perioperative management and anesthetic techniques**

1. Local, monitored anesthesia care, or regional or general anesthesia.
2. *Induction:* standard induction is indicated. In pregnant patients a rapid sequence induction is used, utilizing fentanyl 2 to 3 μg/kg, succinylcholine 1 mg/kg, or vecuronium 0.1 mg/kg. In nonpregnant patients, mask ventilation may be appropriate.
3. *Maintenance:* standard maintenance, inhalational agent/O_2/opioid. Muscle relaxation is not required. *Position:* lithotomy.
4. *Emergence:* standard

E. **Postoperative implications**

1. *Complications:* peroneal nerve injury due to the lithotomy position, nausea and vomiting, bleeding, postdural headache, and premature labor
2. *Pain management:* oral analgesics if the patient is not pregnant

E. In Vitro Fertilization

❖ ❖ ❖

A. Introduction
Laparoscopic in vitro fertilization and embryo transfer are frequently performed for the treatment of infertility. This outpatient procedure is indicated for the treatment of tubal disease, endometriosis, and idiopathic infertility.

B. Preoperative assessment and patient preparation
1. *History and physical examination:* this procedure is frequently performed on healthy patients. Assessment should be thorough.
2. Patient preparation
   a. Laboratory tests: *hemoglobin and hematocrit, other tests as indicated*
   b. Intravenous therapy: *one 18-gauge intravenous tube*

C. Room preparation
1. *Monitoring equipment:* standard
2. *Additional equipment:* no special considerations
3. Drugs
   a. Miscellaneous pharmacologic agents: *opioid, short acting nondepolarizing muscle relaxant, anesthetic agent*
   b. Intravenous fluids: *calculate for minimal blood loss, crystalloids at 2 mL/kg per hour. Estimated blood loss is less than 50 mL.*
   c. Blood: *no special considerations*
   d. Tabletop: *standard*

D. Perioperative management and anesthetic techniques
1. General anesthesia is most common and preferred. Local, regional, subarachnoid block, or epidural techniques can be utilized.
2. *Induction:* standard induction, as indicated. Outpatient procedure is a consideration
3. *Maintenance:* standard maintenance, inhalation agent/O_2/opioid. Consider complications of pneumoperitoneum (i.e., hypercapnia, hypoxia, pneumothorax, ventilation-perfusion mismatch, increased inspiratory pressures, dysrhythmias, altered cardiac output, and hemorrhage). *Position:* supine with Trendelenburg.
4. *Emergence:* standard

E. Postoperative implications
Complications include abdominal and referred shoulder discomfort

F. Pelvic Exenteration

❖ ❖ ❖

A. Introduction
Pelvic examination is a procedure that is performed for the treatment of advanced, recurrent, radioresistant cervical carcinoma. It is

considered a radical surgical approach because all pelvic tissues, including the cervix, bladder, lymph nodes, rectum, uterus, and vagina, are resected. Vaginal reconstruction and appropriate colon and urinary diversions are also performed.

B. Preoperative assessment and patient preparation

1. History and physical examination
   a. Cardiac: *underlying cardiac history, including treatment of cardiotoxic chemotherapy, should be assessed*
   b. Respiratory: *assess for history of smoking or other lung diseases*
   c. Neurologic: *assess for pre/co-existing diseases, evaluate, and document*
   d. Renal: *assess for and correct any electrolyte abnormality*
   e. Gastrointestinal: *bowel preparation and decompression is instituted; evaluate for appropriate hydrations*
   f. Endocrine: *assess for pre/co-existing disease and steroid therapy*
2. Patient preparation
   a. Laboratory tests: *complete blood count, electrolytes, blood urea nitrogen, creatinine, calcium, magnesium, phosphate, prothrombin time, partial thromboplastin time, urinalysis, and renal function tests*
   b. Diagnostic tests: *chest radiography, arterial blood gases, pulmonary function tests, echocardiography, electrocardiography, computed tomography of the pelvis, other tests as indicated by the history and physical examination*
   c. Premedication: *anxiolytics as indicated*
   d. Intravenous therapy: *two 14- to 16-gauge intravenous tubes, central line; consider a pulmonary arterial catheter*

C. Room preparation

1. *Monitoring equipment:* standard with urinalysis catheter, arterial line, central venous pressure and pulmonary arterial catheters
2. *Additional equipment:* fluid warmer and Bair Hugger
3. *Drugs:* standard
4. *Miscellaneous pharmacologic agents:* opioid, anxiolytic, nondepolarizing muscle relaxant, local anesthetic, and antibiotic
5. *Intravenous fluids:* calculate for major blood loss, 10 to 15 mg/kg per hour. Estimated blood loss is 1000 to 4000 mL.

D. Perioperative management and anesthetic technique

1. General anesthesia with epidural
2. *Induction:* standard, as indicated
3. *Maintenance:* inhalational agent/O_2/opioid. Consider local anesthetic via an epidural catheter. Use long-acting nondepolarizing muscle relaxants. Maintain normocarbia, mean arterial pressure of 60 to 88 mm Hg, pulmonary capillary wedge pressure of less than 20 mm Hg, urinary output at 0.5 to 1 mL/kg per hour; transfuse for a hematocrit over 30%. *Position:* both lithotomy and supine positions are used throughout the procedure.
4. *Emergence:* the patient generally is transported to the intensive care unit for 2 to 3 days; postoperative ventilation may be necessary. If the patient is hemodynamically stable, extubation may be considered.

E. Postoperative implications
1. *Complications:* bleeding, fluid maintenance due to large fluid shifts and mobilizations, and peroneal nerve damage due to the lithotomy position
2. *Pain management:* epidural, opiates, or both

G. Gynecologic Lymph Node Biopsy

◆ ◆ ◆

A. Introduction
Laparotomy is performed for diagnosing and treating suspected gynecologic malignancies. The abdominopelvic and peritoneal cavities are explored, the pelvic and para-aortic lymph nodes are dissected, and cytologic washings and tissue samples are obtained. The specimens are sent to the pathology department for inspection, diagnosis, and accurate staging, if malignant. Specific and individualized surgical intervention is then performed. Surgical procedures include tumor debulking, unilateral or bilateral salpingo-oophorectomy, hysterectomy, and pelvic exenteration.

B. Preoperative assessment and patient preparation
1. History and physical examination
   a. Cardiac: *assess for pre-existing disease and evaluate as indicated*
   b. Respiratory: *assess for pre-existing disease and evaluate as indicated*
   c. Neurologic: *assess for pre-existing disease and document*
   d. Renal: *correct any fluid and electrolyte abnormalities*
   e. Gastrointestinal: *assess for abdominal distention; bowel preparation is required*
2. Patient preparation
   a. Laboratory tests: *complete blood count, electrolytes, blood urea nitrogen, creatinine, prothrombin time, partial thromboplastin time, urinalysis*
   b. Diagnostic tests: *chest radiography, electrocardiography, computed tomography of the abdomen and pelvis*
   c. Medications: *evaluate previous medications, chemotherapy, and other cardiotoxic agents that may have been given. Preoperatively administer anxiolytics as indicated.*
   d. Intravenous therapy: *two 14- to 16-gauge intravenous tubes; consider a central line*

C. Room preparation
1. *Monitoring equipment:* standard with urinalysis catheter; consider an arterial line and a central venous pressure catheter
2. *Additional equipment:* nasogastric tube, fluid warmer, Bair Hugger

3. Drugs
   a. Miscellaneous pharmacologic agents: *opioid, anxiolytic, nondepolarizing muscle relaxant, local anesthetic, and antibiotic*
   b. Intravenous fluids: *calculate for major blood loss, crystalloids at 6 to 8 mL/kg per hour. Estimated blood loss is 250 to 1500 mL.*
   c. Blood: *type and cross-match for 2 to 4 units of packed red blood cells*
   d. Tabletop: *standard*

D. Perioperative management and anesthetic technique
   1. General anesthesia with epidural
   2. *Induction:* standard, as indicated
   3. *Maintenance:* inhalational agent/O_2/nondepolarizing muscle relaxants. *Position:* supine.
   4. *Emergence:* standard with extubation unless the patient is hemodynamically unstable

E. Postoperative implications
   1. *Complications:* bleeding, fluid maintenance due to large fluid shifts and mobilizations
   2. *Pain management:* epidural or patient-controlled anesthesia

SECTION XI

PEDIATRICS
A. Myringotomy

* * *

A. Introduction

Myringotomy is a common outpatient procedure in children. Myringotomy is usually associated with the insertion of ventilation tubes into the tympanic membrane as a treatment for recurrent otitis media. Typically, a small incision is made with use of a microscope in the tympanic membrane, and fluid is suctioned via a transcanal approach.

B. Preoperative assessment

Other than a history of frequent and recurrent otitis media, this patient population is generally healthy.

1. History and physical examination
   a. *A careful family history should be obtained preoperatively, including any history of family problems with anesthesia*
   b. Respiratory: *many pediatric patients presenting for myringotomy have a history of frequent upper-respiratory-tract infections. If currently exhibiting signs and symptoms of upper-respiratory-tract infections, these children are at greater risk for laryngospasm intraoperatively and postoperatively. Because this procedure is elective, it is commonly recommended to postpone the procedure until the signs and symptoms of upper respiratory tract infections have subsided.*
   c. Dental: *inspection of the airway and questioning of the parents should identify any loose teeth*
2. Patient preparation
   a. Laboratory tests: *as indicated from the history and physical examination*
   b. Diagnostic tests: *as indicated from the history and physical examination*
   c. Medications: *midazolam 0.2 to 0.3 mg/kg orally may be given with 20 to 30 mL of apple juice as a premedication*

C. Room preparation

1. *Monitoring equipment:* standard
2. Additional equipment—none
3. Standard emergency drugs (including atropine, lidocaine, and succinylcholine)
4. Pediatric standard tabletop
5. Intravenous fluids: *depending on the age of patient, expected length of procedure, and history and physical findings, an intravenous tube may be available for emergency use but is not started routinely. If necessary, use*

a 20- or 22-gauge peripheral tube, normal saline or lactated Ringer's solution at 2 to 4 mL/kg per hour.

D. Perioperative management and anesthetic techniques

1. Mask general anesthesia is usually adequate for uncomplicated myringotomy of otherwise healthy patients
2. *Induction:* mask inhalation induction with halothane, N_2O, and O_2. If an existing intravenous tube is present, routine intravenous induction is appropriate. Routine intravenous induction is preferred with older children and adults.
3. *Maintenance:* standard maintenance with halothane, N_2O, and O_2. No need for muscle relaxation, and opiates are not routinely used. If the patient is an adult, isoflurane or desflurane would be preferred to halothane.
4. *Emergence:* airway is maintained until the patient is fully awake. In older children and adults, antiemetics should be considered.

E. Postoperative implications

Nausea and vomiting can be treated with metoclopramide, droperidol, or ondansetron. Note that these patients are often sensitive to sounds in the immediate postoperative period.

B. Pediatric Intra-Abdominal Procedures

❖ ❖ ❖

A. Introduction

Abdominal procedures may be indicated for a variety of reasons: pyloric stenosis, necrotizing enterocolitis, omphalocele, gastroschisis, megacolon, biliary atresia, intestinal atresia, incarcerated hernia, malrotation and volvulus, imperforate anus, and exstrophy of the cloaca or bladder.

B. Preoperative assessment and patient preparation

1. History and physical examination
   a. Cardiac: *other anomalies (patent ductus arteriosis, ventricular septal defect) may lead to congestive heart failure or murmur. The patient may have a labile blood pressure and hypovolemia from dehydration.*
   b. Respiratory: *premature infants may have immature respiratory centers and apneic/bradycardic episodes from hypoxemia. Respiratory compromise is possible with a large abdominal mass.*
   c. Neurologic: *premature infants may be prone to seizure disorders, myelomeningocele, hydrocephalus; hypoxemia may predispose to intracranial hemorrhage*
   d. Renal: *Wilms' tumor may lead to hematuria and other genito-urinary anomalies*

    e. Gastrointestinal: *the patient may have esophageal/gastric reflux,*
       jaundice, anemia from hepatic disease, diarrhea with malabsorption
       states, a colostomy, bowel preparation, intestinal compression
    f. Endocrine: *hypochloremia and hypokalemia, metabolic alkalosis from*
       vomiting, and neuroblastomas are associated with increased
       catecholamine production
  2. Patient preparation
    a. Laboratory tests: *vary with pathology, procedure, and the history and*
       physical examination—hemoglobin and hematocrit, type and cross-
       match, electrolytes, glucose, liver function tests, prothrombin time,
       partial thromboplastin time
    b. Premedication: *midazolam 0.2 to 0.5 mg/kg orally if at least 1 year*
       old, 30 minutes prior to procedure
C. Room preparation
  1. *Monitoring equipment:* standard; depending on procedure and health
     status, consider an arterial line, central venous pressure catheter,
     pulmonary arterial catheter, Foley catheter, peripheral nerve
     stimulation
  2. *Additional equipment:* heated humidified circuit, heating pad, hot
     lamps, fluid warmers
  3. *Position:* supine
  4. *Fluids:* therapy to address fluid deficit, maintenance, third-space loss,
     and blood loss. Insensible losses may be elevated because of
     phototherapy light or radiant heaters.
    a. *Deficit volume is calculated by multiplying the number of hours since*
       the last fluid intake by hourly maintenance
    b. *Maintenance is calculated by 4 mL/kg per hour for 0 to 10 kg;*
       40 mL/kg per hour plus 2 mL/kg per hour for every kilogram above
       10 for those weighing 10 to 20 kg; 60 mL/kg per hour plus 1 mL/kg
       per hour for every kilogram over 20 kg for those weighing more than
       20 kg
    c. *Third-space loss depends on the site and extent of surgery. Replace*
       with isotonic solutions. For peripheral/superficial: 1 to 3 mL/kg per
       hour. For abdominal/chest/hip: 3 to 4 mL/kg per hour. For
       extensive intra-abdominal: 6 to 10 mL/kg per hour.
    d. *Replace blood when hematocrit is <30% and hemoglobin is <10 g/dL*
D. Perioperative management and anesthetic technique
  1. General anesthesia
  2. *Induction:* decompress the stomach prior to induction. Preoxygenate
     for 2 to 3 minutes. Administer atropine 0.02 mg/kg prior to
     laryngoscopy. Use rapid sequence or awake intubation. Upper-
     extremity intravenous intubation is preferred for inferior vena cava
     compression potential. The endotracheal tube should lead at 20 to
     30 cm H_2O.
  3. *Maintenance:* volatile inhalation agents. Avoid nitrous oxide
     because it distends the bowel. Decreases in central venous pressure
     of 4 mm H_2O or more are associated with vena cava compression.
     Use long- or intermediate-acting muscle relaxants. Use narcotic
     generously, fentanyl 5 to 25 μg/kg per hour, depending on whether
     postoperative ventilation is planned. Keep the oxygen saturation

(SpO$_2$) at 95% to 97%. Avoid hypovolemia. The surgeon may infiltrate the site with local anesthetic prior to closure. Note positive inspiratory pressure (PIP) prior to abdominal closure.
   4. *Emergence:* neostigmine 70 μg/kg and atropine 0.02 mg/kg if postoperative ventilation is not desired. Suction the stomach prior to extubation. Extubate awake.
E. Postoperative implications
   1. Postoperative ventilation may be needed
   2. Residual anesthesia can contribute to postoperative apnea
   3. Peristalsis is usually delayed; may need total parenteral nutrition
   4. Sepsis
   5. Abdominal third-space loss can continue immediately postoperatively—increase the intra-abdominal pressure, bowel ischemia, decrease renal perfusion

C. Congenital Diaphragmatic Hernia

❖   ❖   ❖

A. Introduction
   This condition results from abdominal viscera herniating into the chest through a defect in the diaphragm; the left side is affected more frequently. It occurs in 1 of 2000 to 1 of 3000 neonates; half are stillborn or die immediately. Stillborn babies have a 95% incidence of other anomalies. Live births have a 20% incidence of anomalies (patent ductus arteriosis is common). Herniated abdominal contents occupy the thoracic cavity and compromise lung development, leading to hypoplasia and mediastinal shift. The contralateral lung also has decreased amounts of alveoli. Symptoms usually are present after birth (dyspnea, cyanosis, dextrocardia, bowel sounds in the chest, bulging chest, decreased breath sounds). Infants may have to be intubated after delivery and placed in the neonatal intensive care unit.
B. Preoperative assessment and patient preparation
   1. History and physical examination
      a. Cardiac: *check for other anomalies (patent ductus arteriosis). Mediastinal shift may compress the great vessels.*
      b. Respiratory: *pulmonary shunting and right-to-left shunting. Pneumothorax of the contralateral lung may occur from high positive inspiratory pressure (PIP). Check serial arterial blood gases, EtCO$_2$, oxygen saturation (SpO$_2$), chest radiographs, ventilator setting. Adequate ventilation may correct acidosis.*
      c. Neurologic: *infants may be paralyzed while intubated in the neonatal intensive care unit. Severe hypoxia can lead to neurologic damage.*

d. Renal: *peripheral perfusion may be increased by dopamine or inotropes*

e. Gastrointestinal: *a nasogastric tube should be placed for intermittent suction to prevent further distention and pulmonary compression*

2. Patient preparation

a. Laboratory tests: *arterial blood gases, complete blood count, electrolytes*

b. Diagnostic tests: *chest radiography with bowel-gas pattern and mediastinal shift*

C. Room preparation

1. *Monitoring equipment:* standard. The internal jugular vein can be used for the central venous pressure catheter. Contralateral side precordial to monitor pneumothorax. Venous access in the lower extremities is not recommended because of possible vena cava compression.

2. *Additional equipment:* all warming devices to prevent hypothermia, which increases oxygen consumption and desaturation

3. *Position:* supine. Abdominal incision is usual, but the transthoracic or thoracoabdominal approach may be used.

D. Perioperative management and anesthetic technique

1. General anesthesia

2. *Induction:* rapid sequence or awake intubation

3. *Maintenance:* need a high oxygen concentration. Avoid nitrous oxide because it can diffuse across the viscera and increase lung compression. High-dose narcotics with low concentrations of volatile anesthetics may be used. High ventilation rates are used for adequate oxygenation. High pressure may increase the incidence of pneumothorax. Perform frequent arterial blood gases, keep the arterial carbon dioxide pressure at 25 to 30 mm Hg. With sudden hemodynamic compromise, suspect contralateral pneumothorax and place a chest tube.

4. *Emergence:* infants usually remain intubated, paralyzed, and ventilated in the neonatal intensive care unit

E. Postoperative implications

1. Depend on the severity of pulmonary hypertension and hypoplasia. Some infants show a "honeymoon" period followed by deterioration with right-to-left shunting, hypoxia, hypercapnia, acidosis, pulmonary hypertension, and death.

2. High-frequency oscillation may be used to reduce pulmonary arterial pressure

3. Patent ductus arteriosis may be ligated

4. The infant may need extracorporeal membrane oxygenation. The internal jugular vein may be cannulated with one venovenous cannula, or the internal jugular and common carotid may be cannulated with two venoarterial cannulas. The infant is kept paralyzed.

5. Prostaglandins may be used to decrease pulmonary vascular resistance

COMMON PROCEDURES

6. Tolazoline (Priscoline) relaxes vascular smooth muscle with alpha-adrenergic blockade
7. Intravenous medication can be used for hemodynamic support

D. Pediatric Herniorrhaphies

• • •

A. Introduction

Inguinal repair is the most common procedure performed in children. Premature infants are more likely to have incarcerations, mostly because of failure of the processus vaginalis to obliterate. The procedure is performed through an inguinal crease incision. Complications of hernia repairs are rare. Umbilical hernias are more common in blacks and may close spontaneously (95% to 98% by age 5). Repair is performed through a transverse infra-umbilical incision. Intraperitoneal exploration is rarely done.

B. Preoperative assessment

1. History and physical examination
   a. Cardiac: *routine*
   b. Respiratory: *prolonged ventilation and immature lungs are more susceptible to tracheomalacia, subglottic stenosis, and bronchopulmonary dysplasia*
   c. Neurologic: *premature infants may display transient apneic and bradycardic episodes in response to hypoxemia. Premature infants are more prone to seizure disorders. Complications from general anesthesia may occur from effects on the immature central nervous system.*
   d. Renal: *routine*
   e. Gastrointestinal: *the patient may have abdominal compression if the umbilical hernia is large. Consider rapid sequence induction for incarcerated hernia and bowel obstructions.*
   f. Endocrine: *premature infants are more prone to hypoglycemia. Check the blood glucose level.*
2. Patient preparation
   a. Laboratory tests: *as indicated from the history and physical examination*
   b. Diagnostic tests: *none*
   c. Medications: *midazolam 0.2 to 0.5 mg/kg orally 30 minutes before surgery for children over 1 year of age*

C. Room preparation

1. *Monitoring equipment:* standard
2. *Additional equipment:* use pediatric circle or bain circuit. Warm and humidify gases. Warming pad may be used on the table.
3. *Position:* supine
4. *Fluids:* 0.9 normal saline or lactated Ringer's solution at 4 mL/kg per hour for 1 to 10 kg of weight. Add 2 mL/kg per hour for 11

to 20 kg. Dextrose solutions may be used for infants less than 1 month old.

5. *Blood:* negligible loss

D. Perioperative management and anesthetic technique

1. General anesthesia, mask or endotracheal tube. Caudal block may be performed after induction for postoperative pain.

2. *Induction:* mask with halothane/oxygen/nitrous. Obtain IV after induction. Atropine (0.02 mg/kg IV) prior to laryngoscopy. Vecuronium 0.1 mg/kg or atracurium 0.4 mg/kg. If the child is healthy and more than 1 year old, the mask may be used. If applicable, caudal block with bupivacaine 0.25% with epinephrine 1:200,000, 1 mL/kg after induction (onset of 15 minutes).

3. *Maintenance:* caudal block will decrease the amount of volatile agent. Increase the maximum allowable concentration prior to incision to avoid laryngospasm.

4. *Emergence:* extubate fully awake. Intravenous reversal, neostigmine 0.07 mg/kg and atropine 0.02 mg/kg.

E. Postoperative complications

Postoperative apnea can occur in infants at 50 to 60 weeks of gestational age, especially if premature.

COMMON PROCEDURES

E. Pediatric Anesthesia Care Plan

Name:
Diagnosis:
Allergies:
Med/Surg Hx:

Sex: M F Age: Wt (kg)
Procedure:
Meds:

Anesthesia Complications: Y N

Labs:

Hgb ⟨ WBC
Hct

Na ⟨ Cl ⟨ BUN ⟨ PT
K ⟨ CO$_2$ ⟨ Cr ⟨ BS ⟨ PTT
Plt

FLUIDS

A. Maintenance:

1st 10 kg [4mL/kg per h] ____
2nd 10 kg [2mL/kg per h] ____
> 20 kg [1mL/kg per h] ____
• Total maintenance: [____]

B. NPO Deficit: [Maintenance x NPO°] [____]

C. Surgical Loss: [mL/kg per h] [____]

Incision: • Min 3–5 mL/kg per h • Mod 5–10 mL/kg per h
• Large 8–20 mL/kg per h

TOTAL [____]

IVF [LR or D5 .45%]	1st h	2nd h	3rd h	4th h	5th h

Est Blood Vol (Premie 90 mL/kg • 0–2 y/o 85 mL/kg • 2–16 y/o 80 mL/kg) **Accept Blood Loss** = EBV x (Actual Hct–low Hct/Actual Hct)

Replacement: **Whole Blood** (5 mL/kg ↑Hgb by 1 g • **RBC's** (3 mL/kg ↑Hgb by 1 g) • **Albumin 5%** (10 mL/kg)

AIRWAY

Blade: _____ [Miller 0: preterm & neonate • Miller 1: neonate –age 2 • Miller 1.5: age 2–5 • then Miller 2]

Tubes: _____ [Tube size = (age/4) + or (age + 16)/4]

Length: _____ cm [Length to Lip = (age/2 + 12)]

FGF: _____ L/m (MV x 2.5) MV = RR X TV (TV = 6 mL/kg) Minimal 5 L/m for all children

Circuit: ◊ Newborn JR 0.5 L ◊ 1–3 y/o JR 1.0 L ◊ 3–5 y/o Circle 2.0 L ◊ >5 y/o Circle 3.0 L
(JR = Jackson-Reese)

334

Drugs & Dosages

Drug	IV mg/kg	IM mg/kg	PO mg/kg	Nasal mg/kg
Succinyl ↓1 y/o	1–2	2–4		
Succinyl ↑1 y/o	1–1.5	2–4		
Atropine	.01	.02		
Robinul	.005–.006			
Pentothal	4–6			
Brevitol		7.7		
Ketamine	1–2	3–6	6	3
Versed		.08–.5	.5–.75	.2–.5
Tylenol			10–15	
Fentanyl	.001–.002			
Morphine	.2	.1–.2		
Demerol	.5–2	1–2		
Tracrium	.5			
Pavulon	.05–.1			
Neostigmine	.03–.07			
Edrophonium	.5–.75			
Narcan	.01			
Epinephrine	.01			
Lidocaine	1–1.5			
Na Bicarb	1–2 mEq			
Ca Chloride	20			

Endotracheal Drugs [ALIEN]: Atropine, Lidocaine, Isoproterenol, Epinephrine, Naloxone • Defibrillation 2–4 J/kg • Cardioversion 0.5–1 J/kg

Developed by Ronald Manningham

COMMON PROCEDURES

MISCELLANEOUS
A. Burns

♦ ♦ ♦

A. Introduction

Patients who sustain full-thickness burns are seen in the operating room, probably repeatedly, for debridement and grafting. The initial assessment of the emergency burn patient is begun as for any trauma patient and begins with airway intubation. Keep in mind that airway edema happens rapidly in a burn patient, and intubation after the edema occurs is difficult. Burn patients must be aggressively fluid-resuscitated in the first 48 hours.

B. Preoperative assessment

1. *Cardiac:* assess for any pre-existing cardiac problems. In the acutely burned patient, there is a large increase in circulating catecholamines, which will manifest as tachycardia and possibly as increased blood pressure.

2. *Respiratory:* intubate the patient if there are any signs of upper-airway burn. This could include oral burns, cough productive of soot, and stridor. Assess arterial blood gases with a carboxyhemoglobin level. Intubate with controlled ventilation. Burn patients are also prone to adult respiratory distress syndrome. They may need higher minute ventilation and increasing amounts of positive end-expiratory pressure. Assess neck mobility; there may be sufficient edema or scar formation to cause an unexpected difficult intubation.

3. *Neurologic:* assess and document preoperative neurologic function as accurately as possible

4. *Renal:* relative hypovolemia from increased permeability causes renal hypoperfusion. Also, cellular debris can cause acute renal failure.

5. *Gastrointestinal:* all emergency burn patients are considered to be on a full stomach. Many will develop a paralytic ileus. They are also predisposed to develop a "stress ulcer."

6. *Endocrine:* there is an increased level of stress hormones, leading to hyperglycemia and insulin resistance. There is also a substantial increase in the basal metabolic rates due to increasing catecholamines.

7. *Hematologic:* Coagulopathies have been associated with both the burn process and the relative clotting factor dilution that occurs with volume resuscitation

C. Patient preparation

Complete blood count, electrolytes, blood urea nitrogen, creatinine, glucose, urinalysis, prothrombin time, partial thromboplastin time (D-dimer or fibrin split products if disseminated intravascular coagulation is suspected), type and cross-match (number of units depends on the area to be debrided/grafted), chest radiography, arterial blood gases (with carboxyhemoglobin if indicated). Other tests as suggested by the history.

Begin volume replacement with crystalloid, or both preoperatively. If patient condition permits, an anxiolytic (such as benzodiazepene) and narcotic may be useful preoperatively.

D. Room preparation

1. *Monitors:* standard. Needle electrodes may be needed for electrocardiography; a nerve stimulator may be needed if intact skin is not available. Blood pressure can be measured on the lower extremities; an arterial line or a cuff can be placed over the burned area with a sterile lubricated dressing after consultation with the burn specialist. Most patients with burns of more than 40% to 50% require arterial line, central line, and pulmonary arterial catheter if hemodynamically unstable.

2. *Additional equipment:* blood and fluid warmers. A heated circuit may be used. Room temperature should be increased. Burn patients are extremely poikilothermic.

3. *Positioning:* various positioning or a change of positioning intraoperatively, depending on area being worked on

4. *Drugs and tabletop:* depolarizing muscle relaxants (succinylcholine) can cause life-threatening hyperkalemia (especially on postburn days 4 to 70) and are contraindicated in the burn patient. Burn patients also have an increased need for nondepolarizing relaxants because of up-regulation of ACH receptors. Most surgeons request that antibiotics be given intraoperatively.

E. Perioperative management and anesthetic techniques

Unless the burn is over a small body surface area percentage, most cases are done under general anesthesia. The choice of induction agent depends on the patient condition. Thiopental or propofol is appropriate in the hemodynamically stable patient. If the patient is already intubated, a narcotic/inhaled induction may be indicated. In the hemodynamically unstable patient, ketamine or oxygen/paralysis may be mandated.

The biggest concerns intraoperatively are for fluid and blood replacement and maintenance of body temperature and respiratory parameters. Often, an epinephrine solution is applied for hemostasis. Preoperatively, it is helpful to calculate the maximum epinephrine dosage.

Whenever airway or head and neck injury is possible, the patient remains intubated. Burn patients may require a large amount of narcotic titrated for their pain.

F. Postoperative implications

Pain management, prevention of respiratory complications, and fluid management are the top priorities.

B. Cardioversion

◆　◆　◆

A. Introduction
Synchronized cardioversion is the electrical conversion of a
tachyrhythmia, such as atrial fibrillation, atrial flutter, or
supraventricular tachycardia, unresponsive to intravenous drugs, to a
normal sinus rhythm. A synchronized electrical shock is released
through the chest wall, depolarizing the myocardium and
simultaneously making it refractory, thereby enabling the sinoatrial
node to resume its function as primary pacemaker.

B. Preoperative assessment and patient preparation
1. *History and physical examination:* standard
2. *Diagnostic tests:* 12-lead electrocardiography
3. Preoperative medication and intravenous therapy
   a. *One may desire to hold the daily dose of digoxin*
   b. *One 18-gauge intravenous tube with minimal fluid
      replacement*

C. Room preparation
1. Monitoring equipment
   a. *The procedure usually is performed away from the main operating
      room. All anesthetizing equipment must be available.*
   b. *Artificial cardiac pacing*
2. *Pharmacologic agents:* atropine, lidocaine
3. *Position:* supine

D. Anesthetic techniques
1. Sedation
2. *Intravenous sedation:* midazolam, methohexital (Brevital), propofol
   in sedative doses until the patient's lid reflex is gone

E. Perioperative management
1. *Induction:* preoxygenate the patient with the use of nasal cannula or
   face mask
2. *Maintenance:* as soon as consciousness is lost, the synchronized
   charge should be delivered with the R-wave on the
   electrocardiogram to avoid causing ventricular fibrillation
3. *Emergence:* support the airway and maintain ventilation until
   consciousness is regained

F. Postoperative implications
Monitor the electrocardiogram; complex ventricular arrhythmias may
appear, especially if the patient was on digoxin.

Bibliography
Barash PG, Cullen BF, Stoelting RK. *Clinical Anesthesia*. Philadelphia, PA: J.B.
Lippincott; 1992.

Miller RD. *Anesthesia*. New York, NY: Churchill Livingstone; 1990.

Stoelting RK, Dierdorf SF. *Anesthesia and Co-Existing Disease*. New York, NY:
Churchill Livingstone; 1993.

C. Trauma

✦ ✦ ✦

A. Introduction

Trauma is the fifth leading cause of death in the developed world. Mortality is related to the age and prior condition of the patient, type and severity of the trauma, and rapidity and quality of the emergency treatment received.

B. Preoperative assessment

Often there is only a few minutes to gather information before beginning an anesthetic on a trauma patient. Many times the patient cannot answer any questions and no person familiar with the history is available. If able, the most important questions to ask the trauma patient first are: "Do you have any allergies?", "Do you take medicine for or have any health problems?", and "Have you ever had surgery before?" Ensure blood availability with the appropriate operating room staff members.

1. *Cardiac:* assess for symptoms of shock, monitor continuous electrocardiogram (even preoperatively—may signal a contusion), assess the chest wall for obvious contusion
2. *Respiratory:* assess breath sounds, assess for crepitus, patterns of respiration. Chest radiography is recommended if time permits.
3. *Neurologic:* assess for Glasgow Coma Scale; assume a cervical spine injury until it is definitely ruled out. Assess the level of consciousness and pupillary response. Keep in mind that drug and alcohol intoxication will affect the examination.
4. *Renal:* assess color and amount of urine. Decreased cardiac output or direct renal trauma can lead to acute renal failure.
5. *Gastrointestinal:* all trauma patients are considered to be on a full stomach. Gastric emptying slows or stops at time of the trauma. The presence of a nasogastric tube also provides a "wick" that allows gastric fluid to be aspirated.
6. *Endocrine:* the release of stress hormones transiently elevates blood sugar levels
7. *Hematologic:* severe physical stress can lead to coagulopathies, as can dilution of clotting factors during massive volume resuscitation
8. *Patient preparation:* If time permits, the following laboratory tests should be performed: complete blood count, electrolytes, urinalysis, blood urea nitrogen, creatinine, glucose, partial thromboplastin time and prothrombin time. Type and cross-match for at least 4 units. Chest radiography and 12-lead electrocardiography are desirable in any patient with an obvious chest injury. Computed tomography of injured organs (brain, chest, abdomen) is helpful but often impossible because of time constraints. Cervical spine films should also be adequately visualized before lifting cervical spine precautions. Premedications are avoided in the trauma patient.

C. Room preparation

All monitoring modalities must be immediately available and include arterial line, arterial blood gas measurement, pulmonary artery catheters, blood warmers, and patient warming equipment. The full range of standard and emergency resuscitative drugs must be immediately available. Position is usually supine unless otherwise indicated.

D. Anesthetic technique

General anesthesia with minimal depressant drugs is used until the patient's status and extent of injury can be determined. Immediate establishment of the airway is the priority. Anesthetics are introduced depending on the stability of the patient.

E. Perioperative management

1. *Induction:* administration of 100% oxygen and immediate establishment of the airway are necessary. If facial or head and neck trauma is evident, then a fiberoptic technique or tracheostomy may be required.

   If central nervous system trauma is suspected, then taking precautions to prevent increased intracranial pressure is appropriate.

2. *Maintenance:* oxygen and muscle relaxants are required until the patient is assessed and stabilized. Introduce anesthetics as appropriate. Aggressive management of fluid, electrolyte, blood gas, blood loss, and coagulation status is required.

3. *Emergence:* Continued ventilation and management of all major systems are required in the immediate postanesthesia period.

F. Postoperative implications

Continued ventilation and observation of cardiac, respiratory, renal, and coagulation status are required for at least the first 24 hours after surgery. The patient is transferred to the critical care unit for long-term management of multiple sequelae.

D. Laser Procedures Involving the Airways

◆ ◆ ◆

A. Introduction

Laser is an acronym for "light amplification of the stimulated emission of radiation."

Laser procedures of the airway usually involve the CO_2 laser, because such lasers can excise lesions precisely and cause minimal edema. Tumor debunking of lesions found in the lower trachea and bronchi may require the Nd:YAG laser, which produces its effects at greater depth. There are many hazards of lasers to both the patient and members of the health care team. Damage can be caused to the lips and skin. Fire and explosion are possible with the use of lasers and volatile anesthetics. Toxins produced by the use of laser on tissues may be mutagenic. They may also cause infection, acute bronchial inflammation, and altered gas exchange. Because the airway will be shared by the surgeon and the anesthesia provider, much communication and cooperation is necesary.

B. Preoperative assessment
1. History and physical examination
   a. *A careful history should be obtained with a great deal of emphasis on airway and respiratory concerns. A thorough airway assessment is necessary. This should include thyromental distance, airway classification, cervical range of motion, dentition, phonation, hoarseness, shortness of breath, and edema. The need for awake fiberoptic intubation should be considered. Often, these patients have long smoking histories and may present with chronic obstructive pulmonary disease. Such findings should be noted on the history and physical examination. A complete respiratory assessment should be performed and documented.*
   b. *Nutritional status should be evaluated because this patient population may have undergone chemotherapy or radiation therapy for treatment of airway lesions*
   c. *Renal status should also be evaluated for similar reasons*
2. Patient preparation
   a. Laboratory tests: *Bendon history and physical.*
   b. Diagnostic tests: *pulmonary function tests may be recommended for chronic obstructive pulmonary disease; with chest radiographs, note tracheal duration*
   c. Medications: *preoperative sedation, if administered, should be done so cautiously and should be avoided entirely in patients with severe airway obstruction. Additional sedation could cause complete airway obstruction. An antisialagogue should be given to enhance visualization and to decrease secretions.*

C. Room preparation
1. *Monitoring equipment:* standard
2. Additional equipment
   a. *Standard emergency drugs (including lidocaine, atropine, succinylcholine)*
   b. *Eyes must be protected. The patient's eyes should be taped closed and covered with wet gauze. Others in the room should wear goggles (clean for CO_2 lenses, green for argon, and amber for Nd:YAG lasers).*
   c. *Materials for emergency cricothyroidotomy and tracheostomy should be available and in the room during induction. A surgeon experienced in tracheostomy should be present during induction for the patient with a compromised airway. Jet ventilation equipment should also be readily available.*
   d. *Appropriate endotracheal tubes should be available to decrease the risk of airway fire. This may include metal tubes, red rubber, polyvinyl chloride (PVC), or silicone tubes. PVC tubes are thought to be the least flammable; however, they melt more easily compared with red rubber or silicone tubes. Metal tubes are known to kink and leak. Some advocate PVC tubes and filling the cuff with sterile water or methylene blue–tinted sterile water rather than air (if punctured, one would know immediately). Still, some practitioners advocate wrapping*

PVC tubes with metallic tape to decrease the risk of airway fill; however, this makes the tube rigid and prone to kinking. It also makes for rough edges, which could cause airway trauma. Silicone produces a toxic ash when burnt and is therefore generally not used. Regardless of the endotracheal tube chosen, one should use the lowest fractional inspired oxygen possible as to decrease the risk of airway fire. If an airway fire should occur, ventilation should be stopped and the O_2 source should be discontinued. Flood the area with water. Remove the burned endotracheal tube. Mask-ventilate and reintubate the patient. Bronchoscopy, laryngoscopy, chest radiography, and arterial blood gas measurements should be performed to determine injury and to provide therapy. The patient should be monitored for at least 24 hours. Short-term steroids may be administered, as should antibiotics and ventilatory support as needed.

    e. *Long breathing circuits may be needed if the operating table is to be turned*

    f. Intravenous fluids: *18-gauge or larger tube, normal saline or lactated Ringer's solution at 2 to 4 mL/kg per hour*

D. Perioperative management and anesthetic technique

  1. General anesthesia with endotracheal intubation is appropriate. Some advocate local anesthesia with heavy sedation for certain minor base procedures of the upper airway. However, the patient must not move, and remember that sedation may lead to complete airway obstruction.

  2. *Induction:* standard intravenous induction if the patient has airway obstruction. With airway obstruction or an awake patient, fiberoptic bronchoscopy may be performed, and the airway may be secured prior to induction. Muscle relaxants should be avoided until the airway is secured.

  3. *Maintenance:* isoflurane, desflurane, air and O_2 is standard. Avoid N_2O because it is combustible. Avoid fractional inspired oxygen above 0.40 to decrease the risk of airway fire.

  4. *Emergence:* use awake extubation because there may be some airway edema. Avoid coughing, bucking, and straining on the endotracheal tube to prevent further edema.

E. Postoperative implications

Nausea and vomiting can be treated with metoclopramide, droperidol, or ondansetron.

PART 3

DRUGS

Name
Adenosine (Adenocard)

Classification
Antiarrhythmic

Indications
Supraventricular tachycardia

Dose
6-mg bolus given over 1 to 2 sec followed by normal saline line flush; may increase to 12-mg bolus if arrhythmia persists past 2 min. May repeat 12-mg bolus once. How supplied: 3 mg/mL 2-mL and 5-mL vials.

Onset and Duration
Onset 10–20 sec; duration 1 min.

Adverse Effects
Flushing, dyspnea, chest pain, headache, nausea, cough, malaise

Precautions and Contraindications
Adenosine should not be used in patients receiving methyl xanthine therapy, i.e., aminophylline, theophylline. Dipyridamole (Persantine) inhibits cellular uptake of adenosine. Use with caution in asthmatics. Contraindicated in patients with second- or third-degree heart block.

Anesthetic Considerations
An excellent agent for use under anesthesia in lieu of or preceding administration of calcium channel blockers for long-term suppression.

Name
Albuterol sulfate (Proventil, Ventolin)

Classification
Beta$_2$-adrenergic agonist, sympathomimetic, bronchodilator

Indications
Treatment of asthma and other forms of bronchospasm

Dose
Inhaler (metered dose): 2 deep inhalations 1–5 min apart; may be repeated every 4–6 hr. (Daily dose should not exceed 16–20 inhalations. Each metered aerosol actuation delivers approximately 90 μg per puff.) P.O.: 2–4 mg t.i.d. to q.i.d. (total dose not to exceed 16 mg). Syrup: 2 mg/5mL is available.

Onset and Duration
Onset: Inhalation: 5–15 min; P.O.: 15–30 min. Peak effect: Inhalation: 0.5–2 hr; P.O.: 2–3 hr. Duration: Inhalation: 3–6 hr P.O.: 4–8 hr.

Adverse Effects
Tachycardia, arrhythmias, hypertension, tremors, anxiety, headache, nausea, vomiting, hypokalemia

Contraindications
Safe use not established during pregnancy. Cautious use in patients with cardiovascular disease, hypertension, hyperthyroidism. Monitor glucose and electrolyte levels.

Anesthetic Considerations
Tolerance/tachyphylaxis can develop with chronic use. Additive effects with epinephrine and other sympathomimetics. Antagonized by beta-receptor antagonists.

Name
Alfentanil HCl (Alfenta)

Classification
Opioid agonist; produces analgesia and anesthesia

Dose
Induction: I.V. 50–150 μg/kg; Infusion: 0.1–3 μg/kg per minute.

Onset and Duration
Onset: I.V. 1–2 min; I.M. < 5 min, epidural 5–15 min. Duration: I.V. 1–15 min; I.M. 10–60 min; epidural 30 min.

Adverse Effects
Bradycardia, hypotension, arrhythmias. Respiratory depression. Euphoria, dysphoria, convulsions. Nausea and vomiting, biliary tract spasm, delayed gastric emptying. Muscle rigidity. Pruritus.

Contraindications
Reduce dose in elderly, hypovolemic, high-risk surgical patients and with concomitant use of sedatives and other narcotics. Crosses the placental barrier, and usage in labor may produce depression of respiration in the neonate. Resuscitation may be required; have naloxone available.

Anesthetic Considerations
Circulatory and ventilatory depressant effects potentiated by narcotics, sedatives, volatile anesthetics, nitrous oxide; ventilatory depressant effects potentiated by amphetamines, monamine oxidase, phenothiazine, tricyclic antidepressants; analgesia enhanced by alpha$_2$-agonists; reduced clearance and prolonged respiratory depression with concomitant use of erythromycin; muscle rigidity in higher dose range can be sufficient to interfere with ventilation.

DRUGS

Name
Alprostadil, PGE 1 (Prostin VR$_R$)

Classification
Prostaglandin E

Indications
Neonates: to maintain temporary patency of the ductus arteriosus until corrective or palliative surgery can be performed.

Dose
Children: Continuous infusion into large vein 0.05 to 0.1 μg/kg per minute initially; when a therapeutic response occurs, decrease to lowest possible dose to maintain response (maximum dose 0.4 μg/kg per minute). Dosage forms: 500 μg/ml 1-mL ampules (refrigerate at 2–8°C). Must be diluted in D$_5$W or normal saline for continuous infusion to final concentration of 5–20 μg/mL.

Onset and Duration
Onset 30 minutes; elimination t$_{1/2}$ 5–10 min.

Adverse Effects
Apnea (10%–12%), fever (14%), flushing (10%), bradycardia and seizures (4%). Thrombocytopenia (<1%), disseminated intravascular coagulation (1%), anemia, tachycardia, hypotension (4%), diarrhea (2%), gastric outlet obstruction secondary to antral hyperplasia (related to cumulative dose).

Precautions and Contraindications
Apnea is most frequent in infants under 2 kg within the first hour of administration; ventilatory assistance may be required. Contraindicated in neonates with respiratory distress syndrome. Use with caution in patients with bleeding tendencies due to alprostadil's ability to inhibit platelet aggregation. In all neonates, monitor arterial pressure; should arterial pressure fall significantly, decrease the rate of infusion.

Name
Aminocaproic acid (Amicar)

Classification
Hemostatic agent; prevents the conversion of plasminogen to plasmin

Indications
Control of clinical bleeding where hyperfibrinolysis is a contributing factor. Hyperfibrinolysis should be confirmed by laboratory values such as prolonged thrombin time, prolonged prothrombin time, hypofibrinogenemia, or decreased plasminogen levels. Also: open-heart surgery; postoperative hematuria following transurethral prostatic resection, suprapubic prostatectomy, and nephrectomy; hematologic disorders such as aplastic anemia, abruptio placentae, cirrhosis, neoplastic diseases, and

prophylaxis in hemophiliacs pre- and post-tooth extraction and other bleeding in the mouth and nasopharynx. Reduction of blood loss in trauma and shock; possible prevention of ocular hemorrhaging and bleeding in subarachnoid hemorrhage.

Dose

Acute bleeding: 5 g infused during the first hour, followed by a continuous infusion of 1 g/hr for 8 hr or until bleeding is controlled.

Chronic bleeding: 5 g preoperatively intravenous piggyback (IVPB) over 1 hr, then 5 g IVPB every 6 hr. Do not exceed 30 g in 24 hr. Decrease dose by 15%–25% in patients with renal disease.

Children: 100 mg/kg IVPB over 1 hr, then 30 mg/kg per hour until bleeding is controlled. (Maximum dose 18 g/m^2 in 24 hr.)

Dosage forms: 250 mg/mL 20 mL parenteral vial (5g).

Administration: Dilute each dose in a proper volume of D_5W normal saline, or lactated Ringer's solution.

Onset and Duration

Onset 1–72 hr; $t_{1/2}$ 1–2 hr in patients with normal renal function. No single concentration fits all. It must be diluted. Consult package insert, i.v. reference, or pharmacy.

Adverse Effects

Convulsions, myopathy, rarely muscle necrosis, nausea, vomiting. Rapid infusion associated with hypotension, bradycardia, arrhythmias.

Precautions

A definitive diagnosis of hyperfibrinolysis must be made before administration. Caution when using in cardiac, renal, or hepatic disease. Administration in presence of renal or ureteral bleeding is not recommended because of ureteral clot formation and possible risk of obstruction.

Contraindications

Owing to the substantial risk of serious or fatal thrombus formation aminocaproic acid is contraindicated in patients with disseminated intravascular coagulation unless heparin is given concurrently.

Name

Aminophylline

Classification

Bronchodilator

Indications

Chronic therapy for bronchial asthma. Reversal of bronchospasm associated with chronic obstructive pulmonary disease.

Dose

Loading dose: For patients not already receiving a theophylline preparation, I.V. 5–6 mg/kg (given over 20–30 min) or P.O./rectal 6 mg/kg.

DRUGS

Maintenance: I.V. 0.5 mg/kg per hour; P.O. 2–4 mg/kg every 6–12 hr. Therapeutic range: 10–20 μg/mL.

Dose

Dosage forms: Injection 25 mg/mL; Tablets 100 mg, 200 mg; Tablets (sustained release) 225 mg; Oral solution 105 mg/5 mL; Rectal solution 60 mg/mL (rectal solution not marketed in U.S.); Rectal suppositories 250 mg, 500 mg. Dilution for infusion loading dose: dilute 500 mg in 500 mL D$_5$W or normal saline (1 mg/mL). Children 9–16 years: 1 mg/kg per hour for 12 hr, then 0.8 mg/kg per hour. Children 6 months–9 years: 1.2 mg/kg per hour for 12 hr, then 1 mg/kg per hour.

Onset and Duration

Onset: I.V.: few min; P.O. within 30 min. Duration P.O. 4–8 hr.

Adverse Effects

Palpitations, sinus tachycardia, supraventricular and ventricular tachycardia, flushing, tachypnea, seizures, headache, irritability, nausea, vomiting, hyperglycemia.

Elevated serum levels in patients receiving cimetidine, quinolone antibiotics, macrolide antibiotics, and in patients with cardiac failure or liver insufficiency. Decreased serum levels with phenobarbital, phenytoin, rifampin, and smokers. Frequent monitoring of plasma concentrations. Toxicity occurs with plasma levels greater than 20 μg/mL. Avoid rapid infusions, which may cause hypotension, arrhythmias, and possibly death.

Anesthetic Considerations

Potentiates pressor effects of sympathomimetics and may produce seizures, cardiac arrhythmias, cardiorespiratory arrest, ventricular arrhythmias with excessive plasma levels or in patients receiving volatile anesthetics. Use isoflurane or enflurane in patients who must be given aminophylline or other exogenous sympathomimetic drugs before or during surgery. Use of halothane may potentiate cardiac dysrhythmia.

Name

Amiodarone (Cordarone)

Classification

Class III antiarrhythmic

Indications

Treatment of life-threatening ventricular arrhythmias that do not respond to other antiarrhythmic (i.e., recurrent ventricular fibrillation and hemodynamically unstable ventricular tachycardia). Selective treatment of supraventricular arrhythmias.

Dose

Loading: P.O.: 800–1600 mg/day for 1–3 wk. Maintenance: P.O.: 200–600 mg/day. Therapeutic level 1.0–2.5 μg/mL. Dosage form: Tablets 200 mg. I.V. 100–300 mg.

Onset and Duration
Onset 2–4 days; $t_{1/2}$ between 2 weeks and months. Duration 45 days.

Adverse Effects
Arrhythmias, pulmonary fibrosis or inflammation, hepatitis or cirrhosis, corneal deposits, hyperthyroidism, hypothyroidism, peripheral neuropathy, cutaneous photosensitivity.

Contraindications
Amiodarone increases serum levels of digoxin, warfarin, quinidine, procainamide, phenytoin, diltiazem. The likelihood of bradycardia, sinus arrest, and atrioventricular block increases with concurrent beta-adrenergic antagonist and calcium channel–blocker therapy.

Anesthetic Considerations
Antiadrenergic effects enhanced in the presence of general anesthetics manifesting as sinus arrest, atrioventricular block, low cardiac output, or hypotension. Drugs that inhibit the automaticity of the sinus node such as halothane and lidocaine could accentuate effects of amiodarone and increase the likelihood of sinus arrest. The potential need for a temporary artificial cardiac (ventricular) pacemaker and administration of sympathomimetics such as isoproterenol should be considered in patients receiving this drug.

Name
Amrinone lactate (Inocor)

Classification
Positive inotrope (phosphodiesterase inhibitor)

Indications
Short-term management of congestive heart failure

Dose
Loading dose: 0.75 mg/kg over 2–3 min. A second bolus may follow after 30 minutes. Maintenance is by continuous infusion of 5–10 mg/kg/per minute (maximum 24-hour dose 10 μg/kg). Dosage forms: Injection 5 mg/mL. Dilution for infusion: 500 mg in 500 mL normal saline solution.

Onset and Duration
Onset within 5 min; duration 30 min to 2 hr.

Adverse Effects
Hypotension, arrhythmia, thrombocytopenia, abdominal pain, hepatic dysfunction. Use with caution in hypotensive patients. Avoid exposure of ampule to light. Do not mix in solutions containing dextrose or furosemide. Use with caution in patients with allergies to bisulfites. Fluid balance, electrolyte concentrations, and renal function should be monitored carefully during treatment. Monitor platelet counts chronically.

DRUGS

Anesthetic Considerations

Alternative to conventional inotropes. Useful when both inotropic and vasodilating properties desired and/or to lower pulmonary vascular resistance.

Name

Atracurium (Tracrium)

Classification

Nondepolarizing skeletal muscle relaxant

Indications

Relaxation of skeletal muscles during surgery; adjunct to general anesthesia or mechanical ventilation; facilitation of endotracheal intubation.

Dose

Initially for paralyzing: I.V. 0.3–0.5 mg/kg. Maintenance: I.V. 0.08–0.1 mg/kg. Dosage form: Injection 10 mg/mL.

Onset and Duration

Onset: <3 min; duration 20–35 min; elimination: plasma (half-man elimination, ester hydrolysis), hepatic, renal. The primary metabolite is laudanosine, a cerebral stimulant, excreted primarily in the urine.

Adverse Effects

Vasodilation, hypotension, sinus tachycardia, sinus bradycardia, hypoventilation, apnea, bronchospasm, laryngospasm, dyspnea, inadequate block, prolonged block, rash, urticaria.

Precautions and Contraindications

Use with caution in patients with conditions in which histamine release may prove hazardous, in patients with myasthenia gravis, bradycardia, or electrolyte disturbances, and in pregnant or nursing women.

Anesthetic Considerations

Monitor response with peripheral nerve stimulator. Reverse effects with anticholinesterase. Pretreatment doses may induce sufficient neuromuscular blockade to cause hypotension in some patients.

Name

Atropine sulfate

Classification

Competitive acetylcholine antagonist at muscarinic receptor

Indications

Symptomatic bradycardia, asystole, cardiopulmonary resuscitation (CPR). Antisialogogue. For vagolytic effects to block bradycardia during surgery from stimulation of the carotid sinus, traction on abdominal viscera, or extraocular muscles. Blockade of muscarinic effects of anticholinesterases. Adjunctive therapy in the treatment of bronchospasm, peptic ulcer disease.

Dose

Adults: sinus bradycardia, CPR: I.V., I.M., SQ, via endotracheal tube (diluted in 10 mL sterile water or normal saline: 0.5–1.0 mg every 3–5 min as indicated (maximum dose 40 μg/kg). Preoperative: 0.4 mg I.M., SQ, or P.O. 30–60 min preinduction.

Blockade of muscarinic effects of anticholinesterases: 7–10 μg/kg with edrophonium, 15–30 μg/kg with neostigmine, 15–20 μg/kg with pyridostigmine.

Bronchodilation: Inhalation: 0.025 mg/kg every 4–6 hr. Dilute to 2–3 mL normal saline and deliver by compressed air nebulizer. (maximum dose 2.5 mg/dose). Pediatric bronchodilatory dose is 0.05 mg/kg diluted in normal saline 3 or 4 times daily.

Children: sinus bradycardia, CPR: I.V., I.M., SQ, or via endotracheal tube 0.02 mg/kg every 5 min up to a maximum of 1 mg in children and 2 mg in adolescents (minimum dose 0.1 mg).

Preoperative: P.O., I.M., SQ 0.02 mg/kg for neonates, 0.1 mg for children weighing 3 kg, 0.2 mg for those weighing 7–9 kg, and 0.3 mg for those weighing 12–16 kg.

Dosage forms: Injection: 0.05, 0.1, 0.3, 0.4, 0.5, 0.8, and 1 mg/mL
Inhalation solution: 0.2, 0.5%.
Tablets: 0.4, 0.6 mg.

Onset and Duration

Inhibition of salivation occurs within 30 min–1 hr and peaks in 1–2 hr following P.O. or I.M. administration. Increase in heart rate occurs within 5–40 min after I.V. or I.M. administration. Duration is 15–30 min after I.V. administration and 2–4 hr following I.M. administration.

Plasma $t_{1/2}$ is 2–3 hr.

Adverse Effects

Transient bradycardia due to a weak peripheral muscarinic cholinergic agonist effect in small doses (<0.5 mg in adults), tachycardia (high doses), urinary hesitancy, retention, mydriasis, blurred vision, increased intraocular pressure, decreased sweating, excitement, agitation, drowsiness, confusion, hallucinations, dry nose and mouth, allergic reactions, constipation. Children and the elderly are more susceptible to adverse effects.

Precautions and Contraindications

Avoid where tachycardia would be harmful, i.e., thyrotoxicosis, pheochromocytoma, or coronary artery disease. Avoid in hyperpyrexial states because it inhibits sweating. Contraindicated in acute-angle glaucoma, obstructive disease of the gastrointestinal tract, obstructive uropathy, paralytic ileus or intestinal atony, and acute hemorrhage where cardiovascular status is unstable. Use with caution in patients with tachyarrhythmias, hepatic or renal disease, congestive heart failure, chronic pulmonary disease (since a reduction in bronchial secretions may lead to formation of

DRUGS

bronchial plugs), autonomic neuropathy, hiatal hernia, gastroesophageal reflux, gastric ulcers, gastrointestinal infections, ulcerative colitis.

Anesthetic Considerations

Additive anticholinergic effects may occur when atropine is given concomitantly with meperidine, some antihistamines, phenothiazines, tricyclic antidepressants, and antiarrhythmic drugs that possess anticholinergic activity (e.g., quinidine, disopyramide, procainamide)

Name

Bretylium (Bretylol)

Classification

Class III antiarrhythmic

Indications

Ventricular fibrillation and other ventricular arrhythmias resistant to initial lidocaine or procainamide treatment.

Dose

I.V. loading I.M. ventricular tachycardia: 5–10 mg/kg over 1 min or may be repeated in 1–2 hr. IV loading ventricular fibrillation: 5–10 mg/kg over 1 min (every 15–30 min to maximum 30 mg/kg). Infusion: 1–2 mg/min. Therapeutic level: 0.5–1.0 μg/mL. Dosage form: 50 mg/mL.

Onset and Duration

Onset antifibrillatory: few minutes; I.V./I.M. suppression of ventricular arrhythmia: 20 min to 2 hr. Duration: I.V./I.M. 6–24 hr.

Adverse Effects

Hypotension, transitory hypertension and arrhythmias, anginal attacks, shortness of breath, dizziness, syncope, nausea, vomiting, diarrhea, rash, hiccups.

Contraindications

Use with caution on patients with pheochromocytoma, aortic stenosis, pulmonary hypertension.

Anesthetic Considerations

Tricyclic antidepressants may prevent uptake of bretylium by adrenergic nerve terminals. Treat severe hypotension with appropriate fluid therapy and vasopressor agents such as dopamine or norepinephrine.

Name

Bumetanide (Bumex)

Classification

Loop diuretic

Indications

Treatment of edema of cardiac, hepatic, or renal origin. Hypertension, pulmonary edema. Usually reserved for patients who do not respond to thiazide diuretics or in whom a rapid onset of diuresis is desired.

Dose
Initial dose: 0.5–1 mg I.V. over 1–2 min. If response is not adequate following the initial dose, a second or third dose may be administered at intervals of up to 2–3 hr, up to a maximum of 10 mg/day. Children: Dosage forms: 0.5, 1, 2 mg tablets; 0.25 mg/mL solution for injection in 2 mL, 4 mL, and 10 mL vials.

Onset and Duration
I.V.: few minutes; Peak effect: 15–30 min. Duration: 4 hr with normal doses of 1–2 mg and up to 6 hr with higher doses. Elimination $t_{1/2}$ 1–1.5 hr.

Adverse Effects
Transient leukopenia, granulocytopenia, thrombocytopenia, hypotension, chest pain, dizziness. Electrolyte abnormalities such as hyperuricemia, hypomagnesemia, hypokalemia, hypochloremia, azotemia, hyponatremia, and metabolic alkalosis. Hyperglycemia, diarrhea, pancreatitis, nephrotoxicity, muscle cramps, arthritic pain, ototoxicity (less frequent than with furosemide).

Precautions and Contraindications
Anuria, hypersensitivity to bumetanide, severe fluid and electrolyte imbalance, hepatic coma, if increase in blood urea nitrogen or creatinine occurs. Patients allergic to sufonamides may have hypersensitivity to bumetanide.

Anesthetic Considerations
Loop diuretics may increase the neuromuscular blocking effect of tubocurarine, probably because of their potassium depleting effects.

Name
Bupivacaine HCl (Marcaine, Sensorcaine)

Classification
Amide-type local anesthetic

Indications
Regional anesthesia

Dose
Infiltration/peripheral nerve block: <150 mg (0.25%–0.5% solution). Epidural: 50-100 mg (0.25%–0.75% solution) Children: 1.5–2.5 mg/kg (0.25%–0.5% solution), caudal: 37.5–150 mg (15–30 mL of 0.25% or 0.5% solution). Children: 0.4–0.7 mL/kg, spinal bolus/infusion: 7–17 mg (0.75% solution) Children: 0.5 mg/kg, with minimum of 1 mg. Do not exceed 400 mg in 24 hours. Maximum single dose is 175 mg.

Onset and Duration
Onset: Infiltration: 2–10 min. Epidural: 4–7 min. Spinal: <1 min. Peak effect: Infiltration and epidural: 30–45 min. Spinal: 15 min. Duration: Infiltration/spinal/epidural: 200–400 min (prolonged with epinephrine).

DRUGS

Adverse Effects

Hypotension, arrhythmias, cardiac arrest, respiratory impairment, arrest, seizures, tinnitus, blurred vision, urticaria, anaphylactoid symptoms. High spinal: urinary retention, lower-extremity weakness and paralysis, loss of sphincter control, backache, palsies, slowing of labor.

Precautions and Contraindications

Use with caution in patients with hypovolemia, severe congestive heart failure, shock, and all forms of heart block. Not recommended for obstetrical paracervical block or in concentrations above 0.5% due to incidence of intractable cardiac arrest. Contraindicated in patients with hypersensitivity to amide-type local anesthetics.

Anesthetic Considerations

Prior use of chloroprocaine may interfere with action. I.V. access is essential during major regional block. Toxic plasma levels of bupivacaine may cause cardiopulmonary collapse and seizures.

Name

Chloroprocaine HCl (Nesacaine)

Classification

Ester-type local anesthetic

Indications

Regional anesthesia. Local anesthesia including infiltration, epidural (including caudal), peripheral nerve block, sympathetic nerve block.

Dose

Infiltration and peripheral nerve block: <40 ml (1%–2% solution). Epidural: bolus 10–25 mL (2%–3% solution), approximately 1.5–2 mL for each segment to be anesthetized. Repeat doses at 40–60 min intervals. Infusion: 30 mL/hr (0.5% solution). Caudal: 10–25 mL (2%–3% solution). Children: 0.4–0.7 mL/kg (L2–T10 level of anesthesia). Repeat doses at 40–60 min intervals.

Onset and Duration

Rate of onset and potency of local anesthetic action may be enhanced by carbonation. Onset: Infiltration/epidural: 6–12 min. Peak effect: Infiltration/epidural: 10–20 min. Duration: Infiltration/epidural: 30–60 min (prolonged with epinephrine).

Adverse Effects

Hypotension, arrhythmias, bradycardia, respiratory depression, arrest, seizures, tinnitus, tremors, urticaria, pruritus, angioneurotic edema. High spinal: backache, loss of perianal sensation and sexual function, permanent motor, sensory, autonomic (sphincter control) deficit in lower segments, slowing of labor.

Precautions and Contraindications
Caution in patients with severe disturbances of cardiac rhythm, shock, heart block, or impaired hepatic function. Inflammation or infection at injection site. Elderly, pregnant. Contraindicated in patients with hypersensitivity to local anesthetics, para-aminobenzoic acid/parabens. **Do not use for spinal anesthesia.**

Anesthetic Considerations
Reduce doses in obstetric, elderly, hypovolemic, high-risk patients, and those with increased intra-abdominal pressure. **Do not use for spinal anesthesia.**

Name
Cimetidine (Tagamet)

Classification
Histamine (H_2) antagonist

Indications
Treatment of duodenal or gastric ulcers, gastroesophageal reflux disease. Prophylaxis of aspiration pneumonitis in patients at high risk during surgery.

Dose
Prophylaxis of aspiration pneumonitis: Adults: 300–400 mg P.O. 1.5–2 hr before induction of anesthesia with or without a similar dose the preceding evening. When a more rapid onset of effect is needed, I.V.: dilute 300–400 mg in D_5W or normal saline to a volume of at least 20 mL, and inject over a period not less than 5 min. A slower infusion over 15–30 minutes may be preferable owing to association of occasional severe bradycardia and hypotension with rapid infusion. Children younger than 12 years of age; use not indicated. Dosage forms: Tablets: 300 mg, 400 mg. Parenteral injection: 150 mg/mL.

Onset and Duration
Peak plasma levels: 1–2 hr P.O. Elimination $t_{1/2}$ 2 hr. Plasma cimetidine levels that suppress gastric acid secretion by 50% were maintained 4–5 hours following I.V. injection.

Adverse Effects
Mental status changes such as delirium, confusion, depression primarily in elderly or hepatic- or renal-impaired patients. Leukopenia, thrombocytopenia and gynecomastia reported rarely (1%). Hypotension, severe bradycardia associated with rapid I.V. infusion. Serum creatinine and liver enzymes may rise during treatment, although hepatotoxicity and renal dysfunction are usually reversible.

Precautions and Contraindications
Caution suggested in renal or hepatic insufficiency. Microsomal metabolism of many drugs may be inhibited. Contraindicated in patients allergic to cimetidine or other H_2 antagonists.

DRUGS

Anesthetic Considerations

Cimetidine inhibits the hepatic mixed-function oxidase system; therefore, it may prolong the half-life of many drugs, including diazepam, midazolam, metaprolol, propranolol, theophylline, lidocaine, and other amide local anesthetics. Ranitidine may be the drug of choice in patients receiving lidocaine local or regional anesthesia.

Name

Clonidine (Catapres, Dixatrit)

Classification

Central-acting alpha$_2$-adrenergic agonist; reduces sympathetic outflow by directly stimulating alpha receptors in the medulla vasomotor center.

Indications

Hypertension; epidural and spinal anesthesia; symptomatic control of alcohol, opiate, nicotine, and benzodiazepine withdrawal; diagnosis of pheochromocytoma; growth-hormone stimulation test; cancer pain; Tourette's syndrome; attention deficit disorder; migraines.

Dose

Maintenance: 0.2–0.6 mg/day P.O. in two divided doses. Hypertensive emergencies: 0.15 mg I.V. over 5 min. Transdermal patch every 7 days (maximum dose 2.4 mg/day). Same doses for renal impairment.

Onset

I.V. or P.O.: 30–60 min. Peak effect: 2–4 hr. May take too long for true HTN crisis.

Duration

Antihypertensive: 6–10 hr. Dose-dependent.

Adverse Effects

Rebound hypertension, atrioventricular block, bradycardia, congestive heart failure, orthostatic hypotension, sedation, nightmares, constipation, dry mouth, pruritus, urinary retention, contact dermatitis.

Precautions and Contraindications

Avoid in conduction or sinoatrial disorders, hypersensitivity to clonidine, pregnancy, severe renal or hepatic disease. Concomitant administration of tricyclic antidepressants may increase dose.

• If dose held or changing to transdermal application, watch for rapid increase in blood pressure from unopposed alpha stimulation.
• Crosses the placenta easily. Should be discontinued 8–12 hr prior to delivery.

Anesthetic Considerations
Severe rebound hypertension from abrupt withdrawal with neurological sequelae and myocardial infarction. Labetalol has been successfully used in treatment of hypertensive crisis. Continue on day of surgery.

• Hepatic elimination 50%.
• Reduces perioperative requirements of narcotics and volatile agents.

Name
Cocaine HCl (Cocaine)

Classification
Topical anesthetic and vasoconstrictor, ester-type local anesthetic

Indications
Used for topical anesthesia and vasoconstriction of mucous membranes (oral, laryngeal, and nasal).

Dose
Topical: 1.5 mg/kg (1%–4% solution). Nasal: 1–2 mL each nostril (1%–10% solution). Concentrations >4% increase potential for systemic toxic reactions. Maximum safe dose: 1.5 mg/kg.

Onset and Duration
Onset: <1 min. Peak effect: 2–5 min. Duration: 30–120 min. Rapidly absorbed from all areas of application.

Adverse Effects
Seizures, sloughing of nasal mucosa, arrhythmias, tachycardia, hypertension; increases maximum allowable concentration of inhalation anesthetics.

Contraindications
Topical use only; not for intraocular or I.V. use. Potentiates other sympathomimetics; therefore, use reduced doses, if any at all, in patients receiving pressors, or ketamine. Use with caution in patients with nasal trauma.

Anesthetic Considerations
Hypertension, bradyarrhythmias, tachyarrhythmias, ventricular fibrillation, tachypnea, respiratory failure, euphoria, excitement, seizures, sloughing of corneal epithelium. Use with caution in patients with history of drug sensitivities or drug abuse (high addiction potential) and pregnancy. Prolonged use can cause ischemic damage to nasal mucosa. Contraindicated for intraocular or I.V. use. Sensitizes the heart to catecholamines (epinephrine and monoamine oxidase inhibitors may increase cardiac arrhythmias, ventricular fibrillation, hypertensive episodes). Potentiates arrhythmogenic effects of sympathomimetics. High addiction potential.

DRUGS

Name
Codeine

Classification
Opioid agonist

Indications
Pre- and postoperative analgesia

Dose
P.O.: 15–60 mg every 4 hr; I.M./S.C.: 15–60 mg every 4 hr.

Onset and Duration
Onset: P.O.: 30–60 min; I.M./SQ: 20–60 min. Duration: P.O.: 2–4 hr; I.M./SQ: 2–3 hr.

Adverse Effects
Sedation, clouded sensorium, euphoria, dizziness, seizures with large doses, hypotension, bradycardia, nausea, vomiting, constipation, dry mouth, ileus, urinary retention, pruritus, flushing.

Precautions and Contraindications
Use with caution in head injury, increased intracranial pressure, increased cerebrospinal fluid pressure, hepatic or renal disease, hypothyroidism, Addison's disease, acute alcoholism, seizures, severe central nervous system depression, bronchial asthma, chronic obstructive pulmonary disease, respiratory depression, shock, and the elderly. Patients with known hypersensitivity to the drug.

Anesthetic Considerations
General anesthetics, other narcotic analgesics, tranquilizers, sedatives, hypnotics, alcohol, tricyclic antidepressants, or monoamine oxidase inhibitors increase central nervous system depression.

Name
Cyclosporine (Sandimmune)

Classification
Immunosuppressant

Indications
Prevent rejection of organ/tissue (kidney, liver, heart, allograft) in combination with steroid therapy.

Dose
Initial: P.O. 15 mg/kg as single dose 4–24 hr prior to transplantation, continue for 1–2 wk. Taper to maintenance dose: 5–10 mg/kg per day. I.V.: 0.5–6 mg/kg as single dose 4–12 hr prior to transplantation, continue until patient able to take oral medication.

Onset and Duration
Onset: 1–6 hours (variable). Duration: 1–4 days after. After oral adminis-tration, onset is variable. The terminal $t_{1/2}$ of the drug is 10–27 hr.

Adverse Effects
Hypertension, hirsutism, tremor, acne, gum hyperplasia, headache, blurred vision, diarrhea, nausea, paresthesia, mild nephrotoxicity or hepa-totoxicity.

Precautions and Contraindications
History of hypersensitivity to cyclosporine or polyoxyethylated castor oil. Caution with impaired hepatic, renal, cardiac function, malabsorption syndrome, and pregnancy.

Anesthetic Considerations
Altered lab values: May elevate blood urea nitrogen, serum creatinine, serum bilirubin, SGOT(AST), SGPT(ALT), and LDH. May prolong the duration of neuromuscular blockade by nondepolarizing muscle relaxants.

Name
Dantrolene sodium (Dantrium)

Classification
Skeletal muscle relaxant

Indications
Treatment of malignant hyperthermia (MHT). Prophylaxis of malignant hyperthermia in patients with a family history. Control of spasticity secondary to multiple sclerosis, spinal cord injury, cerebral palsy, or stroke.

Dose
Adults: Malignant hyperthermia: 1 mg/kg rapid I.V. bolus. Repeat every 5–10 min until symptoms are controlled. The dose may be repeated to a cumulative dose of 10 mg/kg. Oral doses of 4–8 mg/kg per day for 1–3 days may be administered in three or four divided doses to prevent recurrence of the manifestations. Prophylaxis of MHT: 2.5 mg/kg I.V. bolus 10–30 min pre-induction, then 1.25 mg/kg I.V. bolus 6 hr later. Dosage forms: Capsules: 25, 50, 100 mg. Parenteral injection: 20 mg. Administration: Reconstitute by adding 60 mL preservative-free sterile water for injection to each 20 mg vial and shake vial until clear. Avoid diluent that contains a bacteriostatic agent. Protect from light and use within 6 hr. For direct I.V. injection. Avoid extravasation.

Onset and Duration
Effective blood concentrations: 100–600 ng/mL. I.V. blood concentra-tions of the drug remain at approximately steady-state levels for 3 or more hours after infusion is completed. Mean $t_{1/2}$ 5–9 hr. Onset: P.O.: 1–2 hr; I.V.: less than 5 min.

Adverse Effects

Hepatotoxicity (hepatitis) 0.5%, with mortality reported as high as 10%. Muscle weakness, tachycardia, erratic blood pressure, fatigue, central nervous system (CNS) depression, visual and auditory hallucinations, bowel obstruction, hematuria, crystalluria, urinary frequency, phlebitis, pericarditis, pleural effusion, postpartum uterine atony, myalgias.

Precautions

Monitor liver function at beginning of therapy. Observe for hepatotoxicity, hepatitis. Owing to increased risk of hepatotoxicity use with caution with severely impaired cardiac or pulmonary function and in women or patients over 35.

Contraindications

Contraindicated in active hepatic disease such as hepatitis or cirrhosis, when spasticity is used to maintain motor function, and in lactation.

Anesthetic Considerations

Enhanced CNS and respiratory depression with other CNS depressants. Avoid concomitant use of calcium channel blockers, which can precipitate hyperkalemia and cardiovascular collapse.

Name

Desflurane (Suprane)

Classification

Inhalation anesthetic

Indications

General anesthesia

Dose

Titrate to effect for induction or maintenance of anesthesia. Minimum alveolar concentration (MAC), 6%. Dosage forms: Volatile liquid.

Onset and Duration

Onset: Loss of eyelid reflex 1–2 min; Duration: Emergence time 8–9 min.

Adverse Effects

Hypotension, arrhythmia, respiratory depression, apnea, dizziness, euphoria, increased cerebral blood flow and intracranial pressure, nausea, vomiting, ileus, hepatic dysfunction, malignant hyperthermia.

Precautions and Contraindications

Contraindicated in patients with known or suspected genetic susceptibility to malignant hyperthermia. Changes in mental function may persist beyond the period of anesthetic administration and the immediate postoperative period.

Anesthetic Considerations
Abrupt onset of malignant hyperthermia may be triggered by desflurane; early signs include muscle rigidity, especially in the jaw muscles, and tachycardia and tachypnea unresponsive to increased depth of anesthesia. Crosses the placental barrier.

Name
Desmopressin (DDAVP)

Classification
Synthetic vasopressin analogue

Indications
Treatment of neurogenic diabetes insipidus, nocturnal enuresis, and in hemophilia A or von Willebrand's disease to increase Factor VIII activity. Reduction of perioperative blood loss following cardiac surgery.

Dose
Preoperative: 30 min prior. Diabetes insipidus: 2–4 μg I.V. or SQ daily in two divided doses; Intranasal: 10–40 μg (0.1–0.4 mL) in one to three doses.

Pediatrics: 3 mos–12 yr: hemophilia A or von Willebrand's disease: 0.3 μg/kg I.V. diluted in saline and infused over 15–30 min. In children >10 kg use 50 mL diluent, and in children <10 kg use 10 mL diluent. Repeated doses in less than 48 hr may increase the possibility of tachyphylaxis.

Intranasal: 0.05–0.3 mL daily in single or divided doses. Doses should start at 0.05 mL or less and be individualized since an extreme decrease in plasma osmolarity in the very young may produce convulsions.

Dosage forms: Desmopressin acetate for injection should be stored at 4°C.

Nasal: 10–40 μg. May be divided into 3 doses. Supplied as 10 μg per 0.1 mL or 100 μg per mL.

Injection: 4 μg/mL.

Onset and Duration
Onset: Intranasal: 1 hr. I.V.: 30 min. Duration 8 to 20 hr. Elimination $t_{1/2}$ 3.6 hr.

Adverse Effects
Hypotension, hypertension, transient headache (with higher doses), psychosis, seizures, water retention, hyponatremia, abdominal cramps, nasal congestion, rhinitis, facial flushing, hypersensitivity reactions.

Precautions and Contraindications
Contraindicated in hypersensitivity to desmopressin acetate and in children under 3 months of age. Patients with type IIB von Willebrand's disease should not receive desmopressin since platelet aggregation may be reduced. Owing to increased risk of thrombosis use with caution in patients with coronary artery disease. Fluid intake should be decreased

DRUGS

in those who do not need the antidiuretic effects of desmopressin. Seizure activity may be related to rapid decreases in serum sodium concentrations secondary to desmopressin.

Name
Dexamethasone (Decadron)

Classification
Long-acting corticosteroid

Indications
Croup, septic shock, cerebral edema, respiratory distress syndrome including status asthmaticus, acute exacerbations of chronic allergic disorders, corticosteroid-responsive bronchospastic states, allergic or inflammatory nasal conditions and nasal polyps.

Dose
Initial: 0.5–9 mg I.M. or I.V. daily, depending upon the disease being treated. In less severe diseases, doses lower than 0.5 mg I.M. or I.V. may suffice, whereas in others, doses higher than 9 mg may be required. Cerebral edema: 10 mg I.V. initially followed by 4 mg I.M. every 6 hr. Reduce dose after 2–4 days, then taper over 5–7 days. Corticosteroid-responsive bronchospastic states: Respihaler: Three inhalations 3–4 times daily (maximum 12 inhalations daily). Nasal conditions: Turbinaire: Two sprays each nostril 2–3 times daily (maximum 12 sprays/24 hr). Children: I.M. or I.V. push 6–40 μg/kg or 0.235–1.25 mg/m^2 given one or two times daily. Must be given slowly over 3–5 minutes I.V. push. Dosage forms: Respihaler inhalation: 0.1 mg/spray dexamethasone phosphate. Turbinaire intranasal: 0.1 mg/spray. Solution for injection: 4, 10, 24 mg/mL. Tablets: 0.25, 0.5, 0.75, 1, 1.5, 2, 4, 6 mg.

Onset and Duration
I.V., I.M.: within 8 hr; Inhalation: within 20 min. Elimination $t_{1/2}$: 200 min, however, metabolic effects at the tissue level persist for up to 72 hr.

Adverse Effects
Cushing's syndrome, adrenal suppression, hyperglycemia, hyperthyroidism, hypercalcemia, peptic ulcer, gastrointestinal hemorrhage, increased intraocular pressure, glaucoma, irritability, psychosis, osteoporosis.

Precautions and Contraindications
Contraindicated in patients with peptic ulcer, osteoporosis, psychosis or psychoneurosis, acute bacterial infections, herpes zoster, herpes simplex ulceration of the eye, and other viral infections. Use with caution in diabetes mellitus, chronic renal failure, infectious disease, elderly. Corticosteroids may increase the risk of developing tuberculosis in patients with a positive purified protein derivative test. May increase the risk of development of serious or fatal infection in individuals exposed to viral illnesses such as chicken pox.

Name
Diazepam (Valium)

Classification
Central nervous system agent; benzodiazepine; anticonvulsant and anxiolytic

Indications
Anxiety, alcohol withdrawal, status epilepticus, preoperative sedation, sedation for cardioversion. Used adjunctively for relief of skeletal muscle spasm associated with cerebral palsy, paraplegia, athetosis, stiff-man syndrome, tetanus.

Dose
Status epilepticus: Adults: I.M./I.V. 5–10 mg; repeat if needed at 10–15 min intervals up to 30 mg; repeat if needed in 2–4 hr.

Children: I.M./I.V. <5 yr: 0.2–0.5 mg slowly 2–5 min up to 5 mg, total dose. Children >5 year: 1 mg slowly 2–5 min up to 10 mg; repeat if needed in 2–4 hr.

Anxiety, muscle spasm convulsions, alcohol withdrawal:

Adult: P.O. 2–10 mg b.i.d. to q.i.d.; I.M./I.V. 2–10 mg; repeat if needed in 3–4 hr.

Child: P.O. >6 mos: 1–2.5 mg b.i.d. or t.i.d.

Dosage forms: Tablets: 2, 5, 10 mg; Capsules: (sustained release) 15 mg; Oral solution: 5 mg/5mL and 5 mg/mL; Injection: 5 mg/mL.

Onset
Onset: P.O..: 30–60 min; I.M.: 15–30 min; I.V.: 1–5 min. Peak effect: 1–2 hr. P.O.. Duration: 15 min to 1 hr I.V.: up to 3 hr P.O. $t_{1/2}$ 20–50 hr; excreted primarily in urine. Metabolized in liver to active metabolites.

Adverse Effects
Drowsiness, fatigue, ataxia, confusion, paradoxical dizziness, vertigo, amnesia, vivid dreams, headache, slurred speech, tremor, muscle weakness, electroencephalogram changes, tardive dyskinesia, hypotension, tachycardia, edema, cardiovascular collapse, blurred vision, diplopia, nystagmus, xerostomia, nausea, constipation, incontinence, urinary retention, changes in libido.

Precautions and Contraindications
Contraindicated in acute narrow-angle glaucoma, untreated open-angle glaucoma, during or within 14 days of monoamine oxidase inhibitor therapy. Safe use during pregnancy (category D) and lactation not established.

Anesthetic Considerations
Reduces requirements for volatile anesthetics, potential thrombophlebitis with I.V. administration. Decreased clearance and dosage requirements

DRUGS

in old age. Effects antagonized by flumazenil. May cause neonatal hypothermia.

Name
Digoxin (Lanoxin)

Classification
Inotropic agent

Indications
Treatment of supraventricular arrhythmias, heart failure, atrial fibrillation, and flutter

Dose
Adults: Loading: I.V./P.O. 0.5–1 mg in divided doses (give 50% of loading dose as first dose, then 25% fractions at 4–8 hr intervals until adequate therapeutic response is noted, toxic effects occur, or the total digitalizing dose has been administered). Monitor clinical response before each additional dose. Maintenance: I.V./P.O. 0.0625–0.25 mg.; dosages should be individualized. Elderly adults (greater than 65 yr): P.O. 0.125 mg or less daily as maintenance dose. Small patients may require less.

Children (>2 yr): Loading: P.O. 0.02–0.06 mg/kg divided every 8 hr for 24 hr; I.V. 0.015–0.035 mg/kg divided every 8 hr for 24 hr. Maintenance: P.O. 25%–35% of digitalizing dose daily, divided into 2 doses.

Children 1 mo to 2 yr: Loading: P.O. 0.035–0.060 mg/kg in three divided doses over 24 hr; I.V. 0.02–0.05 mg/kg. Maintenance: P.O. 25%–35% of digitalizing dose daily divided every 12 hr.

Neonates under 1 mo: Loading: P.O. 0.025–0.035 mg/kg divided every 8 hr over 24 hr; I.V. 0.015–0.025 mg/kg. Maintenance: P.O. 25%–35% of digitalizing dose daily divided every 12 hr.

Premature infants: Loading: I.V. 0.015–0.025 mg/kg in three divided doses over 24 hr. Maintenance: I.V. 0.01 mg/kg daily divided every 12 hr.

Dosage forms: Tablets: 0.125, 0.25, 0.5 mg; Capsules: (Lanoxicaps) 0.05, 0.1, 0.2 mg; Oral solution: 0.05 mg/mL; Injection: 0.1 mg/mL, 1-mL ampule (100 μg); 0.25 mg/mL, 2 mL ampule (500 μg).

Onset and Duration
Onset: I.V. 5–30 min; P.O. 30 min to 2 hr. Duration: I.V./P.O. 3–4 days.

Adverse Effects
Enhanced toxicity in hypokalemia, hypomagnesemia, hypercalcemia. Wild range of arrhythmias, atrioventricular block, headache, psychosis, confusion, nausea, vomiting, diarrhea, gynecomastia. Overdosage may cause complete heart block, atrioventricular dissociation, tachycardia, fibrillation.

Contraindication
Contraindicated in ventricular fibrillation

Anesthetic Considerations
Decrease dosage in patients with impaired renal function and the elderly. Monitor serum potassium, calcium, and digoxin levels. Use of synchro-

nized cardioversion in patients with digitalis toxicity should be avoided since it may initiate ventricular fibrillation.

Increased serum levels with calcium channel blockers (e.g., verapamil, diltiazem, nifedipine), esmolol, flecainide, captopril, quinidine, amiodarone, benzodiazapines, anticholinergics, oral aminoglycosides, erythromycin. Succinylcholine may cause arrhythmias in digitalized patients. Additive bradycardia may occur with cardiac depressant anesthetics.

Name
Diltiazem (Cardizem)

Classification
Calcium channel blocker

Indications
Angina pectoris; supraventricular tachycardia

Dose
Bolus I.V. 0.25 mg/kg over 2 min. If needed, follow after 15 min with 0.35 mg/kg over 2 min. Maintenance infusion of 5–15 mg/hr. Adults: P.O.: 30 mg t.i.d. or q.i.d. before meals and at bedtime. Dosage may be gradually increased to maximum 360 mg/day in divided doses. Sustained release capsules: 90 mg P.O. b.i.d. titrate dosage to effect (maximum recommended dosage 360 mg/day). Dosage forms: P.O: 30, 60, 90, 120 mg; sustained release 60, 90, 120, 180, 240, 300 mg; I.V. 5 mg/mL, 5-mL and 10-mL vials.

Onset and Duration
Onset: P.O.: 30 min; I.V. 1–3 min. $t_{1/2}$ 3–5 hr.

Adverse Effects
Hypotension, flushing, atrioventricular block, constipation, pruritus, bradycardia, edema, nausea, vomiting, diarrhea, depression, headache, fatigue, dizziness.

Precautions and Contraindications
Hypotension, coadministration with digoxin, beta-blockers, cimetidine. Potentiates cardiovascular depressant effects of volatile, injectable anesthetic agents.

Name
Diphenhydramine (Benadryl)

Classification
Histamine (H_1) antagonist, ethanolamine class

Indications
Adjuvant with epinephrine in the treatment of anaphylactic shock and severe allergic reactions. Treatment of drug-induced extrapyramidal effects, motion sickness. Antiemetic.

DRUGS

Dose

Antihistamine or antiemetic: 10–50 mg I.M. or I.V. every 2–3 hr (maximum dosage 400 mg/day).

Bennett et al. (1987) recommend increasing the dosing interval to every 6–12 hr in patients with moderate renal failure (glomerular filtration rate 10–50 ml/min).

Children: 1–2 mg/kg up to 150 mg/m^2 per day in up to four divided doses by slow I.V. push (3–5 min).

Dosage forms: Injection: 10 mg/mL, 50 mg/1 mL steri-dose syringe or ampule. Capsules: 25, 50 mg. Elixir and syrup 12.5 mg/15 mL.

Onset and Duration

Onset: P.O. 1 hr. Duration 4–6 hr. Elimination $t_{1/2}$ 4–8 hr.

Adverse Effects

Most frequent is sedation. Dizziness, tinnitus, tremors, euphoria, blurred vision, nervousness, palpitations, hypotension, psychotic reactions, hypersensitivity. Other side effects are probably related to the antimuscarinic actions of diphenhydramine and include dry mouth, cough, urinary retention.

Precautions and Contraindications

Diphenhydramine is contraindicated in patients with a hypersensitivity to it and other antihistamines of a similar chemical structure. Antihistamines are contraindicated in patients on monoamine oxidase–inhibitor therapy. Avoid in patients with narrow angle glaucoma.

Anesthetic Considerations

Concurrent central nervous system depressants may produce an additive effect with diphenhydramine.

Name

Dobutamine HCl (Dobutrex)

Classification

Beta$_1$ adrenergic agonist; also mild beta$_2$- and alpha$_1$-receptor agonist

Indications

Vasopressor; positive inotrope

Dose

Infusion: 0.5–30 μg/kg per min. *Note:* Must be diluted, and an I.V. pump (syringe pump in pediatric patients) must be used.

Onset and Duration

Onset: 1–2 min. Duration: <10 min.

Adverse Effects

Hypertension, bradycardia, arrhythmias, angina, shortness of breath, headache, phlebitis at injection site.

Precautions
Arrhythmias and hypertension at high doses; increased risk of dangerous arrhythmias while using volatile agents. Use with caution in patients with idiopathic hypertrophic subaortic stenosis.

Contraindications
Do not mix with sodium bicarbonate, furosemide, or other alkaline solution; correct hypovolemia before or during treatment.

Name
Dopamine HCl (Intropin)

Classification
Naturally occurring catecholamine

Indications
Vasopressor; positive inotrope

Dose
Infusion: 1–5 μg/kg low dose for urinary support; pressor dose range, 5–20 μg/kg; >20 μg/kg for extreme cases. *Note:* Must be diluted, and an I.V. pump must be used.

Onset and Duration
Onset: 2–4 min.
Duration: <10 min.

Adverse Effects
Nausea, vomiting, tachycardia, angina, arrhythmias, dyspnea, headache, anxiety.

Precautions
Correct hypovolemia as quickly as possible before or during treatment.

Anesthetic Considerations
Avoid or use at greatly reduced dose if patient has received a monamine oxidase inhibitor. Infuse into a large vein; extravasation may cause sloughing. Treat extravasation by local infiltration of phentolamine (~1 mg in 10 mL normal saline).

Name
Doxacurium chloride (Nuromax)

Classification
Nondepolarizing skeletal muscle relaxant

Indications
Adjunct to general anesthesia; skeletal muscle relaxation during surgery

Dose
Paralyzing: I.V. 0.05–0.08 mg/kg.
Pretreatment/maintenance: 0.005–0.01 mg/kg.
Dosage form: 1 mg/mL injection.

DRUGS

Onset and Duration
  Onset: <4 min. Duration: 30–160 min. Elimination: renal.

Adverse Effects
  Hypotension, flushing, ventricular fibrillation, myocardial infarction, bronchospasm, hypoventilation, apnea, depression, anuria, rash, urticaria, inadequate block, prolonged block.

Precautions and Contraindications
  Contraindicated in patients with epilepsy, convulsive disorders, mechanical disorders of ventilation, head injuries, cerebrovascular accident, known hypersensitivity to the drug, significant cardiovascular impairment. Airway and oxygenation must be ensured before administration.

Anesthetic Considerations
  Monitor response with peripheral nerve stimulator. Reverse effects with anticholinesterase. Pretreatment may cause hypoventilation in some patients.

Name
  Doxapram HCl (Dopram)

Classification
  Central nervous system agent; respiratory and cerebral stimulant (analeptic)

Indications
  Postanesthesia and drug-induced respiratory depression and to hasten arousal and return of pharyngeal and laryngeal reflexes. Chronic pulmonary disease associated with acute hypercapnia.

Dose
  Slow I.V.: 0.5–1.5 mg/kg, repeat at 5 min (maximum dose 2 mg/kg).
    Infusion: 5 mg/min until satisfactory respiratory response is obtained, then 1–3 mg/min (maximum total dose 4 mg/kg, including bolus and infusion.)

Onset and Duration
  Onset: 20–40 sec. Peak effect: 1–2 min. Duration: 5–12 min.

Adverse Effects
  Hypertension, chest pain, tachycardia, bradycardia, arrhythmias, cough, laryngospasm, bronchospasm, hiccups, seizures, hyperactivity, headaches, urinary retention, spontaneous voiding, nausea, vomiting, desire to defecate, decreased hemoglobin/hematocrit levels and red blood cell count, leukopenia. Delay administration for at least 10 min after discontinuation of volatile anesthetics because of sensitization of catecholamines. Concomitant use of monoamine oxidase inhibitors or other sympathomimetics may potentiate adverse cardiovascular effects.

Precautions and Contraindications
Head trauma, epilepsy or other seizure disorders, mechanical disorders of ventilation. Cerebrovascular accident, significant cardiovascular impairment, severe hypertension, or known hypersensitivity to the drug. Use cautiously in patients with history of severe tachycardia or cardiac arrhythmia, increased cerebrospinal fluid pressure or cerebral edema, pheochromocytoma, or hyperthyroidism or hypermetabolic states.

Name
Edrophonium chloride (Enlon, Reversol, Tensilon)

Classification
Anticholinesterase agent

Indications
Reversal of neuromuscular blockade; diagnostic assessment of myasthenia gravis and supraventricular tachycardia.

Dose
Reversal: slow I.V. 0.5–1.0 mg/kg (maximum dose 40 mg); with atropine (0.007–0.015 mg/kg) administer prior to the endrophonium.
Assessment of myasthenia/cholinergic crisis: slow I.V. 1 mg every 1–2 min until change in symptoms (maximum dose 10 mg). I.M. 10 mg.

Onset and Duration
Onset: I.V. 30–60 sec; I.M. 2–10 min. Duration: I.V. 5–20 min; I.M. 10–40 min.

Adverse Effects
Bradycardia, tachycardia, atrioventricular block, nodal rhythm, hypotension. Increased oral, pharyngeal, and bronchial secretions. Bronchospasm, respiratory depression, seizures, dysarthria, headaches, lacrimation, miosis, visual changes, nausea, emesis, flatulence, increased peristalsis, rash, urticaria, allergic reactions, anaphylaxis.

Precautions and Contraindications
Use with caution in patients with bradycardia, bronchial asthma, cardiac arrhythmias, peptic ulcer, peritonitis, or mechanical obstruction of the intestines or urinary tract.
Overdosage may induce a cholinergic crisis characterized by nausea, vomiting, bradycardia or tachycardia, excessive salivation and sweating, bronchospasm, weakness and paralysis.
Treatment with discontinuation of edrophonium and administration of atropine 10 μg/kg I.V. every 10 min until muscarinic symptoms disappear.
Owing to the brief duration of action of edrophonium, neostigmine or pyridostigmine is generally preferred for reversal of the effects of nondepolarizing muscle relaxants.

Anesthetic Considerations
Administer with anticholinergic to avoid cholinergic side effects (e.g., bronchoconstriction, bradycardia). Excellent alternative for intraopera-

DRUGS

tive hypertension especially in patients taking angiotensin-converting enzyme inhibitors.

Name
Enalaprilat (Vasotec IV)

Classification
Angiotensin converting enzyme (ACE) inhibitor

Indications
Hypertension

Dose
I.V. 0.625–1.25 mg over 5 min. every 6 hr. Dosage forms: 1.25 mg/mL, 1 ml and 2 mL vials.

Onset and Duration
Onset 10–15 min. Duration approximately 6 hr.

Adverse Effects
Cough, hypotension, renal impairment, angiodema

Precautions and Contraindications
Patients on diuretics may have to adjust dose while on ACE inhibitors. Contraindicated during pregnancy.

Anesthetic Considerations
Useful addition to antihypertensive drug choices for perioperative use.

Name
Enflurane (Ethrane)

Classification
Inhalation anesthetic

Indications
General anesthesia

Dose
Titrate to effect for induction or maintenance of anesthesia. Minimum alveolar concentration 1.7% in 100% oxygen and 0.6% in 70% nitrous oxide. Dosage form: Volatile liquid 125, 250 mL.

Onset and Duration
Onset: loss of eyelid reflex 2–3 min. Duration: emergence 15 min.

Adverse Effects
Hypotension, arrhythmia, respiratory depression, apnea, seizures, dizziness, euphoria, increased cerebral blood flow and intracranial pressure,

nausea, vomiting, hepatic dysfunction, renal dysfunction, malignant hyperthermia, glucose elevation.

Precautions and Contraindications

Anesthetic requirements decrease with age. Contraindicated in patients with seizure disorders and known or suspected genetic susceptibility to malignant hyperthermia. Changes in mental function may persist beyond the period of anesthetic administration and the immediate postoperative period.

Anesthetic Considerations

Abrupt onset of malignant hyperthermia may be triggered by enflurane. Early premonitory signs include muscle rigidity, especially of the jaw muscles, tachycardia, and tachypnea unresponsive to increased depth of anesthesia. Crosses the placental barrier.

Name

Ephedrine sulfate

Classification

Noncatecholamine sympathomimetic with mixed direct and indirect actions

Indications

Hypotension, bradycardia

Dose

I.V.: 5–25 mg × 2 (100–300 μg/kg); I.M.: 26–50 mg; P.O.: 25–50 mg every 3 hr.

Onset and Duration

Onset: I.V. almost immediate; I.M.: a few minutes. Duration: I.V.: 10–60 min.

Adverse Effects

Hypertension, tachycardia, arrhythmias, pulmonary edema, anxiety, tremors, hyperglycemia, transient hyperkalemia and then hypokalemia, necrosis at the site of injection. Tolerance may develop.

Contraindications

Use cautiously in patients with hypertension and ischemic heart disease; unpredictable effect in patients in whom endogenous catecholamines are depleted; may produce an unacceptable degree of central nervous system stimulation, resulting in insomnia.

Anesthetic Considerations

Increased risk of arrhythmias with volatile anesthetic agents; potentiated by tricyclic antidepressants; increases the maximum allowable concentration of the volatile anesthetics.

DRUGS

Name
Epinephrine HCl (adrenaline chloride)

Classification
Endogenous catecholamine

Indications
Inotropic support; treatment of anaphylaxis; increase duration of action of local anesthetic; hemostasis; cardiac arrest; bronchodilation

Dose
Cardiac Arrest: 0.5–1.0 mg I.V. bolus every 5 min as necessary. Inotropic Support: 2–20 μg/min (0.1–1.0 μg/kg per min).

Onset and Duration
Onset: I.V.: immediate. Duration: I.V.: 5–10 min.

Adverse Effects
Restlessness, fear, throbbing headache, tachycardia, tachydysrhythmias, premature ventricular contractions, ventricular tachycardia, ventricular fibrillation, severe hypertension, angina, extension of myocardial infarction, pulmonary edema.

Contraindications
Use with caution in patients with coronary artery disease, hypertension, diabetes mellitus, and hyperthyroidism, and in patients taking monoamine oxidase inhibitors.

Anesthetic Considerations
May be administered through the endotracheal tube.

Name
Esmolol (Brevibloc)

Classification
Cardioselective beta-blocker

Indications
Supraventricular tachycardia (SVT); perioperative hypertension

Dose
SVT: Loading: 50–200 μg/kg per min for 1 minute. Follow by infusion of 50 μg/kg per min for 4 minutes. If desired effect not achieved, repeat loading dose and increase infusion to 100 μg/kg per min. May repeat process up to maximum of 300 μg/kg per min. Dosage forms: 10 mg/mL in 10-mL vial for direct I.V. injection. 250 mg/mL in 10-mL ampule for I.V. infusion. **USE ONLY AFTER DILUTION IN LARGE-VOLUME PARENTERAL FLUID TO PREPARE INFUSION.**

Onset and Duration
Onset 1–2 min. Duration 10–20 min. Peak effect: 5–6 min. Not to be infused for more than 48 hr.

Precautions and Contraindications
During pregnancy monitor K$^+$ levels. Use with caution in patients with atrioventricular heart block or cardiac failure not caused by tachycardia, obstructive pulmonary disease, diabetes.

Adverse Effects
Hypotension, bradycardia, congestive heart failure, bronchospasm, confusion, depression, urinary retention, nausea and vomiting, erythema.

Anesthetic Considerations
May have additive cardiovascular depressant effects when coupled with volatile, injectable anesthetic agents. May enhance actions of nondepolarizing neuromuscular blocking agents such as tubocurarine, rocuronium, pancuronium.

Name
Ethacrynic acid (Edecrin)

Classification
Loop diuretic

Indications
Edema of cardiac, hepatic, or renal origin. Hypertension, pulmonary edema. Usually reserved for patients who do not respond to thiazide diuretics or in whom a rapid onset of diuresis is desired.

Dose
0.5–1 mg/kg slowly over several minutes up to a maximum of 100 mg in a single dose. The usual average dose is 50 mg. Children: 1 mg/kg over 20–30 min. Dosage forms: 50 mg vial, powder for injection. reconstitute by adding 50 mL D$_5$W or normal saline. Tablets: 25, 50 mg.

Onset and Duration
Onset: I.V. 5–15 min. Duration: I.V. 2 hr but may last 6–7 hr. Elimination t$_{1/2}$ 1–4 hr.

Adverse Effects
Fluid electrolyte imbalance including: hypomagnesemia, hypocalcemia, hypokalemia, hypochloremia, metabolic alkaloses, hyperuricemia. Hypoglycemia and hyperglycemia, thrombocytopenia, agranulocytopenia, vertigo, ototoxicity (associated with rapid I.V. injection), pancreatitis, gastrointestinal hemorrhage, hepatotoxicity, hypotension, diarrhea.

Precautions and Contraindications
Contraindicated for use in patients once anuric renal failure is established. Also contraindicated in patients with hypotension, dehydration with low

DRUGS

serum sodium or metabolic alkalosis with hypokalemia, nursing mothers, and infants and severe watery diarrhea. Avoid rapid I.V. injection. Use with extreme caution in patients with impaired renal or hepatic function.

Anesthetic Considerations
Loop diuretics have been reported to increase the neuromuscular blocking effect of tubocurarine, probably because of their potassium-depleting effects.

Name
Etidocaine HCl (Duranest)

Classification
Amide-type local anesthetic

Indications
Regional anesthesia: infiltration, peripheral nerve block, epidural, caudal

Dose
Infiltration/peripheral nerve block: 50–400 mg (1% solution); Epidural: 100–300 mg (1% or 1.5% solution); Caudal: 100–300 mg (10–30 mL of 1% solution). Children: 0.4–0.7 ml/kg (for L2–T10 level of anesthesia). (Maximum dose: 3 mg/kg without epinephrine, 4 mg/kg with epinephrine.)

Onset and Duration
Onset: Infiltration: 3–5 min; epidural: 5–15 min. Peak effect: Infiltration: 5–15 min; epidural 15–20 min. Duration: Infiltration: 2–3 hr, 3–7 hr with epinephrine; epidural: 3–5 hr.

Adverse Effects
Myocardial depression, arrhythmias, cardiac arrest, hypotension, respiratory depression, anxiety, apprehension, euphoria, tinnitus, seizures, urticaria, edema, nausea, vomiting. High spinal: loss of bladder and bowel control.

Precautions and Contraindications
Use cautiously in debilitated, elderly, or acutely ill patients, severe shock, heart block, pregnancy. Contraindicated in patients with hypersensitivity to amide-type local anesthetics.

Anesthetic Considerations
Do not use for spinal anesthesia. Owing to profound motor blockade not recommended for epidural anesthesia for delivery. Benzodiazepines increase seizure threshold.

Name
Etomidate (Amidate)

Classification
Central nervous system agent; nonbarbiturate hypnotic without analgesic activity

Indications
Induction of general anesthesia

Dose
Adult I.V. 0.2–0.6 (usual 0.3) mg/kg over 30–60 sec. Dosage forms: Injection 2 mg/mL, ampules and prefilled syringe.

Onset and Duration
Onset 1 min. Duration 3–10 min. Metabolized in liver, $t_{1/2}$ 75 min; excreted primarily in urine.

Adverse Effects
Myoclonus, tonic movements, eye movements, hypertension, hypotension, tachycardia, bradycardia, and other arrhythmias, postoperative nausea and vomiting, hypoventilation, hyperventilation, transient apnea, laryngospasm, hiccups, snoring, adrenocortical suppression.

Precautions and Contraindications
Contraindicated during labor and delivery. Safe use during pregnancy, in nursing women, and in children under 4 years not established. Cautious use in immunosuppression.

Anesthetic Considerations
Use with caution in patients with focal epilepsy. Use large veins. Myoclonus reduced by premedication with benzodiazepine or opioid.

Name
Famotidine (Pepcid)

Classification
Histamine (H_2) antagonist

Indications
Duodenal or gastric ulcers and gastroesophageal reflux. Prophylaxis of aspiration pneumonitis in patients at high risk during surgery.

Dose
Prophylaxis of aspiration pneumonitis: Adults: 20–40 mg P.O. the evening before surgery and/or the morning of surgery before induction of anesthesia. If a more rapid onset is desired, 2 mL of I.V. famotidine (10 mg/mL) may be diluted to a concentration of 5–10 mL with D_5W, normal saline, or lactated Ringer's solution and given over at least 2 min 1 hr prior to induction. Dosage forms: Tablets: 20, 40 mg. Parenteral injection: 10 mg/mL in 2 mL or 4 mL vials.

Onset and Duration
Peak serum levels occur 1–3 hr P.O. Plasma famotidine concentrations that suppress gastric acid secretion by 50% are maintained for 12 hr following an oral dose of 40 mg, and 7–9 hr after a 20 mg dose.

DRUGS

Adverse Effects
Headache (2%–4.5%), constipation (1.4%), and drowsiness were the most frequently reported. Mental confusion occasionally in the elderly. Potential bradydysrhythmias and hypotension may be associated with rapid infusion. Reversible hepatitis and hepatotoxicity infrequent. Reversible leukopenia, thrombocytopenia, granulocytopenia and aplastic anemia rare.

Contraindications
Caution suggested in hepatic or renal dysfunction (possible dose reductions required). Contraindicated in patients with known hypersensitivity to famotidine or other histamine$_2$ antagonists.

Anesthetic Considerations
Use with caution when administering halothane anesthesia (arrhythmogenic). Maximum dose for prolongation of local anesthetics: 250 μg. Safe alternative to gastric prophylaxis preoperatively.

Name
Fentanyl (Sublimaze)

Classification
Opioid agonist

Indications
Produces analgesia and anesthesia

Dose
Analgesia: I.V. 1–2 μg/kg.
Induction 30 μg/kg. Infusion: 0.2 μg/kg per minute; Epidural bolus 1–2 μg/kg. Infusion: 2–60 μg/hr; Spinal bolus: 0.1–0.4 μg/kg. Dosage form: Injection 0.05 mg/mL. Transdermal patch 100 μg/hr. In conjunction with epidural administration, 1–2 μg/kg. For infusion with epidural 2–60 μg/hr. In conjunction with spinal anesthesia: bolus dose of 0.1–0.4 μg/kg.

Onset and Duration
Onset: I.V. within 30 sec; I.M. <8 min; epidural/spinal 4–10 min. Duration: I.V. 30–60 min; I.M. 1–2 hr; epidural/spinal 4–8 hr.

Adverse Effects
Hypotension, bradycardia. Respiratory depression, apnea. Dizziness, blurred vision, seizures. Nausea, emesis, delayed gastric emptying, biliary tract spasm. Muscle rigidity.

Precautions and Contraindications
Reduce doses in elderly, hypovolemic, high-risk patients, and with concomitant use of sedatives and other narcotics. Crosses the placental barrier; may produce depression of respiration in the neonate. Prolonged depression may occur after cessation of transdermal patch use.

Anesthetic Considerations

Narcotic effects reversed by naloxone (0.2–0.4 mg I.V.). Circulatory and ventilatory depressant effects potentiated by narcotics, sedatives, volatile anesthetics, nitrous oxide; ventilatory depressant effects potentiated by amphetamines, monoamine oxidase inhibitors, phenothiazine, and tricyclic antidepressants; analgesia enhanced by alpha$_2$-agonists. Muscle rigidity in higher dose range sufficient to interfere with ventilation.

Name

Flumazenil (Romazicon)

Classification

Benzodiazepine-receptor antagonist

Indications

Reversal of benzodiazepine-receptor agonist

Dose

I.V. 0.2–1 mg (4–20 μg/kg), titrate to patient response, may repeat at 20 min intervals (maximum single dose 1 mg, maximum total dose 3 mg in any one hour). Dosage form: Injection 0.1 mg/mL.

Onset and Duration

Onset: 1–2 min. Duration: 45–90 min (depends on plasma concentration of benzodiazepine).

Adverse Effects

Arrhythmia, tachycardia, bradycardia, hypertension, angina, flushing, reversal of sedation, seizures, agitation, emotional lability, nausea, vomiting, pain at injection site, thrombophlebitis.

Precautions and Contraindications

Institute measures to secure airway, ventilation, and I.V. access prior to administering flumazenil. Resedation may occur and is more common with large doses of benzodiazepine.

Anesthetic Considerations

Do not use until the effects of neuromuscular blockade have been fully reversed. Administer in a large vein to minimize pain at injection site. Monitor for resedation.

Name

Furosemide (Lasix)

Classification

Loop diuretic

Indications

Edema of cardiac, hepatic or renal origin. Hypertension, pulmonary edema. Usually reserved for patients who do not respond to thiazide diuretics or in whom a rapid onset of diuresis is desired.

DRUGS

Dose

Diuresis: Adult: I.M. or I.V. 20–40 mg as a single dose. IV doses should be injected slowly over 1–2 min. Additional doses of 20 mg greater than the previous dose may be given every 2 hr until desired response is obtained. For I.V. bolus injections do not exceed 1 g/day given over 30 min. Acute pulmonary edema: 40 mg I.V. initially, may repeat in 1 hr with 80 mg if necessary. Children: I.M. or I.V. 1 mg/kg single dose initially, increasing by 1 mg/kg every 2 or more hr until desired response is obtained or to a maximum of 6 mg/kg per day. Dosage forms: Tablets: 20, 40, 80 mg; Injection 10 mg/mL. Oral solutions 10 mg/mL and 40 mg/5 mL.

Onset and Duration

Onset of diuresis usually occurs 5 min I.V. Duration 2 hr. Elimination $t_{1/2}$ widely variable; normal is ½–1 hr but 11–20 hr has been reported in patients with hepatic or renal insufficiency.

Adverse Effects

Dehydration, hypotension, hypochloremic alkalosis, hypokalemia, hypomagnesemia, hyperglycemia, hyperuricemia. Ototoxicity has been reported with too rapid I.V. injection of large doses. Rarely thrombocytopenia, neutropenia, jaundice, pancreatitis, and a variety of skin reactions.

Precautions and Contraindications

Contraindicated in anuria (except for single dose in acute anuria) and pregnancy. Use with caution in patients with severe or progressive renal disease and hepatic disease. Discontinue if renal function worsens. Caution should be used in patients allergic to sulfonamides, and with severe electrolyte imbalance.

Anesthetic Considerations

Monitor electrolytes and fluid balance. Administer carefully in patients taking digitalis. May be associated with enhancement of nondepolarizing neuromuscular blocking drugs.

Name

Glucagon

Classification

Hormone; antidiabetic agent (antihypoglycemic); diagnostic agent

Indications

Treatment of hypoglycemia or beta-blocker overdose; inotropic agent used to relax smooth muscle of gastrointestinal tract for radiologic studies

Dose

Diagnostic aid for radiologic exam: I.V./I.M. 0.25–2 mg before initiation of radiologic procedure. Hypoglycemia: I.V./I.M. SQ: 0.5–1 mg.

Onset and Duration

Onset: <5 min. Peak effect: 5–20 min. Duration: 10–30 min. Hypertension, hypotension, respiratory distress, dizziness, lightheadedness, nausea, vomiting, urticaria, hypoglycemia, hyperglycemia.

Precautions and Contraindications

Hypersensitivity to drug (due to its protein nature). Use cautiously in patients with history of insulinoma or pheochromocytoma. Safe use during pregnancy and in nursing women has not been established.

Anesthetic Considerations

Rapid I.V. administration may cause decrease in blood pressure. Potentiates hypoprothrombinemic effects of anticoagulants. Parenteral glucose must be given because release of insulin may subsequently cause hypoglycemia.

Name

Glycopyrrolate (Robinul)

Classification

Competitive acetylcholine antagonist at muscarinic receptor

Indications

Vagolytic premedication to block bradycardia during surgery from stimulation of the carotid sinus, traction on abdominal viscera, or extraocular muscles. Blockade of muscarinic effects of anticholinesterases. Adjunctive therapy in the treatment of bronchospasm and peptic ulcer disease. Compared with atropine, glycopyrrolate has two times more potent antisialogue activity, less tachycardia and no clinically significant increases in intraocular pressure at doses used preoperatively. It has no sedative effects.

Dose

Adults: Premedication/vagolysis: I.V., I.M., SQ 0.1 to 0.2 mg (4–6 μg/kg) administered 30–60 min preinduction. May repeat in 2–3 min intervals for vagolysis up to 1.0 mg total. Blockade of muscarinic effects of anticholinesterase: 0.2 mg for each 1 mg of neostigmine or 5 mg of pyridostigmine. Bronchospasm: inhalation 0.4 to 0.8 mg every 8 hr. Dilute injectate solution in 2 to 3 mL normal saline and deliver by compressed air nebulizer. Children: Preoperative 2 yrs or older: 4 μg/kg. For oral administration, use injectable solution and dilute in 3–5 mL juice or carbonated cola beverage. Oral absorption is erratic. Intraoperative vagolysis: 0.01 mg/kg I.V. not to exceed 0.1 mg, may repeat in 2–3 min. Dosage forms: Injection: 0.2 mg/mL. Tablets: 1, 2 mg.

Onset and Duration

Onset after P.O., I.M./S.Q., inhalation, and I.V. administration is 1 hr, 15–30 min, 3–5 min, and <1 min, respectively. Duration of antisialogue effect is 7–12 hr depending on route of administration and dose. Duration of vagal blockade is 2–3 hr I.V.; 8–12 hr P.O.

DRUGS

Adverse Effects

Tachycardia (high doses), bradycardia (low doses), headache, urinary hesitancy, retention, mydriasis, blurred vision, increased intraocular pressure, decreased sweating, excitement, agitation, drowsiness, confusion, dry nose and mouth, allergic reactions, constipation.

Precautions and Contraindications

Avoid where tachycardia would be harmful, i.e., thyrotoxicosis, pheochromocytoma, or coronary artery disease. Avoid in hyperpyrexial states because it inhibits sweating. Contraindicated in acute-angle glaucoma, obstructive disease of the gastrointestinal tract, obstructive uropathy, paralytic ileus, intestinal atony, and acute hemorrhage where cardiovascular status is unstable. Use with caution in patients with hepatic or renal disease, congestive heart failure, chronic pulmonary disease (since a reduction in bronchial secretions may lead to formation of bronchial plugs), hiatal hernia, gastroesophageal reflux, gastrointestinal infections, ulcerative colitis.

Anesthetic Considerations

Additive anticholinergic effects may occur with meperidine, some antihistamines, phenothiazines, tricyclic antidepressants, and antiarrhythmic drugs that possess anticholinergic activity (e.g., quinidine, disopyramide, procainamide).

Name

Granisetron (Kytril)

Classification

Selective serotonin receptor antagonist

Indications

Effective single agent used to control nausea and vomiting induced by cisplatin and other cytotoxic agents

Dose

Prophylaxis of chemotherapy-induced nausea and vomiting: 40 μg/kg or 3 mg as a single I.V. infusion over 5 min to 1 hr completed 30 min before the chemotherapy is implemented. Breakthrough nausea and vomiting during the first 24 hr following therapy: two to three repeat I.V. infusions of 40 μg/kg over 5 min with each separated by at least 10 min. Dilute with 20–50 mL 5% dextrose or 0.9% sodium chloride. P.O.: 1 mg twice daily. Pediatric: 10 μg/kg in children 2–16 yr old. Granisetron has not been studied in children less than 2 yr of age.

Onset and Duration

Peak plasma concentrations demonstrate wide interindividual variation. After a 40 μg/kg dose, nausea and vomiting subsides within several minutes. Serum levels decline to less than 10 ng/mL at 24 hr following a single 40 μg/kg infusion. Antiemetic effects last up to 24 hr following I.V. infusion of 40 μg/kg. Elimination $t_{1/2}$ 10 to 11 hr.

Adverse Effects

Headache and constipation are most common. Somnolence, dizziness, diarrhea, flushing, transient elevation of liver enzymes.

Precautions and Contraindications

Previous hypersensitivity to granisetron, liver disease (due to the noted elevation of liver enzymes after repeat administration of granisetron), pregnancy, or breastfeeding.

Anesthetic Considerations

Owing to the elevation of liver enzymes after repeat doses of granisetron, careful preoperative evaluation of liver function tests is necessary to aid in determining if anesthetic agents excreted hepatically should be avoided. Injection should not be mixed in solution with other drugs. No specific antidote for overdose; give symptomatic treatment. Inducers or inhibitors of cytochrome P 450 drug-metabolizing enzymes may change the clearance and duration of granisetron.

Name

Halothane (Fluothane)

Classification

Potent inhalation anesthetic agent

Indications

Induction and maintenance of general anesthesia

Dose

Induction: 1%–4%. Maintenance: 0.5%–1.5%. Supplied: Glass bottle, volatile liquid.

Onset and Duration

Onset: 5–10 min to achieve surgical anesthesia. Duration: up to 1 hr after discontinuation. Dose-dependent; rapid, pleasant induction and smooth.

Adverse Effects

Hypotension, shallow and rapid respiration, arrhythmia (when sympathomimetic agents are used), vomiting, hypoxia, respiratory difficulty, postoperative shivering, liver damage, bradycardia, increased intracranial pressure, malignant hyperthermia.

Precautions and Contraindications

Arrhythmia may be produced by the combination of halothane and catecholamines. May potentiate effects of nondepolarizing muscle relaxants. Avoid second-time use in individuals who show evidence of liver damage. Halothane has been associated with liver dysfunction (hepatitis, jaundice), especially in persons with prior hepatic disease or previous exposure to halothane. Changes in mental function may persist beyond the period of anesthetic administration and the immediate postoperative period.

DRUGS

Anesthetic Considerations
Use cautiously in patients with severe cardiac disease and during pregnancy (drug is a potent uterine relaxant). Have drugs on hand to treat bradycardia and hypotension. Keep patient warm postoperatively to minimize shivering.

Name
Heparin (Liquaemin Sodium, Panheparin)

Classification
Anticoagulant: accelerates the rate at which antithrombin III neutralizes thrombin and factors VII, IX, X, XI

Indications
Prophylaxis and treatment of deep venous thrombosis (DVT) and pulmonary thromboembolism (PE). Acute arterial occlusion, intracardiac mural thrombosis, following myocardial infarction after I.V. thrombolytic treatment, disseminated intravascular coagulation with gross thrombosis, anticoagulation during cardiopulmonary bypass (CPB), prophylaxis of thromboembolism in patients with mitral valve disease or atrial fibrillation. Maintain patency of in-dwelling venipuncture devices (lock flush). Value in cerebral embolism secondary to transient ischemic attacks has not been established.

Dose
Dosage highly individualized, based on daily activated partial thromboplastin time (aPTT) compared with 6 hr after each dosage change. Obtain baseline aPTT and adjust dose according to clinical state. For prophylaxis (i.e., hip surgery, atrial fibrillation, valve disease): the ratio of aPTT to baseline aPTT should be 1.2–1.5; for prosthetic heart valves, DVT, PE, recurrent embolism: 1.5–2.0. For cardiopulmonary bypass, monitor activated clotting time (ACT) and maintain ACT of 400–480 sec. Baseline ACT values are 80–150 sec. ACT should be determined 5 min after heparin administration. Adequate heparinization must be ensured prior to initiation of CPB.

Dosing guidelines: Cardiopulmonary bypass: prior to induction of anesthesia. 300 units/kg of heparin should be prepared in case emergency initiation of CPB is necessary. I.V. bolus 350–400 units/kg. Up to 500 units/kg may be required to maintain ACT >400 sec in heparin-resistant patients. Additional heparin will be needed for prolonged CPB. A 100 unit/kg hourly reinforcement dose is given starting 2 hr after the initial dose. Prophylactic or low dose subcutaneous therapy: 5000 units SQ every 8–12 hr. Baseline aPTT is obtained since bleeding complications are occasionally discovered but routine PTT monitoring is not necessary. For surgical prophylaxis, ideally started 2 hr preoperatively. Full dose continuous I.V. infusion for treatment of DVT or PE is based on ideal body weight.: I.V. bolus loading dose 70 units/kg (3000–10,000 units); I.V. maintenance dose continuous infusion 13–16 units/kg/hr (750–1300 units/hr). For continuous I.V. infusion, 25,000 units heparin may be mixed in 500 mL D$_5$W or normal saline. The resulting solution is 50 units/mL. Dosage forms: Injection: 1000, 2500, 5000, 7500, 10,000, 20,000, and 40,000 units/mL. Lock flush solution: 10, 100 units/mL. Premixed infusion in dextrose: 50 units/mL. Premixed infusion in normal saline: 50, 100 units/mL.

Onset and Duration
Onset immediate or 20–30 min I.V. or SQ, respectively. $t_{1/2}$ 1–2 hr in healthy adults. Half-life and duration increase with increasing doses; prolonged in liver and renal disease.

Adverse Effects
Hemorrhage, thrombocytopenia, white clot syndrome (rare paradoxical thrombosis), necrotizing skin lesions, elevated liver enzymes, osteoporosis, priapism, hypersensitivity.

Precautions and Contraindications
Avoid I.M. injections. Contraindicated in patients with hemophilia, thrombocytopenia, acute bleeding, peptic ulcer, esophagitis, diverticulitis, esophageal varices, arterial aneurysm, gastrointestinal or urinary tract malignancy, vascular retinopathy, recent liver or renal biopsy, acute pericarditis, threatened abortion, infective endocarditis, recent surgery or trauma to brain, eye, or spinal cord, recent regional anesthesia, severe hypertension, recent cerebrovascular accident, recent surgery.

Platelet counts, hematocrit, and occult blood in stool and urine should be monitored during entire course of therapy. Increased risk of bleeding with concomitant aspirin, nonsteroidal anti-inflammatory drugs, dipyridamole, thrombolytic agents, dextran, dihydroergotamine, warfarin. I.V. nitroglycerin may antagonize the effects of heparin, and should be administered via a separate line if possible. Digoxin, nicotine, propranolol, antihistamines, and tetracycline may reduce heparin's effects.

Bleeding and heparin overdosage may be treated with protamine sulfate. 1 mg protamine neutralizes 100 units heparin.

Anesthetic Considerations
Regional anesthesia is contraindicated. Heparin continuous I.V. infusion should be discontinued 4–6 hr preoperatively and aPTT checked to ensure return to baseline.

Name
Hetastarch (Hespan)

Classification
Plasma expander

Indications
Adjunct for plasma volume expansion in shock due to hemorrhage, burns, sepsis, surgery, or other trauma.

Dose
Plasma volume expansion from 500 to 1000 mL. Total dosage does not usually exceed 1500 mL/day (20 mL/kg per day). In acute hemorrhagic

shock, rates approaching 20 mL/kg per hr have been used. Dosage forms: 6% solution in 0.9% sodium chloride, 500-mL I.V. infusion bottle.

Onset and Duration
Average half-life: 17 days

Adverse Effects
Anaphylactic reactions (periorbital edema, urticaria, wheezing) have been reported. Peripheral edema of the lower extremities, chills, mild temperature elevation, muscle pain. Large volumes may alter coagulation times and result in transient prolongation of prothrombin time, partial thromboplastin time, bleeding, decreased hematocrit, and excessive dilution of plasma proteins.

Precautions and Contraindications
Contraindicated in patients with severe bleeding disorders, severe cardiac failure, renal failure with oliguria or anuria. Hetastarch does not have oxygen-carrying capacity, nor does it contain plasma proteins such as coagulation factors. Therefore, it is not a substitute for blood or plasma.

Anesthetic Considerations
Infuse slowly to avoid volume overload. Check coagulation profile.

Name
Hyaluronidase (Wydase)

Classification
Enzyme

Indications
Adjunct to increase absorption and dispersion of other injected drugs; hypodermoclysis; subcutaneous urography.

Dose
Adjunct: 150 units to injection medium containing other medication. Hypodermoclysis (adults and children >3 yr of age): 150 units injected SQ before clysis or injected into clysis tubing near needle for each 1000-mL clysis solution. Subcutaneous urography (patient prone): 75 units SQ over each scapula, followed by injection of contrast medium at same sites.

Onset and Duration
Onset: immediate. Duration: 30–60 min.

Adverse Effects
Rash, urticaria, local irritation

Precautions and Contraindications
Use with caution in patients with blood-clotting abnormalities or severe hepatic or renal disease. Avoid injecting into diseased areas in order to prevent spread of infection.

Name
Hydralazine (Apresoline)

Classification
Direct-acting arterial vasodilator

Indications
Antihypertensive; treatment of congestive heart failure

Dose
I.V. and I.M.: 2.5–40 mg (0.1–0.2 mg/kg); P.O.: 10–100 mg q.i.d. Dosage forms: Injection 20 mg/mL; Tablets 10, 25, 50, and 100 mg

Onset and Duration
Onset: I.V. 5–20 min; I.M. 10–30 min; P.O. 30–120 min. Duration: I.V. 2–4 hr; I.M./P.O. 2–8 hr.

Adverse Effects
Hypotension, paradoxical pressor response, tachycardia, palpitations, angina, dyspnea, nasal congestion, peripheral neuritis, depression, anxiety, headache, dizziness, nausea, vomiting, diarrhea, lupus-like syndrome, rash, urticaria, eosinophilia, hypersensitivity, leukopenia, splenomegaly, agranulocytosis.

Contraindications
Use cautiously in patients with coronary artery disease, mitral valvular rheumatic heart disease, and patients receiving monoamine oxidase inhibitors.

Anesthetic Considerations
May see reduced response to epinephrine. Enhanced hypotensive effects in patients receiving diuretics, monoamine oxidase inhibitors, diazoxide, and other antihypertensives.

Name
Hydrocortisone sodium succinate (A-Hydrocort, Solu-Cortef)

Classification
Corticosteroid (glucocorticoid and mineralocorticoid properties)

Indications
Treatment of choice for steroid replacement therapy. Also used as antiinflammatory and immunosuppressive; however, glucocorticoids (prednisone) are preferred for this use. Adjunctive therapy in anaphylaxis to prevent prolonged antigen–antibody reactions. Adjunctive treatment of ulcerative colitis (enema).

Dose
Adults:
Shock: 500 mg to 2 g (succinate) I.V. every 2–6 hr until condition stabilized. Not recommended beyond 48–72 hr. Adjunctive therapy in

DRUGS

anaphylaxis: hydrocortisone phosphate or succinate I.V. 5 mg/kg initially, then 2.5 mg/kg every 6 hr. Adrenal insufficiency: Acute adrenal insufficiency–precipitated trauma or surgical stress: if adrenocorticotropic hormone testing is not being performed, 200–300 mg I.V. hydrocortisone succinate over several minutes. Then 100 mg I.V. every 6 hr for 24 hr; if the patient is stable, dosage tapering may begin on the second day. Consider steroid replacement in any patient who has received corticosteroid therapy for at least 1 mo in the past 6–12 mo, with 50–100 mg I.V. (succinate) before, during, and after surgery. For intra-articular, soft tissue, intrasynovial injections, use acetate only (acetate is not for I.V. use) 10–50 mg combined with local anesthetic such as procaine. Injections may be repeated every 3–5 days (for bursae) to once every 1–4 wk (for joints). Children: 0.16–1 mg/kg or 6–30 mg/m^2 (phosphate or succinate) I.M. or I.V. one or two times daily. Dose depends on the disease being treated.

Onset and Duration

Onset: I.V. or I.M. 5 min.

Duration approximates duration of hypothalamus–pituitary–adrenal axis suppression (i.e., 30–36 hr); after a single oral dose of hydrocortisone this is 1.25–1.5 days.

Plasma half-life is 1.5 hr.

Adverse Effects

Glaucoma and cataracts with long-term therapy. Muscle weakness, sodium retention, edema, hypokalemic alkalosis, hyperglycemia, Cushing's syndrome, peptic ulcer, increased appetite, delayed wound healing, psychotic behavior, congestive heart failure, hypertension, growth suppression, pancreatitis.

Acute adrenal insufficiency may occur with abrupt withdrawal after long-term therapy. Withdrawal symptoms: rebound inflammation, fatigue, weakness, arthralgia, fever, dizziness, lethargy, depression, orthostatic hypotension, dyspnea, anorexia, hypoglycemia.

Precautions and Contraindications

Contraindicated in systemic fungal infections. May mask or exacerbate infections. Use with caution in patients with ocular herpes simplex, history of peptic ulcer disease. In patients with myasthenia gravis, hydrocortisone interacts with anticholinesterase agents to produce severe weakness.

Anesthetic Considerations

Barbiturates may increase glucocorticoid metabolism, and a hydrocortisone dosage increase may be indicated.

Hypotension from stress of anesthesia and surgery may occur if regular doses of steroids were taken within 2 mo preceding surgery. Supplemental steroids are indicated commencing with preoperative dose and continuing for 3 days if major surgery, or for 24 hr if minor surgery and one dose for a very brief procedure, then taper to normal therapy.

Owing to adrenal suppression etomidate should be avoided in patients with adrenal insufficiency.

Name
Insulin regular (rapid-acting)(Humulin R, Novolin R, Regular Iletin II)

Classification
Antidiabetic agent

Indications
Diabetic ketoacidosis, treatment of diabetes mellitus, hyperkalemia

Dose
Diabetes mellitus: in general, therapy is initiated with regular insulin SQ 5–10 units in adults and 2–4 units in children 15–30 min before meals and at bedtime. Dose and frequency carefully individualized based on every 4–6 hour blood sugar monitoring. After satisfactory control is achieved, an intermediate form of insulin may be substituted; this is given before breakfast in a dose approximately two thirds to three fourths that of the previous total daily dose established for regular insulin.

Perioperative management of insulin-dependent diabetics: half the usual NPH-isophane insulin dose the morning of the day of surgery. It is critical for the patient who is receiving nothing orally and receiving insulin also to receive an I.V. infusion of dextrose 5–10 g/hr (equal to 100–200 mL of a 5% dextrose solution) to prevent hypoglycemia.

Postoperative: sliding scale every 4–6 hr. Individualize to patient.

Blood Sugar	Insulin Regular
<200 mg/dL	0 units
200–250 mg/dL	5 units SQ
250–300 mg/dL	10 units SQ
300–350 mg/dL	15 units SQ

If blood sugar is >350 mg/dL, give Insulin regular 15 units SQ plus I.V. 1–2 units/hr. Monitor blood glucose hourly. Correct electrolyte imbalances (hypokalemia, hypophosphatemia) and acidosis.

DRUGS

Diabetic ketoacidosis: requires insulin by continuous infusion, hourly blood sugar determination, and correction of acidosis, dehydration, and electrolyte imbalances. After renal function is established, potassium replacement therapy may be needed.

Dosage form: Injection: 100 units/mL. U-500 Insulin (500 units/mL) is available but should be used only to fill implanted insulin pumps. It should never be stocked outside the pharmacy.

Onset and Duration

	Onset (hr)	Peak (hr)	Duration (hr)
Regular (rapid) insulin	0.5–1	1–5	5–8
Intermediate insulins	1–4	4–12	24–28

$t_{1/2}$ regular insulin 4–5 min I.V.

Adverse Effects

Dose-related hypoglycemia. Local allergic reactions, lipoatrophy, and resistance may be overcome by switching to more highly purified sources. In general, human insulin is least antigenic and pork is less antigenic than beef–pork or pure beef. Anaphylaxis. Hyperglycemia (rebound or Somogyi effect).

Precautions and Contraindications

Diabetic ketoacidosis is a life-threatening condition requiring prompt diagnosis and treatment.

Change in purity, stength, brand, type, or species source may result in the need for a change in dosage.

Treat hypoglycemia with 0.6 mL/kg 50% dextrose I.V.

Hypersensitivity may occur.

Insulin requirements may increase dramatically with stress, sepsis, trauma, or pregnancy.

Only Regular Insulins (clear insulins) may be administered I.V. Intermediate insulins may **only** be given SQ.

Hypoglycemic action increased by concomitant administration of alcohol, beta-blockers, monoamine oxidase inhibitors, salicylates, sulfonyl ureas.

Hypoglycemic action decreased by thyroid hormones, corticosteroids, dobutamine, epinephrine, furosemide, phenytoin.

Anesthetic Considerations

Blood sugar levels of 120–180 mg/dL should be sought and blood sugar should be monitored frequently intraoperatively. If it is necessary to administer insulin intraoperatively, continuous I.V. infusion may be the best method. If given subcutaneously, variability of skin blood flow during anesthesia may cause unpredictable results.

Large I.V. boluses of insulin can put the patient at risk for dysrhythmias caused by intracellular shifts of potassium, phosphorus, and magnesium.

Name
Isoflurane (Forane)

Classification
Inhalation anesthetic

Indications
General anesthesia

Dose
Titrate to effect for induction or maintenance of anesthesia. Minimum alveolar concentration (MAC) 1.14%. Dosage form: Volatile liquid, 100 mL.

Onset and Duration
Onset: few minutes, dose-dependent. Duration: emergence time 15 min.

Adverse Effects
Hypotension, tachycardia, arrhythmia, coronary-artery steal, respiratory depression, apnea, dizziness, euphoria, increased cerebral blood flow and intracranial pressure, nausea, vomiting, ileus, hepatic dysfunction, malignant hyperthermia, glucose elevation.

Precautions and Contraindications
Contraindicated in patients with known or suspected genetic susceptibility to malignant hyperthermia. Changes in mental function may persist beyond the period of anesthetic administration and the immediate postoperative period.

Anesthetic Considerations
Anesthetic requirements decease with age. Crosses the placental barrier. Abrupt onset of malignant hyperthermia may be triggered by isoflurane; early signs include muscle rigidity, especially of the jaw muscles, tachycardia and tachypnea unresponsive to increased depth of anesthesia caused by digitalis intoxication. Arrhythmias with concomitant use of volatile anesthetics and other sympathomimetics.

Name
Isoproterenol HCl (Isuprel)

Classification
Synthetic sympathomimetic, almost exclusively beta

Dose
I.M./SQ: 0.2 mg; IV: 0.02–0.06 mg; Infusion: 2–20 μg/min; Sublingual: 10 mg; 10–50 mg p.r.n.

Onset and Duration
Onset: I.V.: immediately; Sublingual: 15–30 min. Duration: I.V.: 1–5 min; Sublingual: 1–2 hr.

Adverse Effects

Tachyarrhythmias, hypertension, angina, paradoxical precipitation of Adams-Stokes attacks, pulmonary edema, headache, dizziness, tremors, nausea, vomiting, anorexia; may exacerbate ischemia and/or hypertension when used for chronotropic support.

Precautions and Contraindications

In patients with tachyarrhythmias, tachycardia, or heart block

Name

Ketamine HCl (Ketalar)

Classification

Central nervous system agent; general anesthetic

Indications

Sole anesthetic agent for diagnostic and surgical procedures for short duration. Induction of anesthesia before administration of other general anesthetics.

Dose

Induction: Adult: I.V. 1–4.5 mg/kg slowly over 60 sec.
I.M. 6–12 mg/kg.
Half of initial dose may be repeated as needed.
Dosage form: Injection 10, 50, 100 mg/mL.

Onset and Duration

Onset: 30 sec I.V.; 3–8 min I.M. Duration: 5–10 min I.V.; 12–25 min I.M.

Adverse Effects

Hypertension, tachycardia, hypotension, arrhythmia, bradycardia, respiratory depression, apnea, laryngospasm, tonic or clonic movements, emergence delirium, hypersalivation, nausea, vomiting, diplopia, nystagmus, slight elevation in intraocular tension. Serious emergence reactions.

Precautions and Contraindications

Contraindicated in hypertension, coronary heart disease, or cardiac hypertension, increased intracranial pressure, history of cerebrovascular accident, increased intraocular pressure, psychiatric disorders; for surgery or diagnostic procedures of pharynx, larynx, and bronchial tree. Safe use during pregnancy including obstetrics not established. Cautious use in convulsive disorders.

Anesthetic Considerations

Do not mix with barbiturates in same syringe. Emergence reactions are common in adults with high doses and are reduced by premedication with benzodiazepine. Catecholamine-depleted patients may respond to ketamine with unexpected reductions in blood pressure and cardiac output.

Name
Ketorolac tromethamine (Toradol)

Classification
Nonsteroidal anti-inflammatory

Indications

Short-term (<5 days) management of moderately severe, acute pain that requires analgesia. Generally used in a postoperative setting. Patients should be switched to alternative analgesics as soon as possible. Ketorolac therapy is not to exceed 5 days because of the potential for increased frequency and severity of adverse reactions.

The combined duration of use of Ketorolac I.V./I.M. and P.O. is not to exceed 5 days. Ketorolac P.O. is indicated only as continuation therapy to Ketorolac I.V./I.M.

Dose

I.M.: (**give slowly** and deeply into the muscle)
Patients <65 yr: One dose of 60 mg;
Patients >65 yr, renal-impaired, and/or less than 50 kg: One dose of 30 mg.
I.V.: I.V. bolus over no less than 15 sec
Patients <65 yr: One dose of 30 mg;
Patients >65 yr, renal-impaired, and/or less than 50 kg: One dose of 15 mg.
Multiple-dose treatment (I.V. or SQ):
Patients <65 yr: 30 mg every 6 hr not to exceed 120 mg per day;
Patients >65 yr, renal-impaired, and/or less than 50: 15 mg every 6 hr not to exceed 60 mg per day.

Onset and Duration

Onset: 30 min with maximum effect in 1–2 hr I.V. or I.M. Duration: 4–6 hr.

Adverse Effects

Gastrointestinal: Peptic ulcers, gastrointestinal bleeding, and/or perforation. Renal: Ketorolac and its metabolites are eliminated primarily by the kidneys, which, in patients with reduced creatinine clearance, will result in diminished clearance of the drug. Renal toxicity with ketorolac has been seen in patients with conditions leading to a reduction in blood volume and/or renal blood flow, where renal prostaglandins have a supportive role in the maintenance of renal perfusion. In these patients, administration of ketorolac may cause a dose-dependent reduction in renal prostaglandin formation and may precipitate acute renal failure. Risk of bleeding: ketorolac inhibits platelet function. Hypersensitivity reactions ranging from bronchospasm to anaphylactic shock have occurred, and appropriate counteractive measures must be available when administering the first dose.

DRUGS

Precautions and Contraindications

Fluid retention, edema, retention of sodium, oliguria, elevations of serum urea nitrogen and creatinine have been reported. Therefore, ketorolac should be used only with caution in patients with cardiac decompensation, hypertension, or similar conditions. Ketorolac is contraindicated in patients with active peptic ulcer disease, recent gastrointestinal bleeding or perforation, or in patients with a history of peptic ulcer disease or gastrointestinal bleeding. Ketorolac is contraindicated in patients with advanced renal impairment and in patients at risk for renal failure due to volume depletion. Contraindicated in patients with suspected or confirmed cerebrovascular bleeding, patients with hemorrhagic diathesis, incomplete hemostasis, and those at high risk of bleeding. Ketorolac is contraindicated as a prophylactic analgesic before any major surgery, and is contraindicated intraoperatively when hemostasis is critical. Ketorolac is contraindicated in patients with previously demonstrated hypersensitivity to ketorolac tromethamine or allergic manifestations to aspirin (ASA) or other nonsteroidal anti-inflammatory drugs (NSAIDs) Contraindicated for intrathecal or epidural administration owing to its alcohol content. Contraindicated in labor and delivery because it may adversely affect fetal circulation and inhibit uterine contractions. Because of the potential adverse effects of prostaglandin-inhibiting drugs on neonates, ketorolac is contraindicated in nursing mothers. Contraindicated in patients currently receiving ASA or NSAIDs because of the cumulative risk of inducing serious NSAID-related side effects.

Anesthetic Considerations

Do not use as prophylactic analgesia before any major surgery or intraoperatively when hemostasis is critical, in patients with suspected or confirmed cerebrovascular bleeding, hemorrhagic diathesis, incomplete hemostasis, and at high risk of bleeding, in patients currently receiving ASA or NSAIDs, for epidural or intrathecal administration, concomitantly with probenecid.

Use of ketorolac is not recommended in children.

Ketorolac reduced the diuretic response to furosemide in normovolemic healthy subjects by approximately 20%. Hypovolemia should be corrected before treatment with ketorolac is initiated. Ketorolac possesses no sedative or anxiolytic properties. Concomitant use with opiate-agonist analgesics can result in reduced opiate analgesic requirements. Ketorolac is highly bound to human plasma protein (99.2%)

Name

Labetalol (Normodyne, Trandate)

Classification

Adrenergic antagonist

Indications

Hypertension

Dose

I.V. bolus: 0.15–0.25 mg/kg given over 2 min, may repeat every 10 min up to 300 mg. Continuous infusion: 2 mg/min; titrate to effect P.O.:

100 mg b.i.d. alone or with diuretic. May increase to 200 mg b.i.d. after 2 days. Further dose increase may be made every 1 to 3 days to maximal response. Maintenance dose: 200–400 mg b.i.d.

Onset and Duration
Onset: I.V.: 1–3 min; P.O.: 20–40 min. Duration: I.V.: 0.25–2 hr; P.O.: 4–12 hr.

Precautions and Contraindications
Contraindicated in bronchial asthma, overt heart failure, greater than first-degree heart block, hepatic failure. Cautious use in chronic bronchitis, emphysema, pre-existing peripheral vascular disease, pheochromocytoma, and diabetes.

Adverse Effects
Hypotension, bradycardia, ventricular arrhythmias, congestive heart failure, chest pain, bronchospasm, headache, diarrhea, systemic lupus erythematosus

Anesthetic Considerations
Inhalation anesthetics may enhance hypotensive effects.

Name
Lidocaine HCl (Xylocaine, Xylocaine jelly, Xylocaine viscous oral solution)

Classification
Amide-type local anesthetic; topical anesthetic; antiarrhythmic agent

Indications
Regional anesthesia; topical anesthesia; treatment of ventricular arrhythmias; attenuation of sympathetic response to laryngoscopy/intubation

Dose
Caudal or epidural: 20–30 mL 1% solution (200–300 mg). May also use 1.5% and 2.0% solutions. (maximum dose 200–300 mg/hr [4.5 mg/kg]). With epinephrine for anesthesia other than spinal, maximum safe dose is 500 mg (7 mg/kg.)

Spinal: 1.5–2 mL 5% solution with 7.5% dextrose (75–100 mg).

Antiarrhythmic: Slow I.V. bolus 1 mg/kg (1–2% solution) followed by 0.5 mg/kg every 2–5 min (to maximum dose of 3 mg/kg per hr). Infusion (0.1% solution) 1–4 mg/min (20–50 μg/kg per min). Use only preservative-free forms for I.V.

Local anesthesia: Topical: 0.6–3 mg/kg (2–4% solution). Infiltration/peripheral nerve block: 0.5–5 mg/kg (0.5–2% solution). Transtracheal: 80–120 mg (2–3 mL of 4% solution). Superior laryngeal nerve: 40–60 mg (2–3 mL of 2% solution on each side). Stellate ganglion: 50 mg (5 mL of 1% solution). I.V. regional: Upper extremity: 200–250 mg (40–50 mL of 0.5% solution). Lower extremity: 250–300 mg (100–120 mL of 0.25% solution).

DRUGS

Onset and Duration
Onset: I.V. (antiarrhythmic effects) 45–90 sec. Infiltration: 0.5–1 min. Epidural: 5–15 min. Peak effects: I.V.: (antiarrhythmic effects) 1–2 min. Infiltration and epidural: <30 min. Duration: I.V. (antiarrhythmic effects): 10–20 min. Infiltration: 0.5–1 hr; with epinephrine 2–6 hr. Epidural: 1–3 hr (prolonged with epinephrine).

Adverse Effects
Hypotension, bradycardia, arrhythmias, heart block, respiratory depression, arrest, anxiety, tinnitus, seizures, postspinal headache, palsies, urticaria, pruritus. High spinal: loss of bladder and bowel control, permanent motor, sensory autonomic (sphincter control), deficit of lower segments.

Precautions and Contraindications
Use with caution in patients with hypovolemia, severe congestive heart failure, shock, all forms of heart block, pregnancy. Contraindicated in patients with hypersensitivity to amide-type local anesthetics, supraventricular arrhythmias.

Anesthetic Considerations
Dosage should be reduced for elderly, debilitated, acutely ill patients. Anesthetic solutions containing epinephrine should be used with caution in peripheral or hypertensive vascular disease. Benzodiazepines increase seizure threshold. Do not use preparations containing preservatives for spinal or epidural anesthesia or for I.V. administration. Do not inject solutions containing epinephrine I.V.

Name
Lorazepam (Ativan)

Classification
Benzodiazepine; antianxiety agent; hypnotic; sedative

Indications
Premedication; induction agent; amnesia; temporary relief of insomnia

Dose
I.V. deep I.M.: 1–2 mg (0.05 mg/kg)(maximum dose 4 mg). Dilute with equal volume D_5W or normal saline solution. P.O.: 1–2 mg, 2 to 3 times/day.
 Preoperative medication: 0.05 mg/kg 2 hr before procedure (maximum dosage 4 mg).
 Dosage forms: Tablets 0.5, 1, 2 mg. Injection: 2 mg/mL, 4 mg/mL.

Onset and Duration
Onset: I.V. 1–5 min; I.M. 15–30 min; P.O. 1–6 hr. Duration: 6–24 hr. $t_{1/2}$ 10–15 hr. metabolized to inactive compounds.

Adverse Effects
Hypotension, hypertension, bradycardia, tachycardia, respiratory depression, dizziness, weakness, depression, agitation, amnesia, hysteria, urti-

caria, visual disturbances, blurred vision, diplopia, nausea, vomiting, abdominal discomfort, anorexia.

Precautions and Contraindications

Intra-arterial injection may cause arteriospasm; treat with local infiltration of phentolamine (5–20 mg in 10 mL normal saline). Use with caution in elderly and debilitated patients. Contraindicated in patients with known hypersensitivity to benzodiazepines and narrow-angle glaucoma.

Anesthetic Considerations

Unexpected hypotension and respiratory depression may occur when combined with opioids. Use with caution in elderly patients and patients with limited pulmonary reserve. Not for use in children <12 yr old. Treat overdose with flumazenil. Decreased requirements for volatile anesthetics.

Name

Magnesium sulfate

Classification

Replacement agents; anticonvulsant

Indications

Prevention and control of seizures in toxemia/eclampsia of pregnancy, epilepsy, nephritis, and hypomagnesemia; treatment of acute magnesium deficiency; tocolytic therapy; adjunctive therapy of acute myocardial infarction, torsades de pointes ventricular tachycardia, and hypokalemia-related arrhythmias; laxative.

Dose

Preeclampsia/eclampsia: I.V. 4 g in 250 mL D_5W or NS infused slowly, followed by 2–3 g/hr by continuous infusion. Blood level should not exceed 7 mEq/L. Hypomagnesemic seizures: Mild: 1 g I.V./I.M. every 6 hr for 4 doses. Total parenteral nutrition: I.V. 8–24 mEq/day.

Onset and Duration

Onset: I.V.: immediate; I.M.: <1 hr; P.O.: 1–2 hr. Peak effects: few minutes; I.M.: 1–3 hr. Duration: I.V.: 30 min; I.M.: 3–4 hr.

Adverse Effects

Hypotension, circulatory collapse, heart block, respiratory paralysis, flaccid paralysis, depressed reflexes, hypocalcemia, flushing, sweating, hypothermia.

Precautions and Contraindications

Not for use in patients with heart block or extensive myocardial damage. I.V. administration contraindicated during the 2 hr preceding delivery. P.O. administration contraindicated in patients with abdominal pain, nausea, vomiting, fecal impaction, or intestinal irritation, obstruction, or perforation. Cautious use in patients with impaired renal function,

DRUGS

digitalized patients, concomitant use of other central nervous system depressants, or neuromuscular blocking agents.

Anesthetic Considerations
Potentiates both depolarizing and nondepolarizing muscle relaxants. Periodic monitoring of serum magnesium concentrations is essential during magnesium therapy. Maintain urine output at a minimum of 100 mL every 4 hr. Monitor deep tendon reflexes during magnesium therapy. Stop therapy as soon as desired effect is reached. Monitor respiratory function.

Name
Mannitol (Osmitrol, Resectisol irrigation)

Classification
Osmotic diuretic

Indications
Reduction of intracranial pressure and intraocular pressure; protection of renal function during periods of hypoperfusion (shock, burn, open-heart surgery, kidney transplants, abdominal aortic aneurysm repair); transurethral prostate resection (TURP) irrigation (minimizes hemolytic effects of water and promotes rapid excretion of absorbed irrigants).

Dose
Adults: Reduction of intracranial/intraocular pressure: 1.5–2 g/kg of 15%–25% solution over 30–60 min. When used preoperatively, give 1–1.5 hr preoperatively for maximum pressure reduction.
    Test dose: If marked oliguria or suspected inadequate renal function, 0.2 g/kg or 12.5 g over 3–5 min. If satisfactory response not obtained, may repeat. If response still not obtained, do not use mannitol. Prevention of oliguric renal failure: 50–100 g I.V. over 2 hr. TURP: 2.5–5% irrigation instilled into bladder. Children: 2 g/kg or 60 g/m^2 as 15%–20% solution over 2–6 hr to treat edema and ascites or over 30–60 min to treat cerebral or ocular edema. Dosage forms: Parenteral injection 5, 10, 15, 20, 25%. Urogenital irrigation solution 2.5%–5%.

Onset and Duration
Diuresis in 1–3 hr; reduction of intracranial and intraocular pressure in 15–30 min. Duration 3–8 hr.

Adverse Effects
Most serious are fluid imbalance and electrolyte loss. Pulmonary edema, hypertension, water intoxication, congestive heart failure, skin necrosis with extravasation.

Precautions
Monitor serum osmolarity and electrolytes closely. Discontinue mannitol if low urine output. May crystallize at low temperature. Do not use a solution containing crystals; resolubilize in hot water with periodic shaking.

Contraindications
Pulmonary edema, congestive heart failure, severe dehydration, impaired renal function not responsive to test dose, edema associated with capillary fragility, and acute intracranial bleeding, except during craniotomy.

Anesthetic Considerations
Disrupts blood–brain barrier, enhancing penetration of other drugs into the central nervous system.

Name
Meperidine HCl (Demerol)

Classification
Synthetic opioid agonist

Dose
I.V./I.M.: 25–100 mg I.V.; Infusion 1–20 mg/hr for short duration, titrate to patient's need.

Onset and Duration
Onset: P.O. 1–45 min; I.M. 1–5 min. Duration: P.O./I.V./I.M. 2–4 hr.

Adverse Effects
Hypotension, cardiac arrest, respiratory depression or arrest, laryngospasm. Euphoria, dysphoria, sedation, seizures, psychic dependence. Constipation, biliary tract spasm. Chest-wall rigidity. Urticaria, pruritus.

Precautions and Contraindications
Reduce doses in elderly, hypovolemic, high-risk surgical patients and with concomitant use of sedatives and other narcotics. Severe and occasionally fatal reactions in patients who are receiving or have just received monoamine oxidase inhibitors. Treat with hydrocortisone. Not for long-term use. Toxic metabolite (normeperidine) is very hazardous, especially in the elderly.

Use with caution in patients with asthma, chronic obstructive pulmonary disease, increased intracranial pressure, or supraventricular tachycardia.

Crosses the placental barrier. Use during labor may produce depression of respiration in the neonate. Resuscitation may be required; have naloxone available.

Cerebral irritation and seizures can occur when used in large doses; potentiates central nervous system and cardiovascular depression of narcotics, sedative-hypnotics, volatile anesthetics, and tricyclic antidepressants; severe, sometimes fatal reaction with monoamine oxidase inhibitors; analgesia enhanced by alpha$_2$ agonists; aggravates adverse effects of isoniazid; chemically incompatible with barbiturates.

Anesthetic Considerations
Use with caution when administering halothane because of increased arrhythmogenic potential.

Name

Mephentermine sulfate (Wyamine sulfate)

Classification

Synthetic noncatecholamine that stimulates alpha and beta receptors, both directly and indirectly.

Indication

Hypotension

Dose

I.V./I.M.: 10–45 mg (0.4 mg/kg); Infusion: 0.25–5 mg/min.

Onset and Duration

Onset: I.V.: 1–5 min; I.M.: 5–15 min. Duration: I.V.: 15–30 min; I.M.: 1–2 hr.

Adverse Effects

Hypertension, arrhythmias, anxiety, seizures, euphoria, paranoid psychosis.

Precautions and Contraindications

Use with caution in patients with severe hypertension or hyperthyroidism. May increase uterine contractions, especially during the third trimester of pregnancy. Not recommended for use in pregnant women. Increased risk of arrhythmias with use of volatile agents.

Anesthetic Considerations

Use caution in patients receiving monoamine oxidase inhibitors or tricyclic antidepressants.

Name

Mepivacaine HCl (Carbocaine, Isocaine, Polocaine)

Classification

Amide-type local anesthetic

Indications

Regional anesthesia: infiltration, brachial plexus block, epidural, caudal

Dose

Infiltration: 50–400 mg (0.5–1.5% solution). Brachial plexus block: 300–400 mg (30–40 mL of 1% solution); Epidural: 150–400 mg (15–20 mL of 1–2% solution). Caudal: 150–400 mg (15–20 mL of 1–2% solution); Children: 0.4–0.7 mL/kg. (maximum safe dosage 7 mg/kg with epinephrine).

Onset and Duration

Onset: Infiltration: 3–5 min. Epidural: 5–15 min. Peak effects: Infiltration/epidural: 15–45 min. Duration: Infiltration: 0.75–1.5 hr; 2–6 hr with epinephrine. Epidural: 3–5 hr (prolonged with epinephrine).

Adverse Effects

Myocardial depression, arrhythmias, cardiac arrest, respiratory depression or arrest, anxiety, apprehension, tinnitus, seizures, loss of hearing, urticaria, pruritus. High spinal: loss of bladder and bowel control, permanent motor, sensory, and autonomic (sphincter control) deficit of lower segments.

Precautions and Contraindications

Use cautiously in debilitated, elderly, or acutely ill patients, especially if severe disturbance in cardiac rhythm or heart block. Pregnancy. Contraindicated in patients with hypersensitivity to amide-type local anesthetics.

Anesthetic Considerations

Do not use solutions with preservatives for caudal or epidural block. Not for spinal anesthesia. Not recommended for obstetric anesthesia. Blood concentration may be reduced by rifampin, with production of withdrawal symptoms; severe reaction with monoamine oxidase inhibitors; withdrawal symptoms precipitated by pentazocine in heroin addicts on methadone therapy; potentiates central nervous system and cardiovascular depressant effects of other narcotic analgesics, volatile anesthetics, phenothiazines, sedative hypnotics, alcohol, tricyclic antidepressants. Analgesia enhanced by alpha$_2$ agonists.

Name

Metaraminol bitartrate (Aramine)

Classification

Synthetic noncatecholamine

Indications

Hypertension; stimulates alpha and beta receptors, both directly and indirectly

Dose

I.M./SQ: 2–10 mg; I.V.: 0.5–5 mg.

Onset and Duration

Onset: I.V.: 1–5 min; I.M./SQ: 5–15 min. Duration: I.V.: 10–15 min; I.M./SQ: 1–2 hr.

Adverse Effects

Apprehension, restlessness, dizziness, headache, tremor, weakness, seizures, hypertension, hypotension, precordial pain, palpitations, arrhythmias, bradycardia, premature ventricular contractions, atrioventricular dissociation, nausea, vomiting, decreased urine output, hyperglycemia, flushing, pallor, sweating.

Precautions and Contraindications

Patients with hypertension, thyroid disease, diabetes, or cirrhosis, and in patients receiving digoxin. In patients with peripheral or mesenteric thrombosis, pulmonary edema, hypercarbia, or acidosis.

DRUGS

Anesthetic Considerations
Increased risk of adverse cardiac effects with the use of general anesthetics.

Name
Methadone HCl (Dolophine HCl)

Classification
Synthetic narcotic

Indications
Analgesia; opiate recovery program

Dose
Analgesia: SQ/I.M./P.O.: 2.5–10 mg (0.1 mg/kg) every 4 hr; Epidural bolus: 1–5 mg; Narcotic abstinence syndrome: P.O.: 20–120 mg/day.

Onset and Duration
Onset: I.V.: Several minutes; I.M.: 3–60 min; P.O.: 30–60 min; Epidural: 5–10 min. Duration: I.V./I.M./P.O.: About 6 hr; Epidural: 6–10 hr.

Adverse Effects
Hypotension, circulatory depression, bradycardia, syncope, respiratory depression, euphoria, dysphoria, disorientation, urinary retention, biliary tract spasm, constipation, anorexia, rash, pruritus, urticaria.

Contraindications
Reduce dose in the elderly, hypovolemic, high-risk surgical patient or with use of narcotics and sedative hypnotics.

Anesthetic Considerations
Do not give pentazocine to heroin addicts on methadone. Ineffective for relief of general anxiety. Use with caution in patients with asthma, chronic obstructive pulmonary disease, increased intracranial pressure. Can produce the drug effects of morphine.

Name
Methohexital sodium (Brevital sodium)

Classification
Ultra short-acting barbiturate

Indications
General anesthetic for short surgical procedures; induction of hypnosis; supplementation of other anesthetics

Dose
I.V. induction: 50–120 mg (average 70 mg); 1–1.5 mg/kg usual dose in adults. Dosage forms: Powder for injection: 500, 2.5, 5.0 mg.

Onset and Duration
   Onset few seconds. *Duration* 5–8 min.

Adverse Effects
   Circulatory depression, thrombophlebitis, myocardial depression, cardiac arrhythmia, respiratory depression, central nervous system disturbances, seizures, nausea and vomiting, abdominal pain, rectal irritation (rectal administration), pain at injection site.

Precautions and Contraindications
   Contraindicated in variegate porphyria or acute intermittent porphyria, hypersensitivity to barbiturates. Use with caution in severe cardiovascular disease, hypotension, shock, Addison's disease, hepatic or renal dysfunction, myxedema, increased intracranial pressure, asthma, myasthenia gravis.

Anesthetic Considerations
   May reduce dose when used in conjunction with narcotics. Overdosage may occur from too rapid or repeated injections. Do not mix with atropine sulfate, tubocurarine, or succinylcholine. Incompatible with silicone. Use only if clear and colorless. Not compatible with lactated Ringer's.

Name
   Methoxamine HCl (Vasoxyl)

Classification
   Alpha receptor agonist

Indication
   Hypotension

Dose
   I.V.: 1–5 mg, given slowly; I.M.: 5–15 mg (0.25 mg/kg).

Onset and Duration
   Onset: I.V.: Almost immediately; I.M.: 15–20 min. Duration: I.V.: 15–60 min; I.M. 60–90 min.

Adverse Effects
   Reflex bradycardia, hypertension, hypotension, respiratory difficulty, tremors, dizziness, seizures, cerebral hemorrhage, headache, projectile vomiting, desire to void.

Precautions and Contraindications
   Use with extreme caution in elderly patients and patients with bradycardia, partial heart block, myocardial disease, or severe arteriosclerosis. Contains sulfites and thus may cause allergic-type reactions

Anesthetic Considerations
   Infuse into large veins to prevent extravasation. Treat extravasation with local infiltration of phentolamine (5–10 mg in 10 mL normal saline solution) or with sympathetic block.

DRUGS

Name
Methylene blue (Urolene Blue)

Classification
Antidote; diagnostic agent

Indications
Treatment of idiopathic and drug-induced methemoglobinemia; dye effect for tissue staining; urinary antiseptic (oral route). Antidote to cyanide poisoning

Dose
I.V.: 1–2 mg/kg (inject over several min). P.O.: 65–130 mg t.i.d. with water.

Onset and Duration
Onset I.V. almost immediate. Peak effects: I.V. <1 hr. Duration: I.V./ P.O. varies.

Adverse Effects
Tachycardia, hypertension, precordial pain, cyanosis, confusion, headache, nausea, vomiting, diarrhea, abdominal pain, bladder irritation, stains skin blue, hemolytic anemia, methemoglobinemia, hyperbilirubinemia.

Precautions and Contraindications
Safe use during pregnancy not established. Contraindicated in patients with renal insufficiency, hypersensitivity to methylene blue, G6PD deficiency (hemolysis), and intraspinal injection.

Anesthetic Considerations
Discoloration of urine and feces. Inject slowly to prevent local high concentration from producing additional methemoglobinemia. Monitor intake and output as well as hemoglobin.

Name
Methylergonovine (Methergine)

Classification
Oxytocic (ergot alkaloid); adrenergic antagonist; sympatholytic

Indications
Prevention and treatment of postpartum hemorrhage caused by uterine atony or subinvolution

Dose
I.M.: 0.2 mg every 2–5 hr (for maximum of 5 doses). I.V.: 0.2 mg/mL (over 1 min while monitoring blood pressure and uterine contractions). P.O.: 0.2–0.4 mg every 6–12 hr for 2–7 days.

Onset and Duration
Onset: I.V.: immediate; I.M.: 2–5 min; P.O.: 5–15 min. Peak effects: 3 hr. Duration: I.V.: 45 min; I.M.: 3 hr; P.O.: 3 or more hr.

Adverse Effects
Hypertension, chest pain, palpitations, dyspnea, headache, nausea, vomiting, tinnitus. High doses can produce signs of ergotism.

Precautions and Contraindications
Cautious use in patients with hypertension, sepsis, obliterative vascular disease, hepatic, renal, and cardiac disease. Contraindicated in patients with hypersensitivity to ergot preparations or with pregnancy, toxemia, untreated hypocalcemia.

Anesthetic Considerations
Monitor for hypertension or other adverse effects. Parenteral sympathomimetics or other ergot alkaloids add to pressor effect and may lead to hypertension. I.V. administration is not routine, as it can produce sudden hypertension and CVAs.

Name
Metoclopramide (Reglan)

Classification
Dopamine-receptor antagonist; antiemetic; stimulant of upper gastrointestinal motility

Indications
Diabetic and postsurgical gastric stasis; prevention of chemotherapy-induced emesis; facilitation of small-bowel intubation; gastroesophageal reflux; prevention of postoperative nausea and vomiting

Dose
Adults: 10 mg I.V. slowly over 1–2 min as a single dose. May repeat once. Children: 6–14 yr: 2.5–5 mg I.V.; children <6 yr: 0.1 mg/kg. Dosage forms: 5 mg/mL in 2- and 10-mL vials. P.O. 5-mg and 10-mg tablets; syrup 5 mg/5 mL.

Onset and Duration
Onset 1–3 min. Duration 2–3 hr. $t_{1/2}$ 2.5–5 hr in patients with normal renal function.

Adverse Effects
Drowsiness occurs frequently. Anxiety, restlessness, mental depression, gastrointestinal upset, urticaria, allergic reactions, diarrhea. Extrapyramidal side effects such as opisthotonos, clonic convulsions, oculogyric crisis, facial grimacing, involuntary movement of limbs, and rarely stridor and dyspnea possibly due to laryngospasm occur with 0.2% or less frequency in above doses, but are more common in children. Diphenhydramine

may readily reverse extrapyramidal effects. Butyrophenones and pheno-thiazines may potentiate extrapyramidal side effects.

Precautions

Pregnancy. May exacerbate Parkinson's disease and hypertension. May increase pressure on suture lines following gut anastomosis or closure. Patients should be cautioned that metoclopramide may impair their ability to perform activities requiring mental alertness, including driving or operating machinery. Alcohol and other central nervous system depressants may enhance these effects.

Contraindications

Do not use with monoamine oxidase inhibitors, tricyclic antidepressants, or sympathomimetics. Metoclopramide should not be used in patients with pheochromocytoma, history of seizure disorder, or gastrointestinal hemorrhage, obstruction or perforation.

Anesthetic Considerations

May increase the neuromuscular blocking effects of succinylcholine by inhibiting plasma cholinesterase.

Name

Midazolam (Midazolam hydrochloride, Versed)

Classification

Benzodiazepine; hypnotic; sedative

Indications

Preoperative sedation; induction of anesthesia; long-term sedation in intensive care unit; sedation prior to short diagnostic and endoscopic procedures

Dose

Should be individualized based on the patient's age, underlying pathology, and concurrent indications. Adolescents (<12 years) I.V. 0.5 mg; can be repeated every 5 min until desired effect achieved. Adults: Preoperative sedation: I.M.: 0.07–0.08 mg/kg 30–60 min before surgery. Usual dose approximately 5 mg. I.V.: Initial 0.5–2 mg slow I.V. over 2 min. Usual total dose 2.0–5 mg; decrease doses in elderly. Reduce dose by 30% if other central nervous system depressants are administered concomitantly. Dosage form: Injection 1, 5 mg/mL.

Onset and Duration

I.V.: 1–5 min; I.M.: 15 min; P.O./rectal: <10 min. Duration 2–6 hr. $t_{1/2}$ 1-4 hr; excreted in urine.

Adverse Effects

Tachycardia, hypotension, bronchospasm, laryngospasm, apnea, hypoventilation, vasovagal episodes, euphoria, prolonged emergence, agitation, hyperactivity, pruritus, rash.

Precautions and Contraindications
Contraindicated in patients with intolerance to benzodiazepines or with acute narrow-angle glaucoma, shock, coma, acute alcohol intoxication. Not for intra-arterial injection. Safe use in pregnancy, labor and delivery, by nursing mothers, or by children not established.

Anesthetic Considerations
Cautious use in chronic obstructive pulmonary disease, chronic renal failure, congestive heart failure, and elderly patients. Reduce doses in hypovolemia and with concomitant use of other sedatives or narcotics. Hypotension and respiratory depression may occur when given with opioids; consider smaller doses. Treat overdose with flumazenil.

Name
Milrinone (Primacor)

Classification
Inotropic agent

Indications
Chronic therapy for congestive heart failure; cardiac bypass procedures and heart transplants

Dose
I.V.: loading dose 50 μg/kg over 10 min; maintenance doses 0.375 μg/kg per min, 0.5 μg/kg per min, or 0.75 μg/kg per min. Dosage form: I.V. 1 mg/mL.

Onset and Duration
Onset: I.V. 2 min; P.O. 1–1.5 hr. Duration: 2 hr.

Adverse Effects
Thrombocytopenia, arrhythmia, angina, hypotension, headache, hyperthermia.

Precautions and Contraindications
Contraindicated in hypersensitivity to milrinone or amrinone. Cautious use in renal insufficiency and aortic or pulmonic valvular disease.

Anesthetic Considerations
Attractive alternative to conventional inotropics. May be useful if both inotropic effect and vasodilation are desirable.

Name
Mivacurium (Mivacron)

Classification
Nondepolarizing skeletal muscle relaxant

Indications
Adjunct to general anesthesia; skeletal muscle relaxation during surgery

Dose
I.V. paralyzing 0.07–0.25 mg/kg. Children: 0.1–0.2 mg/kg over 5–15 sec. Dosage forms: 0.5 mg/mL in 5% dextrose; 0.5 mg/mL.

DRUGS

Onset and Duration
Onset: two min. Duration: 6–10 min.

Adverse Effects
Hypotension, vasodilation, tachycardia, bradycardia, hypoventilation, apnea, bronchospasm, laryngospasm, dyspnea, rash, inadequate block, prolonged block.

Contraindications
Contraindicated in patients with hypersensitivity to the drug.

Anesthetic Considerations
Use with caution in patients with sensitivity to the release of histamine. Prolonged neuromuscular blockade may occur in patients with low plasma pseudocholinesterase; reverse effects with anticholinesterase. Monitor response with peripheral nerve stimulator.

Name
Morphine sulfate (Astramorph, Duramorph, Morphine, MS Contin)

Classification
Opioid Agonist

Indications
Premedication; analgesia; anesthesia; treatment of pain associated with myocardial ischemia and dyspnea associated with left ventricular failure and pulmonary edema

Dose
Analgesia: I.V. 2.5–15 mg; I.M./SQ 2.5–20 mg; P.O. 15–30 mg every 4 hr as needed; P.O. extended release 30 mg every 12 hr; Rectal 5–20 mg every 4 hr. Anesthesia induction: I.V. 1 mg/kg; Epidural bolus 2–5 mg; Epidural infusion 0.1–1 mg/hr; Spinal (preservative-free solution only) 0.2–1 mg. Children: I.V. 0.05–0.2 mg/kg; I.M./SQ 0.1–0.2 mg/kg.

Onset and Duration
Onset: I.V. almost immediate; I.M. 1–5 min; P.O. <60 min; epidural and spinal 1–60 min. Duration: I.V./I.M./SQ 2–7 hr; epidural and spinal 24 hr.

Adverse Effects
Hypotension, hypertension, bradycardia, arrhythmias, chest-wall rigidity. Bronchospasm, laryngospasm. Blurred vision, syncope, euphoria, dysphoria. Urinary retention, antidiuretic effect, ureteral spasm. Biliary tract spasm, constipation, anorexia, nausea, vomiting. Pruritus, urticaria.

Precautions and Contraindications
Reduce dose in elderly, hypovolemic, or high-risk surgical patients and with concomitant use of sedatives and other narcotics. Crosses the placen-

tal barrier; usage in labor may produce depression of respiration in the neonate. Resuscitation may be required; have naloxone available.

Anesthetic Considerations
Central nervous system and cardiovascular depressant effects potentiated by alcohol, sedatives, antihistamines, phenothiazines, butyrophenones, monoamine oxidase inhibitors, tricyclic antidepressants. May decrease the effects of diuretics in patients with congestive heart failure. Analgesia enhanced by alpha$_2$ agonists.

Name
Nalmefene HCl (Revex)

Classification
Opiate antagonist

Indications
Complete or partial reversal of drug effects, respiratory depression, or overdose associated with either natural or synthetic opioids

Dose
Reversal of opiate depression: titrate to the desired response at increments of .25 μg/kg every 2–5 min. Doses >1 μg/kg give no additional therapeutic effects. Titrated at a dose of 0.1 μg/kg every 2–5 min in patients with increased cardiovascular risk. Suspected opiate overdose: first dose 0.5 mg/70 kg; second dose 1.0 mg/70 kg if required 2–5 min later. Doses >1.5 mg/70 kg do not provide increased therapeutic effects. Suspicion of opiate dependency: challenge dose 0.1 mg/70 kg. If signs of withdrawal do not appear within 2 min, the recommended dosage guidelines should be followed.

Onset and Duration
Onset: I.V. within 2 min. I.M. or SQ 5–15 min. I.V. administration of a 1 mg dose of nalmephene will block 80% of brain opiate receptors within 5 min. The duration of action and opiate receptor occupancy of nalmefene was shown to be significantly greater than that of naloxone, which has $t_{1/2}$ of 1.1 hr. Duration: equals that of most opioids. This provides the patient with added protection against possible renarcotization. $t_{1/2}$ 10.8 hr. Metabolized in liver via glucuronide conjugation; excreted in the urine. Plasma clearance is reported to be 0.8 L/hr per kg; plasma-protein binding 45%.

Adverse Effects
A higher occurrence of adverse effects is reported with amounts exceeding recommended dosages. Pulmonary edema, hypotension, hypertension, ventricular arrhythmias, bradycardia. Dizziness, depression, agitation, nervousness, tremor, confusion, myoclonus, withdrawal syndrome. Nausea, vomiting, diarrhea, dry mouth. Headache, chills, pruritus, pharyngitis.

DRUGS

Precautions and Contraindications
Decreased plasma clearance in patients with liver or renal disease. The dose of nalmefene should be delivered over 60 seconds in patients with renal failure to minimize associated hypertension and dizziness. Dosage need not be adjusted for one-time administration. Recurrence of respiratory depression is possible even after a positive response to initial administration. Cautious use in patients at increased cardiovascular risk. Acute withdrawal symptoms are associated with administration to opiate-dependent patients. Incomplete reversal of buprenorphine-induced depression. Emergency use only in pregnancy; cautious use in nursing women. Animal studies have shown a potential for seizure induction. Potential risk of seizure increases with the coadministration of nalmefene and flumazenil. Nalmefene is contraindicated in persons who display an allergic response related to the drug's administration. Safety and effectiveness of nalmefene for neonates and children has not been established.

Anesthetic Considerations
No adverse reactions were noted in studies where nalmefene was administered after benzodiazepines, volatile anesthetics, muscle relaxants, or their reversals.

Name
Naloxone HCl (Narcan)

Classification
Opioid antagonist

Indication
Opiate reversal

Dose
I.V./I.M./SQ: 0.1–2 mg titrated to patient response; may repeat at 2- to 3-min intervals; response should occur with a maximum dose of 10 mg. Children: 5–10 μg/kg every 2–3 min as needed.

Onset and Duration
Onset: I.V.: 1–2 min; I.M./SQ: 2–5 min. Duration: I.V./I.M./SQ: 1–4 hr.

Adverse Effects
Tachycardia, hypertension, hypotension, arrhythmias, pulmonary edema, nausea, and vomiting related to dose and speed of injection.

Precautions and Contraindications
Use with caution in patients with pre-existing cardiac disease.

Anesthetic Considerations
Titrate slowly to effect. Patients who have received naloxone HCl should be carefully monitored because duration of action of some opiates may exceed that of this drug.

Name
Naltrexone HCl (ReVia, Trexan)

Classification
Opiate receptor antagonist

Indications
Reversal of toxic effects of opioid drugs; treatment of opiate and alcohol addiction, Tourette's syndrome, tardive dyskinesia, Lesch-Nyhan disease, and dyskinesia associated with Huntington's disease

Dose
P.O.: 25-mg tablet followed by 25 mg in 1 hr if no signs of withdrawal present (withdrawal will begin 5 min after P.O. dose and may last up to 48 hr).
Dosage form: Tablet: 25, 50 mg.

Onset and Duration
Onset: In 5 min; peak effects seen in 1 hr. Duration: 24–72 hr.

Adverse Effects
Headache, nervousness, confusion, restlessness, hallucinations, paranoia, nightmares, nausea, vomiting, diarrhea, abdominal pain and cramping, phlebitis, epistaxis, tachycardia, hypertension, edema, hepatotoxicity, joint and muscle pain, and severe narcotic withdrawal.

Precautions and Contraindications
Contraindication is absolute in patients dependent on narcotics and patients in acute withdrawal and with liver disease or acute hepatitis. Patients addicted to heroin or other opiates should be drug free for 10 days before initiation of therapy to avoid precipitation of withdrawal syndrome. Serious overdose may occur after attempts to overcome the blocking effects of naltrexone.

Anesthetic Considerations
Baseline liver function studies should be performed. Primary active metabolite is subject to glucuronide conjugation. Aspartate transaminase levels may be temporarily elevated after initiation of therapy. Patients taking naltrexone may not respond to opiates administered during anesthesia. Blockade of naltrexone may be overcome by large (fatal) doses of opiates.

Name
Neostigmine methylsulfate (Prostigmin)

Classification
Anticholinesterase agent

Indications
Reversal of nondepolarizing muscle relaxants; myasthenia gravis

Dose
Reversal: Slow I.V. 0.06 mg/kg (maximum dose: 6 mg), with atropine (0.015 mg/kg) or glycopyrrolate (0.01 mg/kg). Myasthenia gravis: P.O.:

DRUGS

15–375 mg daily (3 divided doses); I.M./Slow I.V.: 0.5–2 mg (dose must be individualized).

Onset and Duration
Onset: Reversal: I.V.: <3 min. Myasthenia: I.M.: <20 min; P.O.: 45–75 min.

Adverse Effects
Bradycardia, tachycardia, atrioventricular block, nodal rhythm, hypotension; increased oral, pharyngeal, and bronchial secretions; bronchospasm, respiratory depression, seizures, dysarthria, headaches, nausea, emesis, flatulence, increased peristalsis, urinary frequency, rash, urticaria, allergic reactions, anaphylaxis.

Precautions and Contraindications
Use with caution in patients with bradycardia, bronchial asthma, epilepsy, cardiac arrhythmias, peptic ulcer, peritonitis, or mechanical obstruction of the intestines or urinary tract. Overdosage may induce a cholinergic crisis characterized by nausea, vomiting, bradycardia or tachycardia, excessive salivation and sweating, bronchospasm, weakness, and paralysis; treatment includes discontinuation of neostigmine use and administration of atropine (10 μg/kg I.V. every 3–10 min until muscarinic symptoms disappear.

Anesthetic Considerations
May increase postoperative nausea and vomiting.

Name
Nicardipine (Cardene)

Classification
Calcium channel blocker

Indications
Hypertension; chronic stable angina; vasospastic angina

Dose
Angina: Initially 20 mg P.O. t.i.d.; titrate dosage according to patient response. Usual dosage 20–40 mg P.O. t.i.d. Hypertension: Initially 20–40 mg P.O. t.i.d.; increase dosage according to patient response. I.V. 5 mg/hr, increased by 2.5-mg/hr increments every 15 min, up to 15 mg/hr.

Onset and Duration
Onset: I.V. 1 min; P.O. 30 min to 2 hr; sustained release 1–4 hr. Duration: I.V./P.O. 3 hr.

Adverse Effects
Edema, dizziness, headache, flushing, hypotension.

Contraindications
Hypersensitivity to nicardipine, other dihydropyridines, or other calcium channel antagonists. Symptomatic hypotension, advanced aortic stenosis.

Anesthetic Considerations
Intravenous calcium channel blocker. May be useful in controlling perioperative hypertension.

Name
Nifedipine (Adalat, Procardia)

Classification
Calcium channel blocker

Indications
Hypertension; chronic stable angina; vasospastic angina

Dose
10–30 mg t.i.d. up to 180 mg/day; unlabeled route: sublingual

Onset and Duration
Onset: P.O. 20 min; sublingual 5–20 min. Duration: P.O./sublingual 12 hr.

Adverse Effects
Hypotension, palpitations, peripheral edema. Bronchospasm, shortness of breath, nasal and chest congestion. Headache, dizziness, nervousness. Nausea, diarrhea, constipation. Inflammation, joint stiffness, peripheral edema. Pruritus, urticaria. Fevers, chills, sweating.

Precautions and Contraindications
Monitor blood pressure carefully during initial administration and titration. Use cautiously in the elderly, hypovolemic patients, and those with acute myocardial infarction and unstable angina.

Anesthetic Considerations
Potentiates effects of depolarizing and nondepolarizing muscle relaxants; additive cardiovascular depressant effects with use of volatile anesthetics, other antihypertensives; increases toxicity of digoxin, carbamazepine, oral hypoglycemics. Cardiac failure, atrioventricular conduction disturbances, and sinus bradycardia with concurrent use of beta-blockers; severe hypotension and bradycardia may occur with bupivacaine; concomitant use of I.V. verapamil and dantrolene may result in cardiovascular collapse.

Name
Nitroglycerin (Nitro-Bid, Nitro-Dur, Nitrogard, Nitrostat, Nitrol, Tridil, Nitrocine, Transderm-Nitro, Nitroglyn, Nitrodisc)

Classification
Peripheral vasodilator

Indications
Antianginal; controlled hypotension, treatment of pulmonary edema and congestive heart failure associated with acute myocardial infarction

DRUGS

Dose

Initially, titrated 5 μg/min to 20 μg/min. Thereafter titrate by 10-μg/min steps. I.V. infusion: 5 μg/min. Tablets: 0.15–0.6 mg every 5 min as needed to maximum of 3 doses in 15 min (sustained release-buccal 1–2 mg every 3–5 hr). Place tablet between lip and gum above incisors. Dosage forms: Injection: 0.5 mg/mL and 5 mg/mL tablets: sublingual 0.15 mg, 0.3 mg, 0.4 mg, 0.6 mg. Sustained release-buccal: 1, 2, 3 mg. P.O. sustained release: 2.5, 2.6, 6.5, 9 mg. Capsules: 2.5, 6.5, 9 mg. Aerosol translingual: 0.4 mg/metered dose. Transdermal systems: 2.5, 5, 7.5, 10, 15 mg/24 hr. Ointment: 2% (1 inch contains 15 mg nitroglycerine). Dilution for infusion: 8 mg diluted in 250 mL D_5W or normal saline (32 μg/mL). 50 mg in 250 mL, 100 mg in 250 mL (400 μg/mL).

Onset and Duration

Onset: I.V. 1–2 min; sublingual 1–3 min; P.O. sustained release 20–45 min; Transdermal 40–60 min.

Adverse Effects

Orthostatic hypotension, tachycardia, flushing, palpitations, fainting, headache, dizziness, weakness, nausea, vomiting.

Precautions and Contraindications

Use with caution in hypotension, uncorrected hypovolemia, inadequate cerebral circulation, increased intracranial pressure, head trauma, cerebral hemorrhage, severe anemia.

Anesthetic Considerations

Hypotensive effects potentiated by alcohol, phenothiazines, calcium channel blockers, beta-blockers, other nitrates, and antihypertensives.

May antagonize anticoagulant effect of heparin. Methemoglobinemia at high doses.

Because of light sensitivity, wrap I.V. solution container in foil. Contraindicated in patients with compensatory hypertension such as with arteriovenous shunts, coarctation of aorta, and inadequate cerebral circulation. Monitor plasma thiocyanate concentrations in patients receiving infusions for greater than 48 hr.

Attenuation of hypoxic pulmonary vasoconstriction may occur. Infusion rates of greater than 3μg/kg per min may result in decreased platelet aggregation. Hypotensive effects potentiated by volatile anesthetics, ganglionic blocking agents, other antihypertensives, circulatory depressants. May see elevated mixed venous PO_2.

Name

Nitroprusside sodium (Nipride, Nitropress)

Classification

Peripheral vasodilator

Indications

Hypertension, controlled hypotension, treatment of cardiogenic pulmonary edema, treatment of cariogenic shock.

Dose
Infusion: 10–300 μg/min (0.25–10 μg/kg per min); Maximum dose: 10 μg/kg per min for 10 min, or chronic infusion of 0.5 μg/kg per min.

Onset and Duration
Onset: 30–60 sec. Duration: 1–10 min.

Adverse Effects
May cause reflex tachycardia; cyanide toxicity may occur even in low doses. Treatment: immediately discontinue nitroprusside use, administer oxygen, treat acidosis with bicarbonate, start sodium nitrate 3%, 4–6 mg/kg over 3 min, to produce 10% methemoglobin, which will reversibly bind free cyanide ion. Follow with infusion of sodium thiosulfate (vitamin B_{12}), 150–200 mg/kg.

Precautions and Contraindications
Renal or hepatic failure, which may lead to increased risk of cyanide toxicity. Potential for fetal cyanide toxicity in pregnant patients.

Anesthetic Considerations
Titrate carefully for short periods of deliberate hypotension. Monitor for cyanide toxicity.

Name
Nitrous oxide (N_2O)

Classification
Inhalation anesthetic

Indications
Component of balanced obstetric anesthesia or dental analgesia

Dose
Induction: 70% in an oxygen mixture. Maintenance: 70% in oxygen. Analgesia: 20%–30%. Supplied in steel cylinders (blue) as a colorless liquid under pressure

Onset and Duration
Onset: 1–5 minutes; duration: 5–10 minutes after cessation of continuous inhalation.

Adverse Effects
Primarily caused by lack of oxygen from improper administration technique. Confusion, cyanosis, convulsions. Bone-marrow depression and malignant hyperthermia possible.

Precautions and Contraindications
Caution patient not to drive or operate other machinery until effects of drug have completely disappeared. Inform patient that confusion, vivid

dreams, dizziness, and hallucinations may occur upon termination. Inspired oxygen concentrations of at least 30% should be given.

Anesthetic Considerations
Nonflammable; will support combustion. Noticeable second-gas effect that initially hastens the uptake of other agents when high concentrations are used. Nitrous oxide diffuses into air-containing cavities 34 times faster than nitrogen can leave. Can cause potential dangerous pressure accumulation (i.e., middle-ear perforation, bowel obstruction, pneumothorax). Check endotracheal tube cuff volume and pressure periodically during general anesthesia.

Name
Nizatidine (Axid)

Classification
H_2 receptor antagonist

Indications
Treatment of duodenal or gastric ulcers and gastroesophageal reflux disease. Prophylaxis of aspiration pneumonitis in patients at high risk during surgery.

Dose
For prophylaxis of aspiration pneumonitis in adults: 150 mg P.O. 2 hr prior to the induction of anesthesia; may be given with or without a similar dose the preceding evening. For patients with impaired renal function as evidenced by serum creatinine level greater than 2.5 mg%, a single dose only is needed. Dosage form: 150-mg capsule

Onset and Duration
Peak plasma levels occurred 1–3 hr after oral administration and were below detectable limits in healthy patients 12 hr later. Elimination half-life is 1–2.8 hr.

Adverse Effects
Headache is the most common side effect, followed by gastrointestinal effects and dizziness (4.5%). Rarely, thrombocytopenia, leukopenia, and anemia occur. Somnolence (2%) and mental confusion can occur in the elderly. Incidence of hepatitis: 0.04%–0.15%.

Precautions and Contraindications
Caution suggested in patients with hepatic or renal dysfunction. Contraindicated in patients with known hypersensitivity to nizatidine or other H_2 antagonists.

Anesthetic Considerations
Safe for use during anesthesia.

Name
Norepinephrine bitartrate (Levophed)

Classification
Catecholamine. Potent peripheral vasoconstrictor of arterial and venous beds. Potent inotropic stimulator of the heart (beta$_1$-adrenergic action)

but to a lesser degree than epinephrine or isoproterenol. Norepinephrine does not stimulate beta$_2$-adrenergic receptors of the bronchi or peripheral blood vessels. Systolic and diastolic blood pressures and coronary artery blood flow are increased. Cardiac output varies reflexly with systemic hypertension but is usually increased in hypotensive subjects when blood pressure is raised to an optimal level. On other occasions, increased baroreceptor activity reflexly decreases the heart rate. The drug reduces renal, hepatic, cerebral, and muscle blood flow.

Indications
Vasoconstrictor; inotrope

Dose
Infusion 8–12 μg/min. Use lowest effective dose.

Onset and Duration
Onset: 1 min. Duration: 2–10 min.

Adverse Effects
Bradycardia, tachyarrhythmias, hypertension, decreased cardiac output. Headache. Plasma volume depletion. Administer into large vein to minimize extravasation. Treat extravasation with local infiltration of phentolamine (10 mg in 10 mL normal saline) or sympathetic block.

Contraindications
Contraindicated in patients with mesenteric or peripheral vascular thrombosis.

Anesthetic Considerations
Increased risk of arrhythmias with use of volatile anesthetics or bretylium, or in patients with profound hypoxia or hypercarbia. Pressor effect potentiated in patients receiving monoamine oxidase inhibitors, tricyclic antidepressants, guanethidine, oxytocics. Necrosis or gangrene with extravasation.

Name
Ondansetron HCl (Zofran)

Classification
Gastrointestinal agent; serotonin (5HT3) receptor antagonist; antiemetic

Indications
Prevention of nausea and vomiting associated with cancer chemotherapy; postoperative nausea and vomiting.

Dose
With chemotherapy: I.V. 3 doses: 0.15 mg/kg first dose 30 min before chemotherapy, then 4–8 hr after first dose (may give 8 mg bolus, then 1 mg/hr continuous infusion with maximum dose of 32 mg/day). Perioperative nausea and vomiting: 2–4 mg.

DRUGS

Onset and Duration

Onset: Variable. Most effective if therapy begins before emetogenic chemotherapy. Peak effects: 1–1.5 hr. Duration: 12–24 hr.

Adverse Effects

Tachycardia, angina, dizziness, lightheadedness, headache, sedation, diarrhea, constipation, dry mouth, rash, bronchospasm, hypersensitivity reactions. Cautious use in pregnancy, nursing mothers, and children younger than 3 years old. Contraindicated in patients with hypersensitivity to ondansetron.

Precautions

Use with caution in pregnant or nursing women.

Anesthetic Considerations

Monitor cardiovascular status, especially in patients with a history of coronary artery disease.

Name

Oxytocin (Pitocin, Syntocinon)

Classification

Oxytocic; lactation stimulant

Indications

Initiate or improve uterine contraction at term after dilation of cervix and delivery of fetus; stimulates letdown reflex in nursing mothers to relieve pain from breast engorgement.

Dose

Administration of oxytocin is always via continuous I.V. infusion.

1. *For augmentation of labor:* 10 IU (1 mL) is diluted in 1000 mL of infusate. Infusion rates vary from 1–10 mU/min.

2. *To minimize postpartum bleeding:* rates of 20–100 mU/min are used. Effects appear within 3 minutes, are maximal at about 20 minutes, and disappear within 15–20 minutes after discontinuing the infusion. In practical terms, 20–40 IU is usually added to 1000 mL of fluid and administered to effect.

Promotion of milk ejection: Nasal: 1 spray or drop in one or both nostrils 2–3 min before nursing or pumping breasts.

Onset and Duration

Onset: I.V. immediate; nasal: few mins; I.M. 3–5 min. Peak effects: I.V.: <20 min. IM: 40 min. Duration: IV: 20 min to 1 hr; nasal: 20 min; I.M.: 2–3 hr.

Adverse Effects

Hypersensitivity leading to uterine hypertonicity, tetanic contractions, uterine rupture, cardiac arrhythmias, nausea, vomiting, hypertension, subarachnoid hemorrhage, seizures from water intoxication and hyponatremia.

Contraindications

Cautious use with other vasoactive drugs. Contraindicated in patients with hypersensitivity to oxytocin. Contraindicated in complications of pregnancy: significant cephalopelvic disproportion, fetal distress in which delivery is not imminent, prematurity, placenta previa, past history of uterine sepsis or of traumatic delivery. Nasal preparation contraindicated during pregnancy.

Anesthetic Considerations

Administration should follow delivery of fetus. May increase pressor effects of sympathomimetics. Prolonged I.V. infusion of oxytocin with excessive fluid volume may cause severe water intoxication with seizures, coma, and death. Infuse I.V. only after dilution in large volume parenteral with an infusion pump.

Name

Pancuronium (Pavulon)

Classification

Nondepolarizing skeletal muscle relaxant

Indications

Adjunct to general anesthesia; skeletal muscle relaxation during surgery

Dose

I.V. paralyzing: 0.04–0.1 mg/kg.
Pretreatment/maintenance: 0.01–0.02 mg/kg.
Dosage forms: Injection 1 mg/mL in 10-mL vial; 2 mg/mL in ampules.

Onset and Duration

Onset: 1–3 min. Duration: 40–65 min.

Adverse Effects

Tachycardia, hypertension, hypoventilation, apnea, bronchospasm, salivation, flushing, anaphylactoid reactions, inadequate block, prolonged block.

Contraindications

Contraindicated in myasthenia gravis, bromide hypersensitivity, severe coronary artery disease, or conditions in which tachycardia is undesirable.

Anesthetic Considerations

Pretreatment doses may cause hypoventilation in some patients. Monitor response with peripheral nerve stimulator. Reverse effects with anticholinesterase.

DRUGS

Name
Thiopental sodium (Pentothal)

Classification
Ultra short-acting barbiturate

Indications
Induction of anesthesia or hypnosis; treatment of seizures caused by inhalation or local anesthetics

Dose
Induction: I.V. 3–5 mg/kg.
Maintenance: I.V. 50–100 mg whenever patient moves. Seizures: 75–125 mg (3–5 mL of 2.5% solution) for seizures following anesthesia; 125–250 mg over a 10 min period for seizures due to a local anesthetic. Dosage forms: Injection: 250 mg, 400 mg, and 500 mg syringes; also supplied in vials with diluent, 500 mg and 1 g; also supplied in kits with 1, 2.5, and 5 g. Rectal suspension: 400 mg/g.

Onset and Duration
Onset: 5–20 sec.
Duration: 20–30 min. Plasma $t_{1/2}$ 3 min; elimination $t_{1/2}$ 9 hr.

Adverse Effects
Inadequate doses may increase sensitivity to pain. Profound dose-dependent depression of respiration. Extravascular injection may cause severe pain and tissue necrosis.

Precautions and Contraindications
Contraindicated in variegate porphyria or acute intermittent porphyria. Use with caution during lactation, in asthmatics, or with hypersensitivity to barbiturates.

Anesthetic Considerations
Should be freshly prepared; discard after 24 hr or if precipitate is present. Effect potentiated by injection of contrast media. Reduces maximum allowable concentration of inhalation anesthetics. Do not mix with atropine sulfate, tubocurarine, succinylcholine, or other drugs.

Name
Phenylephrine (Neo-Synephrine)

Classification
Synthetic noncatecholamine that stimulates alpha$_1$-adrenergic receptors

Indications
Treatment of vasoconstrictor, treatment of hypotension, shock, supraventricular tachyarrhythmias, prolongation of duration of local anesthetics.

Dose

50–100 μg I.V. Do not exceed 0.5 mg initial dose or repeat sooner than 15 minutes. I.V. infusion: 20–50 μg/min titrate to effect.

Onset and Duration

Onset: almost immediate. Duration: 15–20 min.

Adverse Effects

Reflex bradycardia, arrhythmias, hypertension, headache, restlessness, reflex vagal action.

Precautions and Contraindications

Use with extreme caution in elderly patients and patients with hyperthyroidism, bradycardia, partial heart block, or severe arteriosclerosis.

Anesthetic Considerations

Infuse into a large vein; treat extravasation with phentolamine (5–10 mg in 10 mL normal saline and/or sympathetic block). Volatile agents may increase the risk of arrhythmias.

Name

Phentolamine (Regitine)

Classification

Alpha-adrenergic blocker

Indications

Controlled hypotension; treatment of perioperative hypertensive crisis that may accompany pheochromocytomectomy; prevention or treatment of dermal necrosis or sloughing after I.V. administration or extravasation of barbiturate or sympathomimetic

Dose

Antihypertensive: I.V./I.M. 2.5–5 mg. Antisloughing infiltration: 5–10 mg (maximum dose 10 mg). Dilute in 10 mL normal saline. Dosage forms: Injection 5 mg/ml; dilution for infusion 200 mg in 100 mL D_5W or normal saline.

Onset and Duration

Onset: I.V. 1–2 min; I.M. 5–20 min. Duration: I.V. 10–15 min; I.M. 30–45 min.

Adverse Effects

Hypotension, tachycardia, arrhythmias, myocardial infarctions, dizziness, cerebrovascular spasm and occlusion, flushing, diarrhea, nausea, vomiting.

Precautions and Contraindications

Use with caution in patients with ischemic heart disease. Phentolamine-induced alpha-receptor blockade will potentiate $beta_2$-adrenergic vasodilation of epinephrine, ephedrine, dobutamine, or isoproterenol.

DRUGS

Anesthetic Considerations
Use with epinephrine, ephedrine, dobutamine, or isoproterenol. May cause paradoxical fall in blood pressure.

Name
Phenytoin (Dilantin)

Classification
Anticonvulsant

Indications
Anticonvulsant; treatment of cardiac arrhythmias from digitalis intoxication, ventricular tachycardia, and paroxysmal atrial tachycardia resistant to conventional methods; treatment of migraine or trigeminal neuralgia

Dose
Anticonvulsant: 10–15 mg/kg I.V. in 50–100 mL normal saline at a rate not exceeding 50 mg/min or 1.5 g/24 hr.

Maintenance: I.V./P.O. 100 mg every 6–8 hr or 300–400 mg once a day. Antiarrhythmic: I.V.: 1.5 mg/kg slow push every 5 min until arrhythmia is suppressed or undesirable effects appear (maximum dosage 10–15 mg/kg per day).

Children: Anticonvulsant: loading dose 10–15 mg/kg 1 gram intravenous piggyback in normal saline up to 20 mg/kg in 24 hours.

P.O. maintenance: 4–8 mg/kg daily in 2 to 3 equally divided doses.

Dosage forms: Injection: 50 mg/mL. Capsules and extended-release capsules: 30, 100 mg. Chewable tablets: 50 mg. Oral suspension: 30 mg/5 mL, 125 mg/5 mL.

Onset and Duration
Onset: 3–5 min I.V. Therapeutic levels are 10–20 μg/mL and can be attained in 1–2 hr after appropriate loading. $t_{1/2}$ highly variable; increases as plasma levels increase; ranges from 8–60 hr (average 22 hr). Patients with liver disease may have highly variable clearance due to saturation kinetics.

Adverse Effects
Often dose-related. Nystagmus (>20 μg/mL), ataxia (>30 μg/mL), and somnolence (>40 μg/mL). Nausea, vomiting, gum hyperplasia, megaloblastic anemia due to folate deficiency. Osteomalacia with chronic therapy, thrombocytopenia, granulocytopenia, toxic hepatitis, rarely exfoliative dermatitis, Stevens–Johnson syndrome, lupus erythematosus (SLE). When given at a rate exceeding 50 mg/min, hypotension, cardiovascular collapse, and central nervous system depression may occur.

Precautions and Contraindications
If a rash occurs during therapy, the drug should be discontinued; if the rash is exfoliative, purpuric, or bullous or if SLE or Stevens–Johnson syndrome is suspected, phenytoin should not be restarted.

Will precipitate in all solutions other than normal saline. Flush line before and after administration. Do not mix with other drugs. Must be administered with in-line 0.22 micron I.V. filter.

Must be administered within 1 hr of mixing owing to short stability. Not useful in infantile febrile seizures.

Plasma levels should be monitored during therapy after steady state is achieved and whenever toxicity is suspected.

Abrupt withdrawal in patients with epilepsy may precipitate status epilepticus.

Safe use during pregnancy has not been established.

Phenytoin should be administered I.V. only with extreme caution to patients with respiratory depression or myocardial depression. I.V. use is contraindicated in patients with sinus bradycardia, sinoatrial block, second- or third-degree atrioventricular block or Adams–Stokes syndrome.

Phenytoin is highly protein-bound and has multiple drug interactions. Serum levels may be increased by diazepam, theophylline, warfarin, cimetidine, acute alcohol intake, halothane. Serum levels are decreased by chronic alcoholism.

Anesthetic Considerations

Phenytoin treatment may increase the dose requirements for all nondepolarizing muscle relaxants except atracurium. Dose-response curves are shifted to the right and the duration is markedly reduced.

Further confusion is generated by the observation that acute administration of phenytoin to a patient receiving vecuronium will augment the blockade. Phenytoin follows Michaelis–Menten kinetics. A small incremental dose can radically increase free drug levels at equilibrium.

Name
Physostigmine salicylate (Antilirium)

Classification
Anticholinesterase agent

Indications
Reversal of prolonged somnolence and anticholinergic poisoning.

Dose
I.V./I.M.: 0.5–2 mg (10–20 μg/kg) at rate of 1 mg/min; repeat dosing at intervals of 10–30 min.

Onset and Duration
Onset: I.V./I.M.: 3–8 min. Duration: I.V./I.M.: 30 min to 5 hr.

Adverse Effects
Bradycardia, bronchospasm, dyspnea, respiratory paralysis, seizures, salivation, nausea, vomiting, and miosis.

Precautions and Contraindications
High doses may cause tremors, ataxia, muscle fasciculations, and ultimately a depolarization block; use with caution in patients with epilepsy,

parkinsonian syndrome, or bradycardia. Do not use in the presence of asthma, diabetes, mechanical obstruction of the intestine or urogenital tract, and in patients receiving choline esters or depolarizing muscle relaxants.

Anesthetic Considerations
Rapid I.V. administration may cause bradycardia and hypersalivation, leading to respiratory problems or possibly seizures. Treatment of cholinergic crisis includes mechanical ventilation with repeated bronchial aspiration and I.V. administration of atropine, 2–4 mg every 3–10 min, until control of muscarinic symptoms is achieved or until signs of atropine overdose appear.

Name
Pipecuronium bromide (Arduan)

Classification
Nondepolarizing skeletal muscle relaxant

Indications
Adjunct to general anesthesia; skeletal muscle relaxation during surgery

Dose
I.V. paralyzing: 0.07–0.10 mg/kg.
Pretreatment and maintenance: 0.01–0.015 mg/kg.
Children: (3 mo to 1 yr) adult dosage on a mg/kg basis.
Dosage forms: Powder for injection 10 mg (10 mL).

Onset and Duration
Onset: <3 min. Duration: 45–120 min. Elimination: Renal.

Adverse Effects
Hypotension, hypertension, bradycardia, myocardial infarction, hypoventilation, apnea, depression, anuria, urticaria, rash, inadequate block, prolonged block, hypoglycemia, hyperkalemia, increased creatinine. Enhanced neuromuscular blockade in patients with myasthenia gravis.

Anesthetic Considerations
Reverse effects with anticholinesterase. Monitor response with peripheral nerve stimulator. Pretreatment doses may cause hypoventilation in some patients. Recommended only for procedures anticipated to last 90 min or longer.

Name
Prilocaine HCl (Citanest)

Classification
Amide-type local anesthetic

Indications
Regional anesthesia: infiltration/peripheral nerve block, topical, epidural, I.V. regional

Dose

    Infiltration/peripheral nerve block: 0.5–6 mg/kg (0.5–2% solution).
    Topical: 0.6–3 mg/kg (2–4% solution).
    Epidural: 200–300 mg (1–2% solution).
    (Maximum safe dosage: 6 mg/kg without epinephrine; 9 mg/kg with epinephrine 1:200,000.)

Onset and Duration

    Onset: Infiltration: 1–2 min. Epidural: 5–15 min. Peak effects: Infiltration/epidural: <30 min. Duration: Infiltration: 0.5–1.5 hr without epinephrine; 2–6 hr with epinephrine. Epidural: 1–3 hr (prolonged with epinephrine).

Adverse Effects

    Hypotension, arrhythmia, collapse, respiratory depression, paralysis, seizures, tinnitus, blurred vision, urticaria, anaphylactoid reactions, methemoglobinemia. High spinal: urinary retention, lower-extremity weakness and paralysis, loss of sphincter control, headache, backache, slowing of labor.

Precautions and Contraindications

    Use with caution in patients with hypovolemia, severe congestive heart failure, shock, all forms of heart block, pregnancy. Contraindicated in patients with hypersensitivity to amide-type local anesthetics, and in infants <6 mo old (low dose may cause methemoglobinemia).

Anesthetic Considerations

    Treat methemoglobinemia with methylene blue (1–2 mg/kg injected over 5 min). In I.V. regional blocks, deflate the cuff after 40 min and not before 20 min.

Name

Procainamide (Procan SR, Pronestyl)

Classification

    Class Ia antiarrhythmic

Indications

    Treatment of lidocaine-resistant ventricular arrhythmias; arrhythmia control in malignant hyperthermia; treatment of atrial fibrillation or paroxysmal atrial tachycardia.

Dose

    Loading: slow I.V. push 100 mg every 5 min (maximum 500 mg). Do not exceed 50 mg/min (children 3–6 mg/kg given over 5 min). Dilute 1000 mg in 50 mL D_5W. I.M. 100–500 mg in doses divided every 3 or 6 hours. Maintenance: Infusion 2–6 mg/min (children 0.02–0.08 mg/kg per min). Therapeutic level 3–10 μg/mL. Dosage form: Injection 100 mg/mL, 500 mg/mL. Dilution for infusion: 2 g in 500 mL D_5W (4 mg/mL).

DRUGS

Onset and Duration
Onset: I.V. immediate; I.M. 10–30 min. Duration: 2.5–5 hr.

Adverse Effects
Hypotension, heart block, arrhythmias, seizures, confusion, depression, psychosis, anorexia, nausea, vomiting, diarrhea, systemic lupus erythematosus (SLE), pruritus, fever, chills.

Precautions and Contraindications
Reduce doses in patients with congestive heart failure and renal failure. Contraindicated in complete heart block, torsades de pointes, SLE. Use cautiously in first-degree heart block and arrhythmias associated with digitalis toxicity.

Anesthetic Considerations
Periodic monitoring of plasma levels, vital signs, electrocardiogram (QRS widening greater than 25% may signify overdosage). Potentiates effect of both nondepolarizing and depolarizing muscle relaxants.

Name
Procaine HCl (Novocaine)

Classification
Ester-type local anesthetic

Indication
Local anesthetic: infiltration, peripheral nerve block, sympathetic nerve block, regional anesthesia

Dose
Infiltration: <500 mg (0.5–2% solution)
Epidural: <500 mg (1–2% solution). Solutions with preservatives may not be used for epidural or spinal block.
Spinal: 50–200 mg (10% solution with glucose 5%).

Onset and Duration
Onset: Infiltration/spinal: 2–5 min; epidural: 5–25 min.
Peak effects: Infiltration/epidural/spinal: <30 min.
Duration: Infiltration: 0.25–0.5 hr (without epinephrine); 0.5–1.5 hr (with epinephrine); epidural/spinal: 0.5–1.5 hr (prolonged with epinephrine).

Adverse Effects
Hypotension, bradycardia, arrhythmias, heart block, respiratory depression or arrest, tinnitus, seizures, dizziness, restlessness, loss of hearing, euphoria, postspinal headache, palsies, urticaria, pruritus, angioneurotic edema. High spinal: loss of bladder and bowel control, permanent motor, sensory, and autonomic (sphincter control) deficits of lower segments.

Contraindications
Caution in patients with severe cardiac disturbances (heart block, arrhythmias) or inflammation/sepsis at injection site. Contraindicated in

patients with hypersensitivity to local anesthetics, paraaminobenzoic acid (PABA)/parabens, or ester-type anesthetics.

Anesthetic Considerations
Central nervous system effects are generally dose-dependent and of short duration. Vasopressors, oxytocics may cause hypertension. Preparations containing preservatives should not be used for epidural and spinal anesthesia. Reduce doses for spinal anesthesia in obstetric, elderly, hypovolemic, and high-risk patients and those with increased intra-abdominal pressure.

Name
Prochlorperazine Maleate (Compazine)

Classification
Gastrointestinal agent, antiemetic, psychotherapeutic, phenothiazine antipsychotic.

Indications
Antiemetic used to control nausea and vomiting; antipsychotic used in the management of manifestations of psychotic disorders of excessive anxiety, tension, and agitation.

Dose
Antiemetic: P.O.: 5–10 mg t.i.d. or q.i.d. Rectal: 25 mg b.i.d. I.V./I.M.: 5–10 mg (at 5 mg/mL per min). Do not administer SQ because of local irritation. Maximum dose: 40 mg/day.

Onset and Duration
Onset: I.V.: A few minutes. I.M.: 10–20 min. P.O.: 30–40 min. Rectal: 60 min. Peak effects: I.V./I.M./P.O.: 15–30 min. Duration: I.V./I.M./P.O./Rectal: 3–4 hr.

Adverse Effects
Extrapyramidal reactions, dystonia, central nervous system depression, hypotension.

Contraindications
Pediatrics, parkinsonian disease

Anesthetic Considerations
May produce additive central nervous system depression when used with anesthetics. Avoid using with droperidol or metoclopramide because of extrapyramidal effects.

Name
Promethazine HCl (Phenergan, Pentazine, Phenazine, Prothazine)

Classification
Phenothiazine: Gastrointestinal agent, antiemetic, antivertigo agent, antihistamine (H_1-receptor antagonist), sedative or adjunct to analgesics

DRUGS

Indications

Motion sickness, nausea, rhinitis, allergy symptoms, sedation, routine preoperative or postoperative sedation, or as an adjunct to analgesics

Dose

I.V. (administer cautiously I.V. because of hazard of phlebitis, necrosis and gangrene of extremities; must dilute with equal volume of compatible diluent and administer slowly. For children, administer no larger dose than 0.5 mg/kg.) I.M., P.O., rectal: 12.5–50 mg. DO NOT administer SQ or intra-arterially owing to risk of necrosis and gangrene of extremities.

Dosage forms: Tablet, 12.5 mg, 25 mg, and 50 mg; syrup, 6.25 mg/5 mL and 25 mg/5 mL; suppositories, 12.5 mg, 25 mg, 50 mg; injection, 25 mg/mL and 50 mg/mL.

Onset and Duration

Onset: I.V.: 150 sec; I.M., P.O., rectal: 15–30 min. Duration: I.V., I.M., P.O., rectal: 2–5 hr.

Adverse Effects

Hypotension, bradycardia, bronchospasm, drowsiness, sedation, dizziness, confusion, extrapyramidal reactions, agranulocytosis, and thrombocytopenia may occur.

Precautions and Contraindications

Central nervous system and circulatory depressant actions of alcohol, sedative-hypnotics, and anesthetics are potentiated. Use is contraindicated in Parkinson's disease and in patients receiving MAO inhibitors.

Anesthetic Considerations

Anesthetic recovery may be prolonged. Do not use in children under 2 years of age.

Name

Propofol (Diprivan)

Classification

Anesthesia induction agent

Indications

Anesthesia induction and maintenance, I.V. sedation, prolonged sedation in critical care

Dose

I.V. bolus: 1.0–2.5 mg/kg. Dilute in suitable I.V. fluid, preferably D_5W. DO NOT dilute final solution to less than 2 mg/mL, to protect suspension. DO NOT use any filter with pore size smaller than 5 μm.

Infusion: 25–200 μg/kg/min.

Dosage form: 10 mg/mL in 20-mL ampules and 50-mL and 100-mL vials

Onset and Duration
Onset: Immediate. Duration: 5–20 min, depending on dose.

Adverse Effects
Hypotension, bradycardia, respiratory depression, prolonged somnolence, vivid dreams, burning on injection, hiccups, disinhibition, and arrhythmias may occur.

Precautions and Contraindications
Reduce the dose or avoid in patients with cardiac compromise, the elderly, and those with respiratory disease, hypotension, or increased intracranial pressure. Watch for respiratory and cardiac depression when co-administering other central nervous system or cardiac depressant drugs. Strict aseptic technique must be used when handling to avoid bacterial growth in the emulsion vehicle. Use is contraindicated in patients with egg or soybean allergy.

Anesthetic Considerations
Minimize pain on injection by giving a small dose of plain lidocaine 1% before injection. Both convulsant and anticonvulsant effects have been reported, so do not use in patients with a history of seizures. Antiemetic properties may be an advantage in patients at risk for postoperative nausea and vomiting.

Name
Protamine sulfate

Classification
Heparin antagonist

Indications
Treatment of heparin overdosage; heparin neutralization after extracorporeal circulation in arterial and cardiovascular surgery

Dose
Dosage based on blood coagulation studies, usually 1 mg protamine for every 100 U of heparin remaining in the patient given slowly I.V. over 10 minutes in doses not to exceed 50 mg.

Because heparin blood concentrations decrease rapidly, the dose of protamine sulfate required decreases based on elapsed time. One half of the usual dose of protamine should be given if 30 min has elapsed since heparin administration, and one fourth of the usual dose should be used if 2 hr or more has elapsed.

Dosage forms: Parenteral injection for I.V. use only: 10 mg/mL, 5-mL ampule or vial. Reconstitute 50-mg vial by adding 5 mL sterile water or bacteriostatic water containing 0.9% benzyl alcohol. Resultant solution contains 10 mg/mL. Protamine solution is intended for I.V. bolus use and not further dilution. If further dilution is desired, however, 5% dextrose or 0.9% NaCl I.V.P.B. may be used and given over 30 min.

Children: Injections preserved with benzyl alcohol may cause toxicity in the neonate.

Onset and Duration

Neutralization of heparin occurs within 5 min and persists approximately 2 hr.

Adverse Effects

Rapid I.V. injection of protamine is associated with hypotension, bradycardia, and flushing. Hypersensitivity, anaphylaxis, dyspnea, noncardiac pulmonary edema, circulatory collapse, pulmonary hypertension, and "heparin rebound" (after the use of protamine in cardiopulmonary bypass) can also occur. A paradoxical anticoagulant effect may occur with total doses greater than 100 mg.

Precautions and Contraindications

Monitor activated partial thromboplastin time or activated coagulation time at least 5–15 min after protamine administration to determine effect. Have equipment readily available to treat shock. Patients with a sensitivity to fish, vasectomized or infertile males, and patients who have previously received either protamine or insulins containing protamine are considered at higher risk for hypersensitivity. If protamine is used at all, pretreatment with a corticosteroid or antihistamine should be considered. Protamine is contraindicated in patients with a history of allergy to protamine.

Name

Propranolol (Inderal, Ipran, others)

Classification

Nonselective beta-adrenergic receptor antagonist

Indications

Hypertension, angina, ventricular and supraventricular arrhythmias, hyperthyroidism, migraines

Dose

I.V.: 0.25-mg increments, up to 3 mg. P.O.: 10–80 mg every 6–8 hr or 80–240 mg/day sustained release.

Dosage forms: Injection: 1 mg/mL (1 mL); tablet: 10 mg, 20 mg, 40 mg, 60 mg, 80 mg, 90 mg.

Onset and Duration

Onset: I.V.: <2 min; P.O.: 30–60 min. Duration: I.V.: 1–4 hr; P.O.: up to 24 hr sustained release.

Adverse Effects

Bradycardia, hypotension, atrioventricular block, bronchospasm, hypoglycemia, claudication, diarrhea, nausea, vomiting, constipation, nightmares, mental depression, insomnia may occur; propranolol may increase plasma triglycerides and decrease high-density lipoproteins.

Precautions and Contraindications
Use is contraindicated in asthmatics and patients with reduced myocardial reserve, peripheral vascular disease, diabetes, congestive heart failure, and shock. If drug is discontinued abruptly, withdrawal may be manifested as increased nervousness, increased heart rate, increased intensity of angina, or increased blood pressure (related to up regulation). Effects may be potentiated by inhalational anesthetics and other cardiodepressant drugs.

Anesthetic Considerations
Esmolol is preferred for intraoperative use owing to more controllable duration. Propranolol may be useful as antiarrhythmic because of membrane-stabilizing properties.

Name
Pyridostigmine bromide (Mestinon, Regonol)

Classification
Anticholinesterase agent for reversal of nondepolarizing muscle relaxants

Dose
Reversal: I.V.: 10–30 mg (0.1–0.25 mg/kg), preceded by atropine (0.015 mg/kg) or glycopyrrolate (0.01 mg/kg) I.V.
Myasthenia gravis: P.O.: 60–1500 mg/day; S.R. 180–540 mg daily or twice daily; to supplement oral dosage preoperatively and postoperatively, during labor and post partum, during myasthenic crisis, or when oral therapy is impractical, give 1/30 the oral dose I.M. or very slowly I.V.
Neonates of myasthenic mothers: 0.05–0.15 mg/kg I.M. Differentiate between cholinergic and myasthenic crisis in neonates. Administration 1 hr before completion of the second stage of labor enables patients to have adequate strength during labor and provides protection to infants in the intermediate postnatal stage.

Onset and Duration
Onset: Reversal I.V.: 2–5 min; myasthenia: I.M. <15 min; P.O. 20–30 min. Duration: Reversal I.V. 90 min; myasthenia: P.O. 3–6 hr, I.M. 2–4 hr.

Adverse Effects
Bradycardia, atrioventricular block, nodal rhythm, hypotension, increased bronchial secretions, bronchospasm, respiratory depression, nausea, vomiting, diarrhea, abdominal cramps, increased peristalsis, increased salivation, muscle cramps, fasciculations, weakness, miosis, and diaphoresis have been reported.

Precautions and Contraindications
Use with caution in patients with bradycardia, bronchial asthma, cardiac arrhythmias, or peptic ulcer and in patients with peritonitis or mechanical obstruction of the intestines or urinary tract.

DRUGS

Anesthetic Considerations

Overdosage may induce a cholinergic crisis characterized by nausea, vomiting, bradycardia or tachycardia, excessive salivation and sweating, bronchospasm, weakness, and paralysis. Treatment of a cholinergic crisis includes discontinuation of pyridostigmine and administration of atropine (10 μg/kg I.V. every 3–10 min until muscarinic symptoms subside).

Name
Ranitidine (Zantac)

Classification
H_2-receptor antagonist

Indications

Treatment of duodenal or gastric ulcers and gastroesophageal reflux; prophylaxis of aspiration pneumonitis in patients at high risk during surgery.

Dose

For patients with normal renal function: 50 mg I.V.P.B. diluted in at least 25 mL D_5W, NS, or suitable diluent, given over 15–20 min at least 1 hr before induction of anesthesia. The drug may be given with or without a similar dose the preceding evening. For patients with impaired renal function, as evidenced by creatinine clearance <50 mL/min, a single dose only is needed 1–4 hr before induction of anesthesia.

Alternatively, 150 mg ranitidine orally may be substituted for 50 mg I.V.P.B. When given orally, however, it is recommended to be given 2 hr preinduction.

Children 2–18 years: 0.1–0.8 mg/kg/dose I.V.P.B. at least 1 hr before induction infused over at least 5 min. Dilute to concentration of 0.5–2.5 mg/mL.

Dosage forms: 150-mg tablets; parenteral injection: 25 mg/mL in 2-mL or 10-mL multidose vials.

Onset and Duration

Mean gastric acid concentration significantly decreases 1 hr after I.V. infusion. Gastric acid inhibitory effects persist 8–12 hours. Elimination half-life is 2–3 hr.

Adverse Effects

Headache (1.8%), fatigue, dizziness, and mild gastrointestinal disturbances are the most frequent. Reversible hepatitis and potential hepatotoxicity has been reported infrequently. Reversible leukopenia, thrombocytopenia, granulocytopenia, and aplastic anemia have been reported rarely. Bradydysrhythmias and hypotension may be associated with rapid I.V. infusion.

Precautions and Contraindications
Hypersensitivity to ranitidine or other H_2-receptor antagonists. Caution is suggested in patients with hepatic insufficiency.

Name
Remifentanil (Ultiva)

Classification
Opiate analgesic, mu-receptor agonist

Indication
Perioperative analgesia

Dose
Infusion only: induction, 0.5–1 μg/kg/min; maintenance, 0.05–0.8 μg/kg/min; postoperative constipation in postanesthesia care unit, 0.025–0.2 μg/kg/min.

Dosage forms: 1-mg powder, 3-mL vial; 2-mg powder, 5-mL vial; 5-mg powder, 10-mL vial.

Supplemental bolus of 0.05 μg/kg may be given during induction and maintenance. Supplemental bolus is not recommended postoperatively because of risk of apnea or significant respiratory depression. Changes in infusion rate take 2–5 min for clinical response to change.

Adverse Effects
Adverse effects are similar to those of other opiate agonists and include nausea, vomiting, hypotension, bradycardia, respiratory depression, apnea, muscle rigidity, and pruritus.

Precautions and Contraindications
Oxygen saturation should be continuously monitored throughout administration. Resuscitative and airway management equipment must be immediately available. Drug should not be admixed with lactated Ringer's injection and lactated Ringer's 15% dextrose but can be co-administered with these solutions in a freely running I.V. line. Do not run remifentanil in the same line with blood, because drug is metabolized by esterase enzymes. The I.V. line should be cleared after discontinuation to prevent inadvertent administration. Use is contraindicated for epidural or intrathecal administration owing to glycine in the vehicle formulation.

Anesthetic Considerations
Drug effects rapidly dissipate after discontinuation of the infusion, so preparation for postoperative care may include longer-acting opiates or

DRUGS

nonsteroidal anti-inflammatory agents. Because the drug is metabolized by nonspecific esterases, no change in kinetics has been noted in patients with cholinesterase deficiencies or renal or hepatic disease. Normal kinetics have been noted in pediatric, geriatric, and obese patients.

Name
Ritodrine HCl (Yutopar)

Classification
Beta$_2$-adrenergic agonist, tocolytic agent, sympathomimetic

Indication
Management of preterm labor (tocolysis)

Dose
Infusion: Prepare in D$_5$W if clinically appropriate or in NaCl 0.9% I.V. solution of 0.3 mg/mL. Start at 0.1 mg/min (20 mL/hr at this concentration) and slowly increase by 0.05 mg/min every 10 to 15 min, up to 0.35 mg/min. Continue infusion for at least 12 hr after cessation of uterine contractions at maximum rate achieved.

P.O.: Start before discontinuation of the I.V. infusion at 10 mg every 2 hr for 24 hr, then 10–20 mg every 4–6 hr (maximum dose should not exceed 120 mg/d).

Dosage forms: Tablet 10 mg; injection, 10 mg/mL in 5-mL ampules and vials; injection, 15 mg/mL in 10-mL vials and 10-mL prefilled syringe; solution for I.V. infusion, 150 mg in D$_5$W 500 mL (0.3 mg/mL).

Onset and Duration
Onset: I.V.: immediate; P.O.: 40–60 min. Duration: 3–6 hr I.V.

Adverse Effects
Beta$_1$ agonist effects are common and include tachycardia, arrhythmias, hypertension, hyperventilation, pulmonary edema, tremors, headache, anxiety, nausea, vomiting and diarrhea, and hyperglycemia. Reactive hypoglycemia may occur in the infant post partum.

Precautions and Contraindications
Pulmonary edema is common with overhydration, so fluid intake should be closely monitored, especially in patients taking corticosteroids. Monitor glucose and electrolyte levels. Use is contraindicated before 20 weeks of pregnancy and in preeclampsia, eclampsia, intrauterine fetal death or fetal distress, uncontrolled maternal diabetes, maternal hyperthyroidism and hypertension, and placental detachment. Questions have been raised as to the clinical benefits related to perinatal morbidity and mortality.

Anesthetic Considerations
Patients may experience wide swings in vital signs secondary to beta-receptor stimulation. Bradycardia and hypotension may occur after cessation of therapy. Glucose, insulin, and potassium levels are commonly altered during therapy and should be evaluated. Mild hypokalemia is

usually not treated. Additive hypertension and tachycardia occur when drug is given with other sympathomimetics. Adverse effects may be antagonized by beta-blocking agents.

Name
Rocuronium (Zemuron)

Classification
Nondepolarizing neuromuscular blocking agent

Indication
Tracheal intubation and intraoperative skeletal muscle relaxation; in critical care to facilitate mechanical ventilation.

Dose
Adults and children: intubation, 0.6 mg/kg. Maintenance: adults—0.1–0.2 mg/kg; children—0.08–0.12 mg/kg I.V.

Onset and Duration
Onset: 60–90 seconds with intubating doses of 3–5 times ED_{95} (0.9–1.5 mg/kg). ED_{95} = 0.3 mg/kg. Duration: 30–120 min depending on dose.

Adverse Effects
Adverse reactions are rare. Prolonged effect occurs in patients with hepatic disease.

Precautions and Contraindications
Use is contraindicated in patients known to have hypersensitivity to rocuronium bromide. Proper airway maintenance capabilities must be ensured before administration.

Anesthetic Considerations
Use of inhalation agents, antibiotics, and magnesium may prolong duration of action. Many clinicians consider it the agent of choice for nondepolarizing rapid sequence induction and when intubating doses are used. No significant cardiac or histamine-releasing effects occur with clinical doses.

Name
Scopolamine (Transderm Scōp)

Classification
Competitive acetylcholine antagonist at muscarinic receptor

Indications
Prevention and treatment of nausea and vomiting induced by motion (motion sickness), premedication, amnesia, sedation, or vagolysis. Greater sedation, amnesia, antisialogogue and ocular effects than atropine and lesser effects on heart, bronchial smooth muscle, and gastrointestinal

tract. Widely used premedicant for cardiac patients in combination with morphine and a major tranquilizer.

Dose
P.O.: 0.4–1.2 mg. Usual adult I.M., I.V., or SQ dose is 0.3 to 0.65 mg 30 to 80 min before induction.

Transderm patch: 1.5 mg/2.5 cm^2; delivers 0.5 mg/72 hr. Apply to postauricular skin.

Children: 0.006 mg/kg or 0.2 mg/m^2 I.M. or I.V. Maximum dose is 0.3 mg.

Dosage forms: 0.3-, 0.4-, 0.86-, and 1-mg/mL parenteral injection; Transderm patch: 1.5 mg/2.5 cm^2.

Onset and Duration
Onset after I.V. administration is almost immediate; onset after P.O. or I.M. administration is about 30 min. Duration is 30–60 min after I.V. and 4–6 hr after I.M. administration. Transdermal systems are designed to provide an antiemetic effect within 4 hr of application with a duration of up to 72 hr.

Adverse Effects
Hallucinations, delirium, and coma may occur in central anticholinergic syndrome. Treatment is with pyridostigmine 15–60 μg/kg. Other effects include paradoxical bradycardia in low doses, mydriasis, blurred vision, tachycardia, drowsiness, restlessness, confusion, anaphylaxis, dry nose and mouth, constipation, urinary hesitancy, retention, increased intraocular pressure, decreased sweating. Children and elderly are more susceptible to adverse effects.

Precautions and Contraindications
Use is contraindicated in patients with acute angle glaucoma, obstructive disease of the gastrointestinal tract, obstructive uropathy, intestinal atony, and acute hemorrhage when cardiovascular status is unstable.

Use with caution when tachycardia would be harmful (i.e., thyrotoxicosis, pheochromocytoma or coronary artery disease). Avoid in hyperpyrexial states because it inhibits sweating. Use with caution in patients with hepatic or renal disease, congestive heart failure, chronic pulmonary disease (because a reduction in bronchial secretions may lead to formation of bronchial plugs), hiatal hernia, gastroesophageal reflux, gastrointestinal infections, and ulcerative colitis.

Anesthetic Considerations
Potentiates sedative effects of narcotics, benzodiazepines, anticholinergics, antihistamines, and volatile anesthetics.

Name
Sodium Citrate (Bicitra)

Classification
Nonparticulate neutralizing buffer

Indications
Prophylaxis of aspiration pneumonitis during anesthesia. Metabolized to sodium bicarbonate and thus acts as systemic alkalinizer. When given

within 60 minutes of surgery sodium citrate is effective in raising the gastric pH above 2.5 in most patients. Theoretically, this should decrease risk of pulmonary damage secondary to aspiration of gastric contents; however, this remains controversial.

Dose
Adults: 15 mL diluted in 15 mL water as a single dose.
  Children: 5–15 mL diluted in 5–15 mL water as a single dose, or 1 mEq/kg as a single dose
  Dosage forms: Sodium citrate dihydrate 500 mg (321.5 mg of citrate) per 5 mL and citric acid monohydrate 334 mg/5 mL. Each 1 mL contains 1 mEq sodium and 1 mEq citrate.

Onset and Duration
Maximally effective when given less than 60 minutes preoperatively.

Adverse Effects
Saline laxative effect results when sodium citrate is given orally. Metabolic alkalosis occurs in large doses in patients with renal dysfunction.

Contraindications
Sodium citrate is contraindicated in patients with severe renal impairment with oliguria, azotemia, or anuria. It is also contraindicated in patients with Addison's disease, heat cramps, acute dehydration, adynamic episodica hereditaria, and severe myocardial disease.

Name
Somatostatin (Zecnil)

Classification
Synthetic somatostatin, growth hormone release inhibiting factor; also inhibits glucagon, insulin, secretin, gastrin, and thyroid-stimulating hormone

Indications
Prophylaxis in preoperative management of patients with carcinoid syndrome and treatment of hypotensive episodes associated with surgical manipulation of carcinoid tumor, gastrointestinal bleeding, malignant diarrhea, enterocutaneous and pancreatic fistulas, and short bowel syndrome. Epidural somatostatin has been effective in treating postoperative pain; intrathecal and intraventricular somatostatin have been employed for terminal cancer pain in limited studies.

Dose
Adults: Continuous infusion required to sustain therapeutic effects. Usual infusion rate is 250 μg/hr, with or without an initial 250-μg bolus. Dilute 3 mg somatostatin in 50 mL D$_5$W or NS and infuse continuously over 12 hr (250 μg/hr) on a syringe pump. (Octreotide [Sandostatin], a long-acting analogue of somatostatin, may also be used. The initial dose is 50 μg SQ, but I.V. injection can be used in an emergency.) Somatostatin

DRUGS

is currently designated an "orphan drug" by the Food and Drug Administration.

Dosage forms: somatostatin (Zecnil) 3 mg lyophilized ampules; octreotide (Sandostatin) 0.1, 0.05, and 0.5 mg/mL injection.

Onset and Duration

Onset: 5–10 min after initiation of infusion. Effects decrease rapidly after discontinuance of infusion to baseline in 1 hr. Plasma half-life is 1 to 3 min. (The half-life of octreotide is 45 min after I.V. and 80 min after subcutaneous administration.)

Adverse Effects

Nausea, vomiting, diarrhea, and abdominal cramps may occur during infusion. Glucose intolerance in nondiabetic patients and reduced insulin requirements in insulin-dependent diabetics have been noted. Less-frequent effects include arrhythmias and hyponatremia.

Precautions and Contraindications

Use is contraindicated in patients with previous hypersensitivity to somatostatin or octreotide. Use with caution in patients with diabetes. Rebound hypersecretion of growth hormone and other hormones usually occurs after infusion is discontinued. Monitor blood glucose levels during therapy. Rebound fistula output is also noted in patients with enterocutaneous fistulas.

Name

Succinylcholine (Anectine, Quelicin, others)

Classification

Depolarizing skeletal muscle relaxant

Indications

Surgical muscle relaxation for short procedures, to facilitate endotracheal intubation

Dose

Aduts: I.V.: 1–1.5 mg/kg, up to 150 total dose. Children: 1.0–2.0 mg/kg I.V. or 2–4 mg/kg I.M. Pretreat with atropine due to incidence of bradycardia.

Dosage form: Injection: 20 mg/mL; powder for infusion: 500 mg (mix in 500 mL for 1 mg/mL solution).

Onset and Duration

Onset: Immediate. Duration: 5–10 min.

Adverse Effects

Numerous side effects have been reported that relate to the skeletal muscle depolarizing action of the drug. These include hyperkalemia, postoperative muscle pain, increased gastric pressure, and increased intraocular pressure. Numerous cardiac arrhythmias have been reported, including sudden cardiac arrest and bradycardia with repeat dosing or with any dose in children. Prolonged paralysis and inadequate recovery may occur with infusion doses. Masseter muscle spasm may be a premonitory sign of malignant hyperthermia along with sudden unexplained tachycardia or an abrupt increase in carbon dioxide elimination. (See Appendix 10 for malignant hyperthermia protocol.)

Precautions and Contraindications; Anesthetic Considerations
Succinylcholine should not be used for routine intubation in children younger than 12 years old owing to reports of sudden cardiac arrest in children with undiagnosed Duchenne's muscular dystrophy and with muscle disorders. Other contraindications include malignant hyperthermia; patients with genetic variants of plasma cholinesterase or cholinesterase deficiencies; myopathies associated with elevated creatine phosphokinase values; most muscle disorders or muscular dystrophies; acute narrow-angle glaucoma; patients with greater than 25% total body surface areas with third-degree burns; severe muscle trauma or muscle wasting; neurologic injury such as paraplegia, quadriplegia, spinal cord injury or cerebrovascular accident; hyperkalemia; severe sepsis; and electrolyte imbalances. Repeated doses at short intervals (<5 min) are associated with bradycardia.

Name
Sufentanil Citrate (Sufenta)

Classification
Opioid agonist; produces analgesia and anesthesia

Dose
Analgesia: I.V./I.M.: 0.2–0.6 μg/kg
Induction: I.V.: 2–10 μg/kg
Infusion: 0.01–0.05 μg/kg/min
Epidural bolus: 0.2–0.6 μg/kg; infusion 5–30 μg/hr (0.2–0.6 μg/kg/hr)
Spinal: 0.02–0.08 μg/kg.

Onset and Duration
Onset: I.V. immediate; epidural and spinal: 4–10 min. Duration: I.V.: 20–45 min; I.M.: 2–4 hr; epidural and spinal: 4–8 hr.

Adverse Effects
Hypotension, bradycardia, respiratory depression, apnea, dizziness, sedation, euphoria, dysphoria, anxiety, nausea, vomiting, delayed gastric emptying, biliary tract spasm, and muscle rigidity have been reported.

Precautions and Contraindications
Reduce doses in elderly, hypovolemic, high-risk patients and those taking sedatives and other narcotics. Sufentanil crosses the placental barrier; usage in labor may produce depression of respiration in the neonate.

Anesthetic Considerations
Narcotic effect is reversed with naloxone (0.2–0.4 mg I.V.). Duration of reversal may be shorter than duration of narcotic effect. Circulatory

DRUGS

and ventilatory depressant effects are potentiated by other narcotics, sedatives, nitrous oxide, and volatile anesthetics; ventilatory depressant effects are potentiated by monoamine oxidase inhibitors, phenothiazines, and tricyclic antidepressants; analgesia is enhanced by alpha$_2$-agonists; skeletal muscle rigidity in higher doses is sufficient to interfere with ventilation; increased incidences of bradycardia occur with the use of vecuronium.

Name
Terbutaline sulfate (Brethine, Brethaire, Bricanyl)

Classification
Beta$_2$-adrenergic agonist, bronchodilator

Indications
Bronchodilator for treatment of asthma

Dose
Bronchodilator: SQ: 0.25 mg (may repeat in 15–30 min. Do not exceed 0.5 mg in 4–6 hr).
Inhalation: 2 breaths separated by 60 sec every 4–6 hr. P.O.: 5 mg t.i.d. (2.5–5 mg, every 6 hr), up to 15 mg/day.
Children less than 12 years old: P.O.: 0.05 mg/kg/dose t.i.d., maximum 0.15 mg/kg/dose or 5 mg day; SQ 5–10 μg/kg/dose every 20 min × 3 doses.
Dosage forms: Injection: 1 mg/mL (1 mL); tablet: 2.5 mg, 5 mg.

Onset and Duration
Onset: SQ: 30–60 min; P.O.: 2–3 hr; inhalation: 1–2 hr. Duration: SQ: 1–4 hr; P.O.: 4–8 hr; inhalation: 2–6 hr.

Adverse Effects
Adverse effects are similar to those of other beta-agonists and include hypertension, tachycardia, arrhythmias, tremors, dizziness, headache, nausea, vomiting, gastrointestinal upset, hypokalemia, and hyperglycemia.

Precautions and Contraindications
Use with caution in patients with hypertension, ischemic heart disease, arrhythmias, congestive heart failure, diabetes mellitus, hyperthyroidism, and seizures. Action is antagonized by beta-adrenergic blocking agents. Tolerance develops with repeated use.

Anesthetic Considerations
Patients may experience wide swings in vital signs secondary to beta-receptor stimulation. Bradycardia and hypotension may occur after cessation of therapy. Glucose, insulin, and potassium levels are commonly altered during therapy and should be evaluated. Mild hypokalemia is usually not treated. Additive hypertension and tachycardia occur when terbutaline is given with other sympathomimetics. Adverse effects may be antagonized by beta-blocking agents.

Name
Tetracaine HCl (Pontocaine)

Classification
Ester-type local anesthetic

Indications
Local, spinal, and topical anesthesia

Dose
Spinal: 2–20 mg adjusted to height (rarely, >15 mg). Decrease usual dose in pregnant women. Dilute with equal volume of sterile dextrose 10% (hyperbaric) to more easily control height. Apply topical spray 2% solution in short spurts of less than 2 sec. Maximum safe dose: 1.5 mg/kg. Inject slowly: not >1 mL/5 sec. Pediatric doses have not been established.

Dosage forms: Injection: 1% (2 mL) for spinal anesthesia; ointment (ophthalmic) 0.5% (3.5 g); solution, ophthalmic: 0.5% (15 mL), topical: 2% (30 mL, 118 mL).

Onset and Duration
Onset: Spinal: 5–10 min; fixing time: 20–30 min. Duration: 1–3 hr, possibly longer if 10–20 μg of epinephrine is added to spinal bolus.

Adverse Effects
Spinal use: hypotension, bradycardia, respiratory depression or apnea, high or total spinal with paralysis, infection secondary to spinal needle placement, headache.

Precautions and Contraindications
Avoid in patients allergic to ester-type local anesthetics such as procaine, chloroprocaine, or cocaine. Tetracaine contains *para*-aminobenzoic acid (PABA), so avoid in patients with allergy to this sunscreen. Drug is reserved for spinal or topical anesthesia only because other local anesthetic drugs are safer for injection or infiltration. Seizures may occur with toxic doses. Monitor vital signs carefully during initial administration. Not for ocular use.

Anesthetic Considerations
Long-standing agent for spinal anesthesia. Use amide local anesthetics such as lidocaine or bupivacaine if allergy is suspected. Watch for high spinal level. Produces a stronger motor block and more relaxation than bupivacaine. Adequate hydration minimizes hypotension. Reduce dose in morbidly obese, obstetric, and elderly patients and those with increased abdominal pressure.

Name
Thiamylal (Surital)

Classifications
Barbiturate, ultra short-acting intravenous sedative-hypnotic anesthesia-inducing agent

DRUGS

Indications

Induction agent for general anesthesia; sole anesthetic for short surgical procedures.

Dose

Induction: 3–5 mg/kg of 2.5% solution intravenously.
Dosage form: Injection, powder: dilute to 10 mg/mL.

Onset and Duration

Onset: Immediate. Duration: 10–30 min depending on dose.

Adverse Effects

Hypotension, respiratory depression, apnea, laryngospasm, bradycardia may occur.

Precautions and Contraindications

Do not use in patients with allergies to any barbiturate or a history of porphyria. Reduce dose or possibly avoid in elderly patients and those with severe cardiovascular disease, shock, or asthma.

Anesthetic Considerations

Actions are nearly identical to those of thiopental. Use with caution in patients with cardiorespiratory compromise or moderate to severe multiorgan failure. Reduce dose in the elderly.

Name

Trimethaphan (Arfonad)

Classification

Autonomic ganglion blocking agent, antihypertensive

Indications

Controlled hypotension during surgery; use during neurologic procedures and abdominal aneurysm repair

Dose

1% solution (500 mg in 500 mL). Infuse 0.3–2 mg/min and adjust to effect.

Onset and Duration

Onset: Immediate. Duration: 5–30 min depending on duration of infusion.

Adverse Effects

Hypotension, tachycardia, histamine release, mydriasis, urinary retention, and dry mouth.

Precautions and Contraindications

Avoid in asthmatics because of frequent histamine release. Excessive hypotension and tachycardia occur especially in hypovolemic patients. Avoid in patients with deficiencies of plasma cholinesterase.

Anesthetic Considerations

Use as a supplement for deliberate hypotensive techniques. Tachyphylaxis develops frequently and can be minimized by infusing slowly for brief periods. Nitroprusside and nitroglycerin are more commonly used.

Name

Vancomycin (Vancocin)

Classification

Antimicrobial agent

Indications

Treatment of documented or suspected methicillin-resistant *Staphylococcus aureus* or beta-lactam–resistant coagulase-negative *Streptococcus*. Documented or suspected staphylococcal or streptococcal infections in penicillin- or cephalosporin-allergic patients.

Prophylaxis of bacterial endocarditis in high-risk patients (rheumatic heart disease, mitral valve prolapse, valvular heart dysfunction, bioprosthetic and allograft valves) who undergo dental, oral, or upper respiratory procedures and who are penicillin or cephalosporin allergic. Also for prophylaxis in penicillin-allergic patients undergoing gastrointestinal, biliary, or genitourinary tract surgery or instrumentation who are at risk of developing enterococcal endocarditis.

Prophylactic therapy for potential infections related to ventricular-peritoneal shunt, vascular graft, or open-heart surgery in penicillin-allergic patients.

Because vancomycin is not absorbed orally, the only indication for oral vancomycin is pseudomembranous colitis.

Dose

Initial I.V. dosage recommendation: Adults: initial I.V. dose 15 mg/kg, followed by 10 mg/kg every 12 hr in patients with normal renal function. Maximum dose is 3 g/day. Patients with mild renal failure (creatinine clearance ≤50 mL/min) should receive vancomycin every 24–72 hr; patients with moderate renal failure (creatinine clearance of 10–50 mL/min) should receive vancomycin every 72–240 hours; and patients with severe renal failure (creatinine clearance <10 mL/min) should receive vancomycin every 240 hr.

Children: Children more than 5 kg and 7 days postnatal age and younger than 13 years of age: 10 mg/kg every 6 hr. Children older than 13 years of age can be dosed as adults.

Peak and trough serum levels should be monitored if therapy extends beyond 24 hr perioperative prophylaxis. Dosage and dosage interval should be adjusted to produce peak levels of 25 to 40 μg/mL and trough levels of 5–10 μg/mL.

Dosage forms: Parenteral injection for I.V. use: 500 mg or 1-g vials. Reconstitute sterile powder by adding 10 mL or 20 mL sterile water to 500-mg or 1-g vials, respectively. Reconstituted solution containing 500 mg or 1 g must be further diluted with at least 100 mL or at least 250 mL D_5W or NS, respectively. Infuse I.V.P.B. over 1–1.5 h.

DRUGS

Onset and Duration

Half-life varies: 4–6 hr reported in patients with normal renal function. Usually given 1 hr before procedure for prophylaxis of endocarditis. Some clinicians suggest dose should be repeated 8–12 hr later in patients with normal renal function. However, the American Heart Association, American Academy of Pediatrics, and the American Dental Association state that a second dose is unnecessary.

Adverse Effects

Red man syndrome (erythema, pruritus, and rash involving face, neck, upper trunk, and arms), hypertension, and tachycardia are associated with rapid infusion. Ototoxity is associated with prolonged serum concentrations >40 mg/mL. Other adverse effects are chills, fever, neutropenia, thrombocytopenia, agranulocytosis, and phlebitis.

Precautions and Contraindications

Monitor renal function tests frequently during therapy. Use with caution in patients with renal impairment or those receiving other nephrotoxic or ototoxic drugs. Use is contraindicated in patients hypersensitive to vancomycin. Avoid in patients with previous hearing loss.

Anesthetic Considerations

Vancomycin potentiation of succinylcholine-induced neuromuscular blockage has been reported. The drug may increase neuromuscular blockade by nondepolarizing muscle relaxants whose dose should be titrated.

Name

Vasopressin (Pitressin)

Classification

Antidiuretic hormone

Indications

Treatment of diabetes insipidus, treatment of bleeding esophageal varices and other types of upper gastrointestinal bleeding, and control of refractory operative bleeding in intrauterine procedures.

Dose

Diabetes insipidus or treatment of abdominal distention in postoperative patients: 5–10 U three to four times daily as needed.

Gastrointestinal hemorrhage: 0.2–1 U/min infused I.V. After 12 hr of hemorrhage control, decrease the dose by half and then stop within next 12–24 hours. I.V. nitroglycerin should be infused concomitantly to control side effects.

Locally to operative site: 20 U in 30 mL NS as a gauze soak.

Children: For diabetes insipidus: 2.5–5 U I.M. or SQ every 6 to 8 hr; titrate based on response.

I.V.: 1–3 mU/kg/hr

Gastrointestinal bleeding: 0.01 U/kg/min.

Dosage forms: 20 pressor U/mL aqueous injection; must be diluted for I.V. infusion in D_5W or NS to a concentration of 100–1000 U/L.

Onset and Duration

Antidiuretic action lasts 2–8 hr after I.M. or SQ administration; the pressor effects last 30–60 min after I.V. injection. Half-life is 10–35 min.

Adverse Effects

Tremor, sweating, vertigo, water intoxication, hyponatremia, metabolic acidosis, abdominal cramps, nausea, vomiting, urticaria, and anaphylaxis; angina in patients with pre-existing cardiovascular impairment.

Precautions and Contraindications

Use is contraindicated in patients with anaphylaxis or hypersensitivity to vasopressin and in those with chronic nephritis with nitrogen retention until reasonable nitrogen blood levels are attained. Use with extreme caution in patients who cannot tolerate rapid retention of extracellular water or who have coronary artery disease. Use a central vein preferably with I.V. infusion owing to possibility of tissue necrosis with extravasation. Monitor patients with epilepsy, migraine, asthma, and heart failure closely. I.V. administration should be used only for emergency treatment of gastrointestinal hemorrhage.

Name

Vecuronium (Norcuron)

Classification

Nondepolarizing muscle relaxant

Indications

Intraoperative muscle relaxation, endotracheal intubation, and facilitation of mechanical ventilation in critical care

Dose

I.V.: 0.05–0.2 mg/kg for paralysis.
Dosage form: Powder for injection 10 mg (5 mL, 10 mL).

Onset and Duration

Onset: 1–3 min. Duration: 30–90 min.

Adverse Effects

Prolonged paralysis occurs in patients with hepatic disease. Apnea ensues immediately on administration, so appropriate airway management and resuscitative equipment must be immediately available. No significant cardiac effects have been noted.

Anesthetic Considerations

Monitor response with a nerve stimulator to avoid excessive dosing. Long-term infusions in critical care may result in prolonged recovery and

DRUGS

inability to reverse due to active metabolites. Corticosteroid therapy in patients with multiorgan failure may exacerbate this effect.

Name
Verapamil (Isoptin, Calan, others)

Classification
Calcium channel blocker

Indications
Supraventricular arrhythmias, hypertension, angina

Dose
I.V.: 2.5–10 mg slowly; may repeat in 30–60 min. P.O.: 120–480 mg/day in divided doses.

Dosage forms: Injection: 2.5 mg/mL (2 mL); tablet: 40 mg, 80 mg, 120 mg; tablet, sustained release: 120 mg, 180 mg, 240 mg.

Onset and Duration
Onset: I.V.: 2–5 min; P.O.: 30–60 min. Duration: I.V.: 30 min to 2 hr; P.O.: 4–12 hr.

Adverse Effects
Hypotension, heart block, tachycardia or bradycardia; ankle edema and constipation with chronic oral use.

Precautions and Contraindications
Significant hypotension may occur in patients with poor left ventricular function. It may exacerbate atrioventricular block or Wolff-Parkinson-White syndrome. Additive depression occurs with other cardiac depressants.

Anesthetic Considerations
Titrate slowly owing to significant cardiac depressant effects, which are additive with anesthetics. Diltiazem infusion may be better option for treatment of intraoperative atrial arrhythmias. Beta-blockers are superior for treatment of sinus tachycardia.

Name
Vitamin K, Phytonadione (Aquamephyton, Mephyton)

Classification
Vitamin, water-soluble

Indications
Prevention and treatment of hypoprothrombinemia caused by drug- or anticoagulant-induced vitamin K deficiency or hemorrhagic diseases of the newborn

Dose

I.V. route should be used for emergencies only. Inject slow I.V. only: not >1 mg/min.

Newborn hemorrhage: I.M., SQ prophylaxis 0.5–1 mg within 1 hr of birth. Treat with 1–2 mg/day.

Anticoagulant reversal: Infants, 1–2 mg every 4–8 hr. Adult P.O., I.V., I.M., SQ: 2.5–10 mg; may repeat I.V., SQ, I.M. dose every 6–8 hr and oral dose in 12–48 hr.

Dosage forms: Tablet: 5 mg; injection: 2 mg/mL in 0.5-mL ampule and 10 mg/mL in 1-mL ampule and 2.5-mL and 5-mL vials.

Onset and Duration

Onset: I.V., I.M., SQ: 1–3 hr. P.O.: 4–12 hr. Duration: 6–48 hr depending on dose and route of administration.

Adverse Effects

Severe anaphylaxis may occur with I.V. use. Severe hemolytic anemia has been reported in neonates given large doses (20 mg).

Precautions and Contraindications

Use intravenous route in emergencies only, owing to possibility of severe anaphylaxis. Vitamin K is ineffective in hereditary hypoprothrombinemia or hypoprothrombinemia secondary to severe liver disease.

Anesthetic Considerations

Monitor prothrombin time. Transfusion of blood or fresh-frozen plasma may be necessary in severe hemorrhagic states.

Name

Tubocurarine chloride

Classification

Nondepolarizing skeletal muscle relaxer

Indications

Adjunct to general anesthetics to provide adequate muscle relaxation

Dose

Neonates: <1 month: 0.3 mg/kg single dose; Maintenance: 0.15 mg/kg as needed. Children and adults: 0.2–0.4 mg/kg single dose. Maintenance: 0.04–0.2 mg/kg. Dosage forms: Injection: 3 mg/mL.

Onset and Duration

Onset <2 min; Duration: 25–90 min; Elimination: renal, hepatic.

Adverse Effects

Hypotension, bradycardia, arrhythmia, respiratory depression, apnea, inadequate block, prolonged block, rash, urticaria.

DRUGS

Precautions and Contraindications

Persons in whom release of histamine is a hazard, hyperthermia, myasthenia gravis, electrolyte imbalance, or acidosis.

Anesthetic Considerations

Monitor response with peripheral nerve stimulator. Use with caution in asthmatics. Reverse effects with anticholinesterase. Pretreatment doses may induce a degree of neuromuscular blockade to cause hyperventilation in some patients.

Name

Warfarin (Coumadin)

Classification

Anticoagulant; depresses formation of vitamin K–dependent clotting factors (II, VII, IX, X) in the liver.

Indications

Treatment or prophylaxis of deep-vein thrombosis or pulmonary thromboembolism. Prophylaxis of thromboembolism in patients with atrial fibrillation, undergoing cardioversion of atrial fibrillation, with prosthetic heart valves, after major surgery requiring prolonged immobilization (total knee or hip replacements), and after myocardial infarction in patients who are at high risk of embolism (those with congestive heart failure, atrial fibrillation, previous myocardial infarction, or history of thromboembolism).

Dose

Warfarin dosing is adjusted according to PT. Standardization of PT results among laboratories is accomplished with the use of an International Normalized Ratio equation:

$$INR = \left(\frac{PT_{Patient}}{PT_{Reference}}\right)^{ISI}$$

where ISI is the International Sensitivity Index.

The typical goal INR is 2 to 3, except for patients with prosthetic valves, in whom 2.5 to 3.5 is the desired goal. Commonly, doses of 5–10 mg/day are tapered to 2–10 mg/day, as indicated by the PT. Consult the pharmacy for institutional guidelines.

Multiple drug interactions may increase or decrease response. Dosage forms: 2, 2.5, 5, 7.5, and 10 mg tabs; 50 mg for parenteral injection with 2 mL diluent.

Onset and Duration

Antithrombogenic effects may not occur for up to 5–7 days after initiation of therapy. Many clinicians recommend that heparin be administered concurrently for 3–7 days until the desired PT is achieved. Duration of action of a single oral dose is 2–5 days. $t_{1/2}$ 0.5–3 days.

Adverse Effects

Dose-dependent bleeding ranging from minor local bleeding or ecchymosis (2%–10%) to major hemorrhagic complications occasionally resulting in death. Major hemorrhage usually involves gastrointestinal or genitourinary tract, but may involve hepatic, cerebral, or pericardial sites. Minor bleeding can be treated with vitamin K I.M. or I.V. 5–10 mg up to 50 mg. Frank bleeding should be treated with administration of fresh whole blood or fresh-frozen plasma (15 mL/kg). Agranulocytosis, leukopenia, thrombocytopenia, necrosis of skin, purple-toe syndrome, neuropathy.

Precautions and Contraindications

Contraindicated in bleeding or patients with hemorrhagic blood dyscrasias, aneurysms, pericarditis or pericardial effusions, uncontrolled hypertension, recent or contemplated surgery of the eye, brain or spinal cord or any traumatic surgery resulting in large open surfaces, recent cerebrovascular accident. Renal and hepatic function should be monitored periodically. PT should be monitored daily initially, then after PT is stabilized, every 4–6 wk. Warfarin is teratogenic and is contraindicated in pregnancy. Risks of hemorrhage may be increased with concomitant use of aspirin, nonsteroidal anti-inflammatory drugs, cimetidine, amiodarone, steroids, chloral hydrate, metronidizole, streptokinase, urokinase, antibiotics, and heparin. Discontinue warfarin promptly in patients with purple-toe syndrome or skin necrosis. Further warfarin is contraindicated in these patients. Numerous drugs may affect patient response to warfarin, especially hepatic-enzyme inducing or reducing drugs and highly protein-bound drugs; consultation with a pharmacist or physician regarding all drugs is recommended. Use with extreme caution in protein C deficiency, congestive heart failure, carcinoma, liver disease, or poor nutritional state.

Anesthetic Considerations

Regional anesthesia is contraindicated. Barbiturates should be avoided if possible as they may decrease warfarin's effect. When emergency surgery is necessary in patients receiving warfarin, fresh-frozen plasma 15 mL/kg or whole blood can restore coagulation to normal.

DRUGS

Generic Name	Trade Name
adenosine	Adenocard
albuterol	Proventil, Ventolin
alfentanil	Alfenta
alprostadil (prostaglandin E$_1$)	Prostin VR Pediatric
aminocaproic acid	Amicar
aminophylline	Elixophyllin, Theodur, Theolair
amiodarone	Cordarone
amrinone	Inocor
atracurium	Tracrium
atropine	
bretylium	Bretylol
bumetanide	Bumex
bupivicaine	Marcaine HCl, Sensorcaine
chloroprocaine	Nesacaine
cimetidine	Tagamet
clonidine	Catapres
cocaine	
codeine	
coumarin (warfarin)	Coumadin
cyclosporine	Optimmune, Sandimmune
tubocurarine chloride	Tubocurarine
dantrolene	Dantrium
dexamethasone	Decadron, Hexadrol
desflurane	Suprane
desmopressin (vasopressin)	DDAVP
diazepam	Valium
digoxin	Lanoxin
diltiazem	Cardizem
diphenhydramine	Benadryl
dobutamine	Dobutrex
dopamine	Intropin
doxacurium	Nuromax
doxapram	Dopram
edrophonium	Enlon, Tensilon
enalapril	Vasotec IV
enflurane	Ethrane
ephedrine	
epinephrine (adrenaline)	
esmolol	Brevibloc
ethacrynic acid	Edecrin
etidocaine	Duranest
etomidate	Amidate
famotidine	Pepcid
fentanyl	Duragesic, Oralet, Sublimaze
flumazenil	Romazicon
furosemide	Lasix
glucagon	
glycopyrrolate	Robinul
granisetron	Kytril
halothane	Fluothane
heparin	
hetastarch	Hespan
hyaluronidase	Wydase

Generic Name	Trade Name
hydralazine	Apresoline
hydrocortisone	Hydrocort, Solu-Cortef
insulin	Humulin, Novolin
isoflurane	Forane
isoproterenol	Isuprel
ketamine	Ketalar
ketorolac	Toradol
labetalol	Normodyne, Trandate
lidocaine	Xylocaine
lorazepam	Ativan
magnesium sulfate	
mannitol	
meperidine	Demerol
mephenteramine	Wyamine Sulfate
mepivacaine	Carbocaine, Polocaine
metaraminol	Aramine
methadone	Dolophine HCl
methohexital	Brevital Sodium
methoxamine	Vasoxyl
methylene blue	Urolene Blue
methylergonovine	Methergine
metoclopramide	Reglan
midazolam	Versed
milrinone	Primacor
mivacurium	Mivacron
morphine	Astramorph PF, Duramorph, Morphine, MS Contin
nalmefene	Revex
naloxone	Narcan
naltrexone	ReVia
neostigmine	Prostigmin
nicardipine	Cardene
nifedipine	Adalat, Procardia
nitroglycerin	Nitro-Bid, Nitro-Dur, Nitrogard, Nitrostat, Nitrol, Nitrocine, Nitroglyn, Nitrodisc, Transderm-Nitro, Tridil
nitroprusside	Nipride
nitrous oxide	
nizatidine	Axid
norepinephrine	Levophed
ondansetron	Zofran
oxytocin	Pitocin, Syntocinon
pancuronium	Pavulon
phentolamine	Regitine
phenylephrine	Neo-Synephrine
phenytoin	Dilantin
physostigmine	Antilirium
pipecuronium	Arduan
prilocaine	Citanest
procainamide	Procan SR, Pronestyl
procaine	Novocain
prochlorperazine	Compazine
promethazine	Phenergan

Generic Name	Trade Name
propofol	Diprivan
propranolol	Inderal
protamine	
pyridostigmine	Mestinon, Regonol
ranitidine	Zantac
ritodrine	Yutopar
rocuronium	Zemuron
scopolamine	
sevoflurane	Ultane
sodium citrate	Bicitra, Shohl solution
somatostatin	
succinylcholine	Anectine, Quelicin
sufentanil	Sufenta
terbutaline	Brethaire, Bricanyl
tetracaine	Pontocaine
thiamylal	
thiopental sodium	Pentothal
trimethaphan	Arfonad
tropisetron	Novoban
vancomycin	Vancocin
vasopressin	Pitressin Synthetic
vasopressin tannate	Pitressin Tannate
vecuronium	Norcuron
verapamil	Calan, Isoptin
vitamin K (phytonadione)	AquaMEPHYTON, Konakion
warfarin	Coumadin

Drug	Route	Dose
Emergency (Resuscitation) Drugs		
Atropine	IV	0.01 mg/kg per dose (minimum 0.1 mg/ dose)
Adenosine	IV	100 μg/kg rapid IV bolus, incremental doses 100 μg/kg every 2 min to a maximum of 300 μg/kg
Calcium chloride	IV	10–20 mg/kg
Calcium gluconate	IV	50–100 mg/kg
Epinephrine	IV	0.01 mg/kg (0.1 mg/kg via ETT)
Lidocaine	IV	1 mg/kg
Sodium bicarbonate	IV	1–2 mEq/kg
Narcotics		
Codeine	IM/PO	0.5–1 mg/kg
Meperidine	IV	0.5–1 mg/kg
Midazolam	IV	0.01–0.02 mg/kg
	IM	0.08 mg/kg
	Intranasally	0.2–0.3 mg/kg
	PO	0.3–0.5 mg/kg
Morphine	IV	0.05–0.1 mg/kg
	IM	0.1–0.2 mg/kg
Sufentanil	IV	10–25 μg/kg
Fentanyl	IV	1–2 μg/kg
Induction Agents		
Propofol	IV	2–3 mg/kg
Ketamine	IV	1–2 mg/kg
	IM	5–7 mg/kg
Methohexital	IV	2–3 mg/kg
Thiopental	IV	3–6 mg/kg
Muscle Relaxants		
Atracurium	IV	0.2–0.5 mg/kg
Pancuronium	IV	0.04–0.15 mg/kg
Succinylcholine	IV	1–2 mg/kg
	IM	2.5–4 mg/kg
Tubocurarine	IV/IM	0.3–0.6 mg/kg
Vecuronium	IV	0.04–0.2 mg/kg
Reversal Agents		
Edrophonium	IV	0.5–1 mg/kg
Neostigmine	IV	0.05–0.07 mg/kg
Pyridostigmine	IV	0.2 mg/kg

The current drugs of choice for the treatment of common arrhythmias are listed below. The dosages and adverse effects of each drug are given in the table that follows. Several reports have indicated that at least some antiarrhythmic agents, given to asymptomatic or mildly symptomatic patients, may increase rather than decrease mortality.

Drugs of Choice for Common Arrhythmias

Arrhythmia	Drug of Choice	Alternatives	Remarks
Atrial fibrillation or atrial flutter*	Digoxin to slow ventricular response	Verapamil, diltiazem or a beta-blocker to slow ventricular response[†]	Digoxin, verapamil, and possibly beta-blockers may be dangerous for patients with Wolff-Parkinson-White syndrome. Amiodarone, flecainide, encainide, and propafenone also are effective for suppression.[†]
Supraventricular tachycardia§	Adenosine or verapamil‖	Esmolol, another beta-blocker, or digoxin for termination	Cardioversion or atrial pacing may be required for some patients. Quinidine, procainamide, disopyramide, diltiazem, propranolol, acebutolol, verapamil, flecainide, encainide, propafenone, or digoxin may be effective for long-term suppression.
Ventricular premature complexes or nonsustained ventricular tachycardia	No drug therapy indicated for asymptomatic patients¶	For symptomatic patients, a beta-blocker	There is no evidence that prolonged suppression with drugs prevents sudden cardiac death. For post-myocardial infarction patients, treatment with a beta-blocker has decreased mortality, and treatment with encainide or flecainide has increased it.
Sustained ventricular tachycardia**,††	Lidocaine for acute treatment	Procainamide, bretylium	Cardioversion is the safest and most effective therapy. A beta-blocker, procainamide, quinidine, amiodarone, disopyramide, or mexiletine can be used for long-term suppression.
Ventricular fibrillation‡‡	Lidocaine	Procainamide, amiodarone, bretylium	Cardiopulmonary resuscitation with rapid defibrillation is essential.

Cardiac glycoside–induced ventricular tachyarrhythmias‡,††,§§	Lidocaine	Phenytoin, procainamide, a beta-blocker	Self-limited if short-acting digitalis has stopped. Digoxin-immune Fab (digoxin antibody fragments—Digibind) should be used to treat life-threatening digoxin or digitoxin intoxication. Avoid cardioversion and bretylium, except for ventricular fibrillation or sustained ventricular tachycardia. A beta-blocker of procainamide can worsen heart block.
Sinus bradycardia, second- or third-degree heart block	Atropine	Isuprel, temporary external pacing	Doses of atropine <0.5 mg can produce paradoxical bradycardia owing to the central and/or peripheral parasympathomimetic effects of low doses. Atropine can be given per ETT.
Torsades de pointes	Magnesium	Cardiac pacing, isoproterenol	Magnesium may be effective even in the absence of hypomagnesemia. Potassium may also be needed, and administration of causative agents (e.g., quinidine) should be discontinued.

* Cardioversion is the treatment of choice for fibrillation or flutter of recent onset with compromised circulation due to excessively rapid ventricular rate. For patients with atrial flutter, atrial pacing can also be effective.

† May be preferred by some patients.

‡ A recent analysis of several older studies suggests that the use of quinidine for this indication may increase mortality. Whether other drugs used for this condition also might increase mortality remains to be determined.

§ Vagotonic maneuvers (e.g., carotid sinus massage, gagging, the Valsalva maneuver, or increasing venous return by straight leg raising) may be tried first.

|| Verapamil is contraindicated for patients receiving intravenous beta-blockers or for those with congestive heart failure, and the agent should be used with caution in patients taking oral quinidine.

¶ Some authorities give lidocaine early during acute myocardial infarction to prevent ventricular fibrillation.

** Cardioversion is preferred by most cardiologists for sustained ventricular tachycardia causing hemodynamic compromise; however, some first try a chest thump or IV lidocaine, or both.

†† Some ventricular tachycardias can be caused or exacerbated by bradycardia or heart block. In the presence of high-grade heart block, antiarrhythmic drugs can cause cardiac standstill. When high-grade heart block is present, therefore, a temporary pacemaker should be inserted before antiarrhythmic drugs are used; pacing may abolish the arrhythmia. When a drug must be used in the presence of heart block, lidocaine or phenytoin is least likely to increase the block.

‡‡ Defibrillation is the treatment of choice; drugs used for the prevention of recurrence.

§§ Potassium chloride can be given carefully (usually, 20 mEq/h IV) to a patient with low normal serum potassium concentrations. Extreme care must be taken to keep serum potassium levels below 5.5 mEq/L. In the presence of heart block not associated with paroxysmal atrial tachycardia, potassium should be withheld if the serum concentration is >4.0 to 4.5 mEq/L because high serum potassium concentrations may increase atrioventricular block.

Modified from Anonymous. Drugs for cardiac arrhythmias. Med Lett Drug Ther 1989;31:790.

APPENDIX 4 Difficult Airway Algorithm

1. Assess the likelihood and clinical impact of basic management problems:
   A. Difficult intubation
   B. Difficult ventilation
   C. Difficulty with patient cooperation or consent

2. Consider the relative merits and feasibility of basic management choices:

   A. Non-surgical technique for initial approach to intubation   vs.   Surgical technique for initial approach to intubation

   B. Awake intubation   vs.   Intubation attempts after induction of general anesthesia

   C. Preservation of spontaneous ventilation   vs.   Ablation of spontaneous ventilation

3. Develop basic primary and alternative strategies:

AWAKE INTUBATION

Airway approached by non-surgical intubation   Airway secured by surgical access*

- Succeed*
- FAIL
  - Cancel case
  - Consider feasibility of other options(a)
  - Surgical airway*

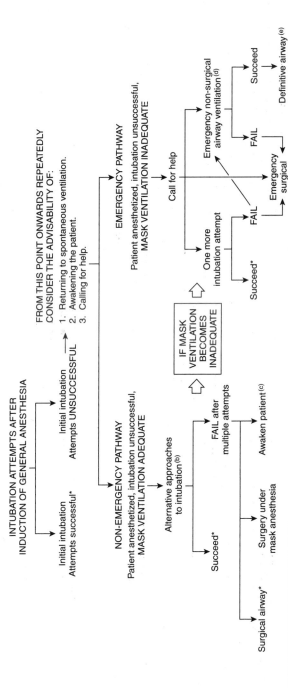

INTUBATION ATTEMPTS AFTER
INDUCTION OF GENERAL ANESTHESIA

Initial intubation
Attempts successful*

Initial intubation
Attempts UNSUCCESSFUL

FROM THIS POINT ONWARDS REPEATEDLY
CONSIDER THE ADVISABILITY OF:
1. Returning to spontaneous ventilation.
2. Awakening the patient.
3. Calling for help.

NON-EMERGENCY PATHWAY
Patient anesthetized, intubation unsuccessful,
MASK VENTILATION ADEQUATE

EMERGENCY PATHWAY
Patient anesthetized, intubation unsuccessful,
MASK VENTILATION INADEQUATE

Alternative approaches to intubation(b)

IF MASK
VENTILATION
BECOMES
INADEQUATE

Succeed*

Surgery under
mask anesthesia

FAIL after
multiple attempts

Awaken patient(c)

Surgical airway*

Call for help

One more
intubation attempt

Succeed*

FAIL

Emergency non-surgical
airway ventilation(d)

Succeed

FAIL

Emergency
surgical
airway*

Definitive airway(e)

*CONFIRM INTUBATION WITH EXHALED CO_2

(a) Other options include (but are not limited to): surgery under mask anesthesia, surgery
    under local anesthesia infiltration or regional nerve blockade, or intubation attempts
    after induction of general anesthesia.
(b) Alternative approaches to difficult intubation include (but are not limited to): use of
    different laryngoscope blades, awake intubation, blind oral or nasal intubation, fiberoptic
    intubation, intubating stylet or tube changer, light wand, retrograde intubation, and surgical
    airway access.
(c) See awake intubation.
(d) Options for emergency non-surgical airway ventilation include (but are not limited
    to): transtracheal jet ventilation, laryngeal mask ventilation, or esophageal-tracheal
    combitube ventilation.
(e) Options for establishing a definitive airway include (but are not limited to): return to
    awake state with spontaneous ventilation, tracheotomy, or endotracheal intubation.

*Reprinted by permission from the American Society of Anesthesiologists' Task Force on Management of the Difficult Airway, Park Ridge, IL.

Universal Algorithm for Adult Emergency Cardiac Care (EEC)

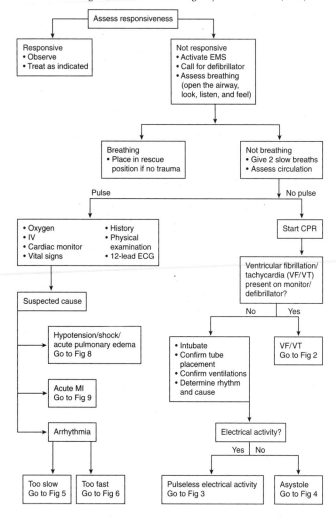

Algorithm for Ventricular Fibrillation and Pulseless Ventricular Tachycardia (VF/VT).

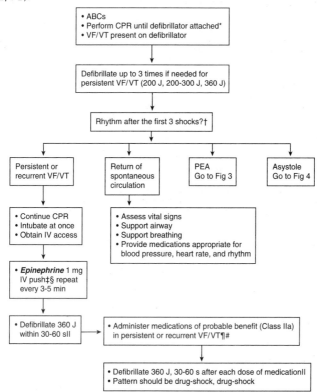

- ABCs
- Perform CPR until defibrillator attached*
- VF/VT present on defibrillator

↓

Defibrillate up to 3 times if needed for persistent VF/VT (200 J, 200-300 J, 360 J)

↓

Rhythm after the first 3 shocks?†

| Persistent or recurrent VF/VT | Return of spontaneous circulation | PEA Go to Fig 3 | Asystole Go to Fig 4 |

Persistent or recurrent VF/VT:
- Continue CPR
- Intubate at once
- Obtain IV access

↓

- **Epinephrine** 1 mg IV push‡§ repeat every 3-5 min

↓

- Defibrillate 360 J within 30-60 sǁ

→

- Administer medications of probable benefit (Class IIa) in persistent or recurrent VF/VT¶#

↓

- Defibrillate 360 J, 30-60 s after each dose of medicationǁ
- Pattern should be drug-shock, drug-shock

Return of spontaneous circulation:
- Assess vital signs
- Support airway
- Support breathing
- Provide medications appropriate for blood pressure, heart rate, and rhythm

---

Class I: definitely helpful
Class IIa: acceptable, probably helpful
Class IIb: acceptable, possibly helpful
Class III: not indicated, may be harmful

* Precordial thump is a Class IIb action in witnessed arrest, no pulse, and no defibrillator immediately available.

† Hypothermic cardiac arrest is treated differently after this point. See section on hypothermia.

‡ The recommended dose of **epinephrine** is 1 mg IV push every 3-5 min. If this approach fails, several Class IIb dosing regimens can be considered:
- Intermediate: **epinephrine** 2-5 mg IV push, every 3-5 min
- Escalating: **epinephrine** 1 mg-3 mg-5 mg IV push (3 min apart)
- High: **epinephrine** 0.1 mg/kg IV push, every 3-5 min

§ **Sodium bicarbonate** (1 mEq/kg) is Class I if patient has known preexisting hyperkalemia

ǁ Multiple sequenced shocks (200 J, 200-300 J, 360 J) are acceptable here (Class I), especially when medications are delayed

¶ • **Lidocaine** 1.5 mg/kg IV push. Repeat in 3-5 min to total loading dose of 3 mg/kg; then use
- **Bretylium** 5 mg/kg IV push. Repeat in 5 min at 10 mg/kg
- **Magnesium sulfate** 1-2 g IV in torsades de pointes or suspected hypomagnesemic state or severe refractory VF
- **Procainamide** 30 mg/min in refractory VF (maximum total 17 mg/kg)

• **Sodium bicarbonate** (1 mEq/kg IV): Class IIa
- if known preexisting bicarbonate-responsive acidosis
- if overdose with tricyclic antidepressants
- to alkalinize the urine in drug overdoses

Class IIb
- if intubated and continued long arrest interval
- upon return of spontaneous circulation after long arrest interval

Class III
- hypoxic lactic acidosis

Algorithm for Pulseless Electrical Activity (PEA)

PEA includes
- Electromechanical dissociation (EMD)
- Pseudo-EMD
- Idioventricular rhythms
- Ventricular escape rhythms
- Bradyasystolic rhythms
- Postdefibrillation idioventricular rhythms

- Continue CPR
- Intubate at once
- Obtain IV access
- Assess blood flow using Doppler ultrasound

↓

Consider possible causes
(Parentheses = possible therapies and treatments)
- Hypovolemia (volume infusion)
- Hypoxia (ventilation)
- Cardiac tamponade (pericardiocentesis)
- Tension pneumothorax (needle decompression)
- Hypothermia
- Massive pulmonary embolism (surgery, *thrombolytics*)
- Drug overdoses such as tricyclics, digitalis, β-blockers, calcium channel blockers
- Hyperkalemia*
- Acidosis†
- Massive acute myocardial infarction (go to Fig 9)

↓

- *Epinephrine* 1 mg IV push,*‡ repeat every 3-5 min

↓

- If absolute bradycardia (<60 beats/min) or relative bradycardia, give *atropine* 1 mg IV
- Repeat every 3-5 min up to a total of 0.04 mg/kg§

Class I: definitely helpful
Class IIa: acceptable, probably helpful
Class IIb: acceptable, possibly helpful
Class III: not indicated, may be harmful
* *Sodium bicarbonate* 1 mEq/kg is Class I if patient has known preexisting hyperkalemia
† *Sodium bicarbonate* 1 mEq/kg:
Class IIa
- if known preexisting bicarbonate-responsive acidosis
- if overdose with tricyclic antidepressants
- to alkalinize the urine in drug overdoses
Class IIb
- if intubated and long arrest interval
- upon return of spontaneous circulation after long arrest interval
Class III
- hypoxic lactic acidosis
‡ The recommended dose of *epinephrine* is 1 mg IV push every 3-5 min.
If this approach fails, several Class IIb dosing regimens can be considered.
- Intermediate: *epinephrine* 2-5 mg IV push, every 3-5 min
- Escalating: *epinephrine* 1 mg-3 mg-5 mg IV push (3 min apart)
- High: *epinephrine* 0.1 mg/kg IV push, every 3-5 min
§ Shorter *atropine* dosing intervals are possibly helpful in cardiac arrest (Class IIb).

Asystole Treatment Algorithm

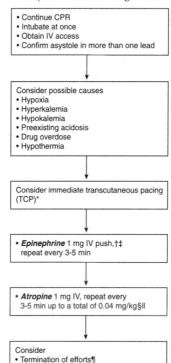

- Continue CPR
- Intubate at once
- Obtain IV access
- Confirm asystole in more than one lead

↓

Consider possible causes
- Hypoxia
- Hyperkalemia
- Hypokalemia
- Preexisting acidosis
- Drug overdose
- Hypothermia

↓

Consider immediate transcutaneous pacing (TCP)*

↓

- *Epinephrine* 1 mg IV push,†‡ repeat every 3-5 min

↓

- *Atropine* 1 mg IV, repeat every 3-5 min up to a total of 0.04 mg/kg§‖

↓

Consider
- Termination of efforts¶

Class I: definitely helpful
Class IIa: acceptable, probably helpful
Class IIb: acceptable, possibly helpful
Class III: not indicated, may be harmful

* TCP is a Class IIb intervention. Lack of success may be due to delay in pacing. To be effective TCP must be performed early, simultaneously with drugs. Evidence does not support routine use of TCP for asystole.

† The recommended dose of *epinephrine* is 1 mg IV push every 3-5 min. If this approach fails, several Class IIb dosing regimens can be considered:
- Intermediate: *epinephrine* 2-5 mg IV push, every 3-5 min
- Escalating: *epinephrine* 1 mg-3 mg-5 mg IV push (3 min apart)
- High: *epinephrine* 0.1 mg/kg IV push, every 3-5 min

‡ *Sodium bicarbonate* 1 mEq/kg is Class I if patient has known preexisting hyperkalemia.

§ Shorter *atropine* dosing intervals are Class IIb in asystolic arrest.

‖ • *Sodium bicarbonate* 1 mEq/kg:
Class IIa
- if known preexisting bicarbonate-responsive acidosis
- if overdose with tricyclic antidepressants
- to alkalinize the urine in drug overdose
Class IIb
- if intubated and continued long arrest interval
- upon return of spontaneous circulation after long arrest interval
Class III
- hypoxic lactic acidosis

¶ If patient remains in asystole or other agonal rhythms after successful intubation and initial medication and no reversible causes are identified, consider termination of resuscitative efforts by a physician. Consider interval since arrest.

Bradycardia Algorithms (with the Patient Not in Cardiac Arrest)

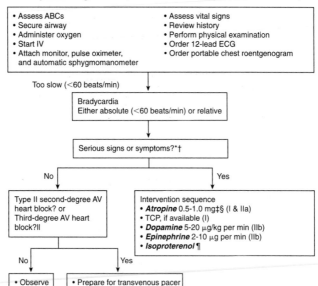

- Assess ABCs
- Secure airway
- Administer oxygen
- Start IV
- Attach monitor, pulse oximeter, and automatic sphygmomanometer

- Assess vital signs
- Review history
- Perform physical examination
- Order 12-lead ECG
- Order portable chest roentgenogram

Too slow (<60 beats/min)

Bradycardia
Either absolute (<60 beats/min) or relative

Serious signs or symptoms?*†

No

Type II second-degree AV heart block? or
Third-degree AV heart block?‖

Yes

Intervention sequence
- *Atropine* 0.5-1.0 mg‡§ (I & IIa)
- TCP, if available (I)
- *Dopamine* 5-20 μg/kg per min (IIb)
- *Epinephrine* 2-10 μg per min (IIb)
- *Isoproterenol* ¶

No

- Observe

Yes

- Prepare for transvenous pacer
- Use TCP as a bridge device#

* Serious signs or symptoms must be related to the slow rate.
   Clinical manifestations include:
   symptoms (chest pain, shortness of breath, decreased level of consciousness) and
   signs (low BP, shock, pulmonary congestion, CHF, acute MI).
† Do not delay TCP while awaiting IV access or for ***atropine*** to take effect if patient
   is symptomatic.
‡ Denervated transplanted hearts will not respond to ***atropine***. Go at once to pacing,
   catecholamine infusion, or both.
§ ***Atropine*** should be given in repeat doses in 3-5 min up to a total of 0.04 mg/kg.
   Consider shorter dosing intervals in severe clinical conditions. It has been suggested
   that atropine should be used with caution in atrioventricular (AV) block at the His-
   Purkinje level (type II AV block and new third-degree block with wide QRS complexes)
   (Class IIb).
‖ Never treat third-degree heart block plus ventricular escape beats with ***lidocaine***.
¶ ***Isoproterenol*** should be used, if at all, with extreme caution. At low doses it is
   Class IIb (possibly helpful); at higher doses it is Class III (harmful).
Verify patient tolerance and mechanical capture. Use analgesia and sedation
   as needed.

Tachycardia Algorithm

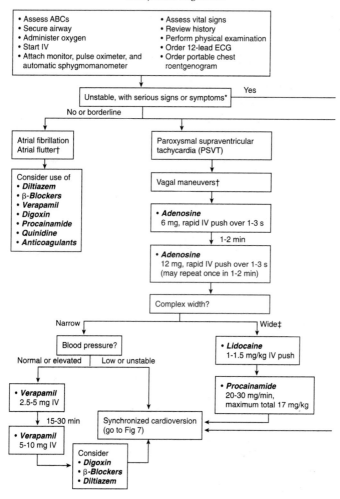

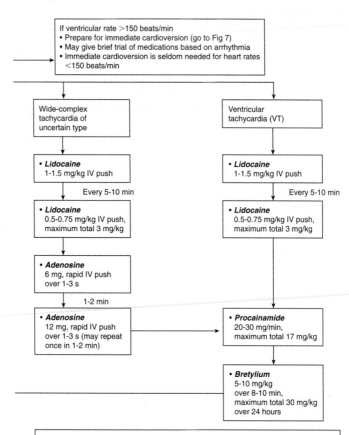

If ventricular rate >150 beats/min
• Prepare for immediate cardioversion (go to Fig 7)
• May give brief trial of medications based on arrhythmia
• Immediate cardioversion is seldom needed for heart rates
  <150 beats/min

Wide-complex
tachycardia of
uncertain type

Ventricular
tachycardia (VT)

• **Lidocaine**
1-1.5 mg/kg IV push

• **Lidocaine**
1-1.5 mg/kg IV push

Every 5-10 min

Every 5-10 min

• **Lidocaine**
0.5-0.75 mg/kg IV push,
maximum total 3 mg/kg

• **Lidocaine**
0.5-0.75 mg/kg IV push,
maximum total 3 mg/kg

• **Adenosine**
6 mg, rapid IV push
over 1-3 s

1-2 min

• **Adenosine**
12 mg, rapid IV push
over 1-3 s (may repeat
once in 1-2 min)

• **Procainamide**
20-30 mg/min,
maximum total 17 mg/kg

• **Bretylium**
5-10 mg/kg
over 8-10 min,
maximum total 30 mg/kg
over 24 hours

*   Unstable condition must be related to the tachycardia. Signs and symptoms may
    include chest pain, shortness of breath, decreased level of consciousness, low blood
    pressure (BP), shock, pulmonary congestion, congestive heart failure, acute
    myocardial infarction.
†   Carotid sinus pressure is contraindicated in patients with carotid bruits; avoid ice
    water immersion in patients with ischemic heart disease.
‡   If the wide-complex tachycardia is known with certainty to be PSVT and BP is
    normal/elevated, sequence can include **verapamil.**

Electrical Cardioversion Algorithm (with the Patient Not in Cardiac Arrest)

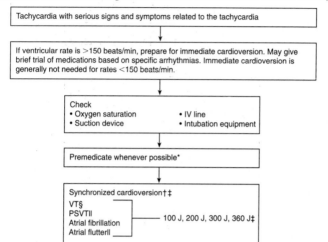

Tachycardia with serious signs and symptoms related to the tachycardia

↓

If ventricular rate is >150 beats/min, prepare for immediate cardioversion. May give brief trial of medications based on specific arrhythmias. Immediate cardioversion is generally not needed for rates <150 beats/min.

↓

Check
- Oxygen saturation
- Suction device
- IV line
- Intubation equipment

↓

Premedicate whenever possible*

↓

Synchronized cardioversion†‡
VT§
PSVT‖
Atrial fibrillation
Atrial flutter‖ —— 100 J, 200 J, 300 J, 360 J‡

---

*   Effective regimens have included a sedative (eg, *diazepam, midazolam, barbiturates, etomidate, ketamine, methohexital*) with or without an analgesic agent (eg, *fentanyl, morphine, meperidine*). Many experts recommend anesthesia if service is readily available.
† Note possible need to resynchronize after each cardioversion.
‡ If delays in synchronization occur and clinical conditions are critical, go to immediate unsynchronized shocks.
§ Treat polymorphic VT (irregular form and rate) like VF:
   200 J, 200-300 J, 360 J.
‖ PSVT and atrial flutter often respond to lower energy levels (start with 50 J).

Algorithm for Hypotension, Shock, and Acute Pulmonary Edema

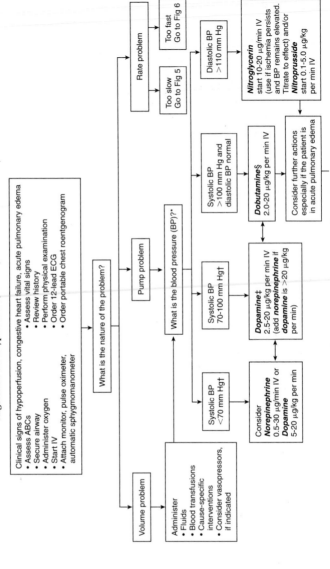

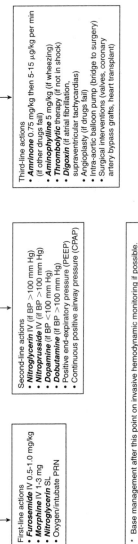

First-line actions
- *Furosemide* IV 0.5–1.0 mg/kg
- *Morphine* IV 1–3 mg
- *Nitroglycerin* SL
- Oxygen/intubate PRN

Second-line actions
- *Nitroglycerin* IV (if BP >100 mm Hg)
- *Nitroprusside* IV (if BP >100 mm Hg)
- *Dopamine* (if BP <100 mm Hg)
- *Dobutamine* (if BP >100 mm Hg)
- Positive end-expiratory pressure (PEEP)
- Continuous positive airway pressure (CPAP)

Third-line actions
- *Amrinone* 0.75 mg/kg then 5–15 µg/kg per min (if other drugs fail)
- *Aminophylline* 5 mg/kg (if wheezing)
- *Thrombolytic* therapy (if not in shock)
- *Digoxin* (if atrial fibrillation, supraventricular tachycardias)
- Angioplasty (if drugs fail)
- Intra-aortic balloon pump (bridge to surgery)
- Surgical interventions (valves, coronary artery bypass grafts, heart transplant)

* Base management after this point on invasive hemodynamic monitoring if possible.

† Fluid bolus of 250–500 mL normal saline should be tried. If no response, consider sympathomimetics.

‡ Move to *dopamine* and stop *norepinephrine* when BP improves.

§ Add *dobutamine* when BP improves. Avoid *dobutamine* when systolic BP <100 mm Hg.

465

Acute Myocardial Infarction Algorithm

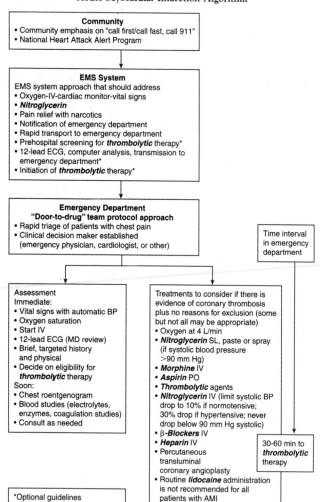

All algorithms in Appendix 5 from Emergency Cardiac Care Committee and Subcommittees, American Heart Association. Guidelines for cardiopulmonary resuscitation and emergency cardiac care. JAMA. 1992;268:2216–2230. Copyright 1992, American Medical Association.

Parameter	Formula	Normal Range
CO	HR × SV	4.0–8.0 L/min
CI	CO ÷ BSA	2.5–4.0 L/min
CVP	cm H_2O = mm Hg × 1.34	2–6 mm Hg
PCWP	—	8–12 mm Hg
MAP	[(DBP × 2) + SBP] ÷ 3	70–105 mm Hg
SVR	[(MAP − CVP) ÷ CO] × 80	800–1200 dynes/cm/sec^{-5}
PVR	[(PAM − PCWP) ÷ CO] × 80	37–250 dynes/cm/sec^{-5}
SV	(CO × 1000) ÷ HR	60–100 mL/beat
SVI	SV ÷ BSA	33–47 mL/beat per m^2
LVSWI	[SVI (MAP − PCWP)] × 0.0136	38–85 g · m^2/beat
RVSWI	[SVI (PAM − PAD)] × 0.0136	7–12 g · m^2/beat
RVEDV	SV ÷ EF	100–160 mL
RVESV	EDV − SV	50–100 mL
RVSV	(CO × 1000) ÷ HR	60–100 mL
EF	(EDV − ESV) ÷ EDV or SV ÷ EDV	40–60%
CPP	MAP − CVP or MAP − ICP	70–80 mm Hg

CO = cardiac output; CI = cardiac index; CVP = central venous pressure; PCWP = pulmonary capillary wedge pressure; MAP = mean arterial pressure; SVR = systemic vascular resistance; PVR = pulmonary vascular resistance; SV = stroke volume; SVI = stroke volume index; LVSWI = left ventricular stroke work index; RVSWI = right ventricular stroke work index; RVEDV = right ventricular end-diastolic volume; RVESV = right ventricular end-systolic volume; RVSV = right ventricular stroke volume; EF = ejection fracture; CPP = coronary perfusion pressure.

Test	Normal Values
Vital capacity (VC)	60–70 mL/kg
Tidal volume (VT) (spontaneous ventilation)	6–8 mL/kg
Minute ventilation ($\dot{V}E$)	80 mL/kg
Functional residual capacity (FRC)	28–32 mL/kg
Forced expiratory volume in 1 second (FEV_1)	>75%
Forced vital capacity (FVC)	60–70 mL/kg
Dead space (VDS)	2 mL/kg
VDS/VT	33%
FEV_1/FVC	>75%

APPENDIX 8 Nomogram for the Determination of Body Surface Area of Children and Adults

To determine the surface area, find the height of the person and the weight on the appropriate scales, and then connect these points with a straight edge. The point at which this line intersects with the line of the surface area scale indicates the surface area of the patient in square meters. (From Boothby WM, Sandiford RB. *Boston Med Surg J*. 1921; 185:337, as shown in Rakel RE. *Conn's Current Therapy*. Philadelphia, PA: W.B. Saunders Co.; 1991.)

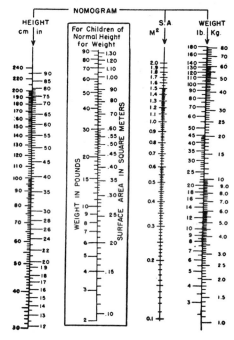

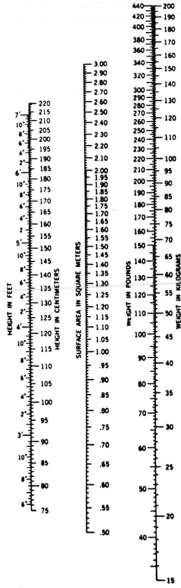

The surface area is estimated by a straight line connecting the height of the patient with his/her weight intersecting the surface area line. If the patient is of average size, the surface area can be estimated from weight alone (see boxed scale in diagram). (From Behrman, RE. *Nelson Textbook of Pediatrics*. 14th ed. Philadelphia, PA; W.B. Saunders Co.; 1992.)

Age	Weight (kg), 50th Percentile	Respiratory Rate (breaths/min)	Heart Rate (beats/min)	Systolic Blood Pressure (mm Hg)
Newborn	3	35–40	120–140	55–70
0–2 mo	4	35–40	120–130	60–80
3 mo	5.5	24–30	120–130	80–90
6 mo	7	24–30	120–130	90–100
12 mo	10.0	22–30	110–120	95 ± 30
2 y	12.0	18–24	100–110	95 ± 25
3 y	14.0	16–22	100–110	95 ± 25
4 y	16.0	14–20	95–105	95 ± 20
5 y	18.0	14–20	95–105	95 ± 20
6 y	20.0	12–20	90–100	105 ± 13
7 y	22.0	12–20	90–100	105 ± 13
8 y	25.0	12–20	90–100	105 ± 13
9 y	28.0	12–20	85–95	105 ± 13
10 y	34.0	12–20	85–95	112 ± 19

Estimating Weight in Kilograms

<1 y: (age [mo]) × 0.5 + 3.5
>1 y: (age [y]) × 2 + 1

Estimating Endotracheal Tube (ETT) Size*

Age	ETT Size	Laryngoscope Blade	Distance (cm)
Newborn	3.0	0–1 (straight)	8–10
6 mo	3.5	1 (straight)	10–11
1 y	4.0	1–1.5 (straight)	11
2 y	5.0	1–1.5 (straight)	12

Over 20 mo: 4.0 + age (y) ÷ 4

Length of insertion   (over 1 y: 12 + age ÷ 2

* This is only a guide; prepare an ETT one size larger and one size smaller than ETT size selected.

Estimated Blood Volume (EBV)

Age	Volume (mL/kg)
Premature	100
Full-term	90
0–2 y	80–85
2–16 y	70–75

Maximum Allowable Blood Loss (MABL)

$$MABL = \frac{EBV \times (initial\ Hct - target\ Hct)}{initial\ Hct}$$

NPO Time

Age (mo)	Clear liquids (h)	Milk/Solids (h)
0–6	2	4
6–36	3	6
>36	8	8

Calculation of Maintenance Fluid Requirements

Weight (kg)	Requirement
0–10	4 mL/kg per h
10–20	40 mL + 2 mL/kg >10
>20	60 mL + 1 mL/kg >20

NPO Deficit

NPO hours × Maintenance: Replace 50% the first hour, 25% the second hour, and 25% the third hour.

LOOK FOR: tachycardia, rigidity, hypercarbia, tachypnea, cardiac arrhythmias, respiratory and metabolic acidosis, fever, unstable/rising blood pressure, cyanosis/mottling, and myoglobinuria.

Acute Phase Treatment

1. Immediately discontinue all volatile inhalation anesthetics and succinylcholine. Hyperventilate with 100% oxygen at high gas flows; at least 10 L/min. The circle system and CO_2 absorbent need not be changed.

2. Administer dantrolene sodium 2–3 mg/kg initial bolus rapidly with increments up to 10 mg/kg total. Continue to administer dantrolene until signs of MH (e.g., tachycardia, rigidity, increased end-tidal CO_2, and temperature elevation) are controlled. Occasionally, a total dose greater than 10 mg/kg may be needed. Each vial of dantrolene contains 20 mg of dantrolene and 3 grams mannitol. Each vial should be mixed with 60 mL of sterile water for injection USP without a bacteriostatic agent.

3. Administer bicarbonate to correct metabolic acidosis as guided by blood gas analysis. In the absence of blood gas analysis, 1–2 mEq/kg should be administered.

4. Simultaneous with the above, actively cool the hyperthermic patient. Use IV cold saline (not Ringer's lactate) 15 mL/kg q 15 min × 3.
   a. Lavage stomach, bladder, rectum, and open cavities with cold saline as appropriate.
   b. Surface cool with ice and hypothermia blanket.
   c. Monitor closely since overvigorous treatment may lead to hypothermia.

5. Arrhythmias will usually respond to treatment of acidosis and hyperkalemia. If they persist or are life threatening, standard anti-arrhythmic agents may be used, with the exception of calcium channel blockers (may cause hyperkalemia and CV collapse).

6. Determine and monitor end-tidal CO_2, arterial, central or femoral venous blood gases, serum potassium, calcium, clotting studies and urine output.

7. Hyperkalemia is common and should be treated with hyperventilation, bicarbonate, intravenous glucose and insulin (10 units regular insulin in 50 mL 50% glucose titrated to potassium level or 0.15 U/kg regular insulin in 1 mL/kg 50% glucose). Life-threatening hyperkalemia may also be treated with calcium administration (e.g. 2–5 mg/kg of $CaCl_2$).

8. Ensure urine output of greater than 2 mL/kg/hr by hydration and/or administration of mannitol or furosemide. Consider central venous or PA monitoring because of fluid shifts and hemodynamic instability that may occur.

9. **Sudden Unexpected Cardiac Arrest in Children:** Children less than about 10 years of age who experience sudden cardiac arrest after succinylcholine in the absence of hypoxemia and anesthetic overdose should be treated for acute hyperkalemia first. In this situation calcium chloride should be administered along with other means to reduce serum potassium. They should be presumed to have subclinical muscular dystrophy and a neurologist should be consulted.

---

* Names of on-call physicians available to consult in MH emergencies may be obtained 24 hours a day through the MH Emergency HOTLINE 1 800 MH HYPER (1-800-644-9737).

For nonemergency or patient referral calls: MHAUS, P. O. Box 1069, Sherburne, NY 13460-1069. tel.: (607) 674-7901. MH INFO-BY-FAX: 1-800-440-9990.

From Emergency Therapy for Malignant Hyperthermia. Sherburne, NY: Malignant Hyperthermia Association of the United States; 1995. Poster.

Post Acute Phase

A. Observe the patient in an ICU setting for at least 24 hours since recrudescence of MH may occur, particularly following a fulminant case resistant to treatment.

B. Administer dantrolene 1 mg/kg IV q 6 hours for 24–48 hours post episode. After that, oral dantrolene 1 mg/kg q 6 hours may be used for 24 hours as necessary.

C. Follow ABG, CK, potassium, calcium, urine and serum myoglobin, clotting studies and core body temperature such time as they return to normal values (e.g., q 6 hours). Central temperature (e.g., rectal, esophageal) should be continuously monitored until stable.

D. Counsel the patient and family regarding MH and further precautions. Refer the patient to MHAUS. Fill out an Adverse Metabolic Reaction to Anesthesia (AMRA) report available through the North American Malignant Hyperthermia Registry (717) 531-6936.

CAUTION: This protocol may not apply to every patient and may require alteration according to specific patient needs.

1. While the anesthesia machine is off, inspect it for
   Identification number
   Valid inspection sticker
   Correct connection of the breathing circuit with no damaged areas
   Intact CO_2 absorber cylinder that is not discolored
   Presence of a cylinder wrench (back of the machine)
   Correct mounting of the cylinders in the yokes
   Damage to vaporizers and the amount of agent, and for whether filled caps are
   tightly sealed.
2. Check the level of O_2 in the cylinder by disconnecting it from the main pipeline
   supply and by opening and then reclosing the cylinder with the cylinder wrench.
   Replace any cylinder of O_2 that shows <600 psig on its pressure gauge.
   Flush the system of O_2 using the O_2 flush valve.
   Check the second O_2 cylinder, if present.
3. Check the level of N_2O in the cylinder by disconnecting it from the main pipeline
   supply, and by opening and closing the cylinder with the cylinder wrench.
   If the N_2O pressure is <745 psig, then the cylinder is less than 25% full and
   must be replaced.
4. While both the N_2O and O_2 are disconnected from the main pipeline, turn off
   the cylinders and turn on the master switch so that the machine is on.
   This drains the machine of O_2, testing the O_2 failure safety valve; alarm will
   sound.
   N_2O level also decreases to zero.
   Before reattachment to the pipeline, be sure to turn the N_2O and O_2 flowmeters to zero.
5. Check the flowmeters by adjusting the flow of the gases through their full range
   and then by evaluating for erratic movements of the floats.
6. Test the ratio protection warning system by turning the N_2O flowmeter gauge
   to a high level and noting whether the O_2 flowmeter level increases. This
   prevents hypoxic mixtures from getting to the patient.
7. Calibrate O_2 monitor:
   Disconnect the O_2 monitor head from the machine and allow it to sit in room
   air for 1 to 3 minutes until the reading is 21%.
   Reconnect the head to the system and flush using the O_2 flush valve several
   times while monitoring whether the reading reaches 100%.
8. Check for high pressure leak:
   Close the pop-off (APL) valve and occlude the system at patient's end.
   Flush the system to inflate the bag, producing in-line pressure of 25 to 35 cm
   H_2O; hold this pressure for approximately 20 seconds while watching for any
   decreases on pressure gauge.
9. Evaluate scavenger system:
   Once the reservoir bag is full at 20 to 30 cm H_2O, open the APL valve and
   push the residual O_2 from the reservoir bag into the scavenger bag. Note
   inflation of the scavenger and then the drainage into the main pipeline system
   by deflating the scavenger bag. This results from the appropriate amount
   of suction in the system.
10. Test ventilator:
    Place the reservoir bag on the patient's end of the breathing circuit, turn
    switching valve to ventilator, and turn on the ventilator.
    Monitor the up-and-down motion of the bellows.
    Evaluate the unidirectional valves on inspiration and expiration.
    Note the filling and emptying of the reservoir bag.
    Be sure to switch the valve back to the bag after performing this test.

Test		Normal Serum Values
ACT		80–120 s
Albumin, total		6.6–7.9 g/dL
	fractional	4.4–4.5 g/dL
Anion gap		8–14 mEq/L
ABG	pH	7.35–7.45
	$PaCO_2$	35–45 mm Hg
	PaO_2	80–100 mm Hg
	HCO_3	22–26 mEq/L
Bilirubin, direct		0–0.4 mg/dL
	indirect	0.1–1.2 mg/dL
BUN		8–20 mg/dL
Ca		4.5–5.5 mEq/L
Cl		100–108 mEq/L
CK, total		
	female	15–57 U/L
	male	24–100 U/L
	MB	0–7 IU/L
	MM	6–70 IU/L
Cr		0.2–1.5 mg/dL
Fibrinogen		195–365
Glucose, fasting		70–100 mg/dL
Hb	female	15–16 g/dL
	male	14–18 g/dL
	glycosylated	5.5–9%
HCT	female	37–47%
	male	42–52%
K		3.8–5.5 mg/dL
LDH		48–115 IU/L
Mg		1.5–2.5 mEq/L
Na		134–145 mEq/L
Phosphorus		1.8–2.6 mEq/L
Platelets		130,000–370,000/mm³
Pseudocholinesterase		8–80 U/mL
PT		11–13.2 s
PTT		22.5–32.2 s
RBC	female	4.2–5.4 million/μL
	fmale	4.7–6.2 million/μL
AST		8–20 U/L
ALT	female	9–24 U/L
	male	10–32 U/L
T_3		90–230 ng/dL
T_4		5–13 μg/dL
WBC		4100–10,900/μL

I. Perform a thorough and complete preanesthesia assessment.

II. Obtain informed consent for the planned anesthetic intervention from the patient or legal guardian.

III. Formulate a patient-specific plan for anesthesia care.

IV. Implement and adjust the anesthesia care plan based on the patient's physiological response.

V. Monitor the patient's physiologic condition as appropriate for the type of anesthesia and specific patient needs.

VI. There shall be complete, accurate, and timely documentation of pertinent information on the patient's medical record.

VII. Transfer the responsibility for care of the patient to other qualified providers in a manner which assures continuity of care and patient safety.

VIII. Adhere to appropriate safety precautions, as established within the institution, to minimize the risks of fire, explosion, electrical shock and equipment malfunction. Document on the patient's medical record that the anesthesia machine and equipment were checked.

IX. Universal precautions shall be taken to minimize the risk of infection to the patient, the CRNA, and other staff.

X. Anesthesia care shall be assessed to assure its quality and contribution to positive patient outcomes.

XI. The CRNA shall respect and maintain the basic rights of patients.

* *Adopted by the American Association of Nurse Anesthetists, June 1989. Revised 1992, 1996. © 1992, 1996, American Association of Nurse Anesthetists. Adapted by permission.*

Bibliography

Barash PG, Cullen BF, Stoelting RK, eds. *Clinical Anesthesia.* 2nd ed. Philadelphia, PA: J.B. Lippincott Co.; 1992.

Braunwald E, ed. *Heart Disease: A Textbook of Cardiovascular Medicine.* 4th ed. Philadelphia, PA: W.B. Saunders Co.; 1992.

Chestnut DH, ed. *Obstetric Anesthesia: Principles and Practice.* St. Louis, MO: C.V. Mosby Co.; 1994.

Firestone LL, Lebowitz PW, Cook CE, eds. *Clinical Anesthesia Procedures of the Massachusetts General Hospital.* 3rd ed. Boston, MA: Little, Brown & Co.; 1988.

Guyton AC, Hall JE. *Textbook of Medical Physiology.* 9th ed. Philadelphia, PA: W.B. Saunders Co.; 1996.

Hardman JG, Limbird LE, eds. *Goodman and Gilman's The Pharmacologic Basis of Therapeutics.* 9th ed. New York, NY: McGraw-Hill Publishing Co.; 1996.

Jaffe RA, Samuels SI, eds. *Anesthesiologists' Manual of Surgical Procedures.* New York, NY: Raven Press; 1994.

Katz J, Benumof JL, Kadis LB, eds. *Anesthesia and Uncommon Diseases.* 3rd ed. Philadelphia, PA: W.B. Saunders Co.; 1990.

Katz J, Steward DJ, eds. *Anesthesia and Uncommon Pediatric Diseases.* 2nd ed. Philadelphia, PA: W.B. Saunders Co.; 1993.

Miller RD, ed. *Anesthesia.* 4th ed. New York, NY: Churchill Livingstone; 1994.

Motoyama EK, Davis PJ, eds. *Smith's Anesthesia for Infants and Children.* 6th ed. St. Louis, MO: C.V. Mosby Co.; 1996.

Nagelhout JJ, Zaglaniczny K, eds. *Nurse Anesthesia.* Philadelphia, PA: W.B. Saunders Co.; 1997.

Omogui S: *Anesthesia Drug Handbook.* 2nd ed. St. Louis, MO: C.V. Mosby Co.; 1995.

Stoelting RK, Dierdorf SE. *Anesthesia and Co-Existing Disease.* New York, NY: Churchill Livingstone; 1993.

Yaffe SJ, Aranda JV, eds. *Pediatric Pharmacology: Therapeutic Principles in Practice.* 2nd ed. Philadelphia, PA: W.B. Saunders Co.; 1992.

INDEX

Note: Page numbers followed by the letter t refer to tables.